DYING AND DEATH IN CANADA

Dying and Death in Canada

Fourth Edition

HERBERT C. NORTHCOTT
AND DONNA M. WILSON

UNIVERSITY OF TORONTO PRESS
Toronto Buffalo London

© University of Toronto Press 2022
Toronto Buffalo London
utorontopress.com

ISBN 978-1-4875-0926-2 (cloth)   ISBN 978-1-4875-0929-3 (EPUB)
ISBN 978-1-4875-0927-9 (paper)   ISBN 978-1-4875-0928-6 (PDF)

Library and Archives Canada Cataloguing in Publication
Title: Dying and death in Canada / Herbert C. Northcott and Donna M. Wilson.
Names: Northcott, Herbert C., 1947– author. | Wilson, Donna M., Ph. D., author.
Description: Fourth edition. | Includes bibliographical references and index.
Identifiers: Canadiana (print) 20210306599 | Canadiana (ebook) 20210306629 |
    ISBN 9781487509279 (paper) | ISBN 9781487509262 (cloth) |
    ISBN 9781487509293 (EPUB) | ISBN 9781487509286 (PDF)
Subjects: LCSH: Death—Canada. | LCSH: Death—Social aspects—Canada. | LCSH:
    Death—Psychological aspects. | LCSH: Grief. | LCSH: Bereavement—Psychological
    aspects. | LCSH: Loss (Psychology)
Classification: LCC BF789.D4 N67 2022 | DDC 306.90971—dc23

We welcome comments and suggestions regarding any aspect of our publications—please feel free to contact us at news@utorontopress.com or visit us at utorontopress.com.

Every effort has been made to contact copyright holders; in the event of an error or omission, please notify the publisher.

University of Toronto Press acknowledges the financial assistance to its publishing program of the Canada Council for the Arts and the Ontario Arts Council, an agency of the Government of Ontario.

 Canada Council **Conseil des Arts**
for the Arts **du Canada**

 ONTARIO ARTS COUNCIL
CONSEIL DES ARTS DE L'ONTARIO
an Ontario government agency
un organisme du gouvernement de l'Ontario

Funded by the   Financé par le
Government   gouvernement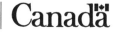
of Canada   du Canada

This book is dedicated to my students, both undergraduate and graduate, who have taught me more than I have taught them.

–HN

I would like to dedicate this book to friends and family who, through their life and also through their dying and death, have brought special meaning to life. I would also like to recognize my nursing career for having helped me realize that dying and death comprise important opportunities for reflection and growth.

–DW

Brief Contents

Contents

Illustrations

Tables

Figures

Images

Acknowledgments

For the 2001 first edition of this book, Wendy Maurier and Michael Stingl reviewed the entire manuscript, Kathryn Wilkins reviewed chapters 3 and 4, and Christy Nickerson conducted library research and also reviewed chapters 4 through 6. All of these reviewers provided helpful suggestions. Chapters 1 through 3 benefited from statistical data analysis and research assistance provided by Corrine Truman. Data access and analysis for chapters 1 to 3 were made possible by a National Health and Research Development Program operational research grant (#6609-2096-96) and the University of Alberta, which provided a Social Science Research grant and EFF (Endowment Fund for the Future) support for an Advancement of Scholarship grant. Chapters 5 and 6 include personal accounts concerning dying and death provided by individuals who remain anonymous; we are very grateful to them for sharing their stories. Finally, the authors thank Barbara Tessman for her excellent editorial work and Peter Saunders of Garamond Press for his support of this project.

For the 2008 second edition of this book, Jennifer Northcott assisted with the literature search to update chapters 4 through 6. The authors are grateful to Betsy Struthers for her excellent editorial work and to Anne Brackenbury of Broadview Press for her support of the second edition.

For the 2017 third edition of this book, the authors thank anonymous reviewers who provided helpful suggestions, Leanne Rancourt for her outstanding editorial assistance, and Anne Brackenbury at the University of Toronto Press for her continuing support of this book. We thank the production staff at the University of Toronto Press, including Beate Schwirtlich and Ashley Rayner. And finally, we are grateful to the anonymous contributors who shared their personal stories, experiences, and insights.

For this 2021 fourth edition, we are grateful to Carli Hansen at the University of Toronto Press for inviting us to do a fourth edition, and for collecting anonymous reviews of the previous edition and of the manuscript for the fourth edition. We thank the anonymous reviewers for their encouraging and helpful suggestions and Samantha Rohrig of The Editing Company for her excellent and helpful copyediting. Many others should also be thanked, including the members of the production team. Finally, we thank the anonymous persons who contributed their stories and insights for this new edition of *Dying and Death in Canada*.

Preface

Dying and death were among the last taboos to be explored by twentieth-century social science beginning in the 1960s. This book focuses on Canada and Canadian studies of dying and death. The first edition was published in 2001, the second edition in 2008, and the third edition in 2017. Initially, the first edition of this book was meant to serve as a supplement to larger texts such as Corr and Corr (2013), DeSpelder and Strickland (2011), Kastenbaum (2012), or Leming and Dickinson (2016), all of which were written outside of Canada but often used in Canada. The Canadian literature on dying, death, and end-of-life care has developed considerably over the past two decades, and the fourth edition of this book provides a comprehensive overview focusing on the Canadian context. Although *Dying and Death in Canada* is written primarily for students who wish to learn about dying and death and for practitioners who work with the dying and the bereaved, it is also relevant for the dying and the bereaved as well as others interested in the topic.

Dying is a process; death is an event. For the dying person, the process of dying culminates in the event of death. For that reason, throughout this book the term "dying" typically precedes the term "death," and discussions of dying typically precede discussions of death. This is in contrast to the more common usage that curiously focuses first on death and adds dying almost as an afterthought.

Dying and death in a society reflect the material and social conditions of that society. For example, dying and death come frequently and early in life in a society where there is widespread poverty, austere living conditions, inadequate nutrition, unclean water, limited sewage and garbage disposal, war or civil unrest, and underdeveloped medical technology and health care delivery systems. In contrast, dying and death typically come late in life in a more "developed" society like Canada in the twenty-first century. How we live influences how and at what age we die. And the society and culture in which we live influences what we think and do about dying and death.

Dying is both a personal experience and a social role given shape and meaning by social practices and cultural definitions (Lucas 1968). Death itself is both a personal event and an event with social significance. The same is true for the bereaved person who loses a loved one to death. The bereaved grieve or mourn in both personal and social ways, since the meaning assigned to dying and death is both personally and socially constructed.

Dying and Death in Canada is divided into three parts. Part 1 explores the causes of dying and death in Canada both historically and at present. It contains two chapters: chapter 1 focuses on factors affecting changes in dying and death among different groups at different times throughout the country's history, while chapter 2 examines trends and causes of dying and death in Canada in the early decades of the twenty-first century.

Part 2 examines the collective constructions of—that is, the social and cultural response to—dying and death in Canada. The social and cultural context is important because it, in part, shapes the meaning individuals assign to the experiences of dying and death. Chapter 3 discusses dying and death from the point of view of Canadian social institutions such as the family, religion, the legal system, the health care system, and the death care industry. Chapter 4 investigates the cultural constructions of the meaning of dying and death and the social rituals that attend death and help to give it a collectively shared meaning.

Part 3 discusses dying and death from the personal points of view of the dying, the bereaved, and caregivers. Chapter 5 examines individual perspectives on dying and death from the point of view of the person who is dying, while chapter 6 discusses dying and death from the point of view of people who are associated with the dying and the dead as surviving family members. Chapter 7 features the voices of professionals who work with the dying and the dead. These professionals provide accounts of their experiences as first responders, including police officers, firefighters, paramedics, emergency medical technicians, and journalists; health care workers, including physicians, nurses, and personal care aides; and death care workers, including medical examiners, funeral directors, and individuals who work at cemeteries and crematoria.

DYING AND DEATH IN CANADA

PART ONE

The Demography and Epidemiology of Dying and Death

CHAPTER ONE

The History of Dying and Death in Canada

Death is inevitable for all living creatures. Death occurs following a process of dying that ranges in length from only a few minutes to many years. The dying process, causes and timing of death, and social responses to death vary considerably from one individual and family to another, from one society to another, and from one historical period to another. This diversity and the finality of death have raised and sustained human interest in dying and death for centuries.

Perhaps the greatest challenge in writing about dying and death historically is finding reliable information from the past. Despite such early efforts as a 1678 Quebec law mandating the keeping of vital statistics (Harding le Riche 1979) and more recent efforts like the development in 1945 of the Vital Statistics Council for Canada (Statistics Canada 2020a), historical information on dying and death in Canada is limited. Long ago, information on any given death was often restricted to a single line on a church's burial roster or a hospital's daily record of discharges (Fair 1994). Personal letters describing dying processes were written by family members and friends, but these provide information about relatively few deaths. Even today, information on dying and death continues to be sparse and incomplete, despite more consistent data collection and sophisticated computerization measures.

Although death is less of a **taboo** subject now, most people today do not dwell on their own death or on the potential death of others close to them. In large part, this avoidance is a natural outcome of death having become a circumstance primarily of old age (Marshall 2013). Death can thus be dismissed by most people as a topic for which little information is needed. Further, dying and death are uncomfortable topics for many people because they bring out fears and, in some cases, unpleasant memories of loss or of dying processes that were not optimal. In short, dying and death are topics that most people would much rather not think about nor personally experience in the near future. Yet death used to be a common life event. Until around the second half of the twentieth century, high death rates and large families meant that bereavement was experienced much more frequently in Canada than it is today (Arnup 2013). The public health movement before the Second World War and advances in health care and the health care system after the Second World War brought about radical changes in dying and death. As a result of these changes, most Canadians came to expect to live a long life.

At the same time that death was becoming increasingly associated with old age, it also became increasingly associated with institutions. Over much of the twentieth century, death was moved from the home, family, and community into the hospital, where the process of dying was largely removed from public scrutiny and consciousness (Wilson, Northcott, et al. 2001; Wilson, Smith, et al. 2002). Then, starting in the 1970s, as more people began reaching very advanced ages, nursing homes also became a frequent place of dying and death (Wilson, Shen, and Birch 2017). Consequently, knowledge of and skills in end-of-life care, once common among family members, became the responsibility of health care providers. It is not surprising, then, that dying and death became neglected topics in everyday conversation and everyday life.

This chapter examines the history of dying and death in Canada. It begins with dying and death among the Indigenous peoples across Canada in the pre-contact era and then reviews the situation in early post-contact Canada before progressing to the twentieth and twenty-first centuries. Trends in life expectancy, historical changes in the causes of death, and historical contexts relevant to dying and death in Canada are discussed.

DYING AND DEATH AMONG INDIGENOUS PEOPLES ACROSS CANADA IN THE PRE-CONTACT ERA

Prior to the arrival of European explorers and settlers, Indigenous groups of First Nations and Inuit peoples lived across Canada, each with its own unique lifestyle and culture. Centuries after contact between the Norse and the Indigenous peoples of Newfoundland and Labrador, Jacques Cartier landed on the Gaspé Peninsula and claimed the land for France in 1534 (Morton 2006). More than half a century later, the first French settlement was founded in Acadia (i.e., Nova Scotia and New Brunswick) in 1604. Given the sheer size of the land and the limited number of Europeans who arrived, many Indigenous groups were not greatly influenced by the Europeans until decades or even centuries after these events. Indeed, almost 250 years after Cartier's landing, fur traders in Western Canada remarked on meeting Indigenous groups that had never before encountered a non-Indigenous person (Bryce 1902).

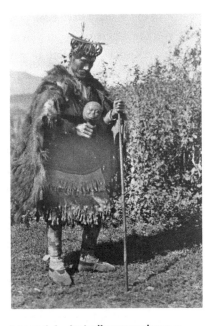

Image 1.1. An Indigenous shaman from the West Coast of Canada
Source: Johnny Lagaxnitz wearing a medicine man costume, 1924, Canadian Museum of History, 62475.

In the pre-contact era, **shamans** and other Indigenous healers provided health care to their people. Since Indigenous health care "was not only physical but spiritual" (Stone 1962, 6), Indigenous healers were adept at gathering and using natural products as medicines and employing a "supernatural article or agency that may be of aid in curing disease" (Stone 1962, 5). Indigenous peoples were aware of and used the medicinal properties of plants, roots, leaves, herbs, bark, and other substances.

Although death frequently came early in life for Indigenous peoples in the pre-contact era, not all deaths were premature; an unknown proportion reached advanced ages. The historian Eric Stone (1962) reported that as a consequence of clean environments, natural foods, continual physical labour, and other positive lifestyle factors, a "considerable" number of Indigenous people reached old age in precolonial North America. Longevity was also noted after the arrival of the Europeans. For instance, an Indigenous woman who died in 1800 at a Hudson's Bay fort in Manitoba was said to have been "upwards of one hundred years old" (Brown 1980, 68). In 1884, three Indigenous men in Western Canada were said to be in their mid-nineties (Carter 1973).

Despite instances of advanced age, existence was precarious for Indigenous peoples. Since food supplies were often limited (Stone 1962), starvation would especially have threatened older people and children. Abandonment of elders may have been practised to some degree when food was limited, or when a person began to require care or assistance, could no longer perform a necessary function, or developed a serious health problem (Burch 1988; Brown 1980; de Beauvoir 1973; Dickason 1984).

It is likely that older Indigenous individuals experienced disorders that commonly affect older people today. Stone (1962) thought Indigenous people long ago tended to develop rheumatism and arthritis as a result of injury, repetitive physical labour, and bouts of scurvy. They also developed eye infections as a result of smoke irritation from cooking and heating fires; colds, pleurisy, and pneumonia; and gastrointestinal problems that were thought to be due to bouts of starvation alternating with times of plenty (Stone 1962). These conditions would have contributed indirectly or directly to death. For example, if older Indigenous people had limitations such as reduced eyesight, arthritis, or loss of teeth, then their ability to procure, prepare, and eat food would have been impaired, and their ability to migrate with a nomadic group would have been compromised. The seriousness of this issue is illustrated by a report that Indigenous people were relieved to leave their weak and disabled dependents at fur-trading forts instead of leaving them behind in the wilderness to fend for themselves until death (Brown 1980). Olive Dickason (1984), a noted Canadian historian, reported that ill infants and elderly Indigenous people were left at early hospitals to be cared for.

Life expectancy among Indigenous peoples would have been considerably lower than today. On the eve of the arrival of the Europeans, Indigenous life expectancy would likely have been only 30 to 40 years, as it was for Europeans at that time. It is not surprising then that Corlett reported in 1935 that cancer seldom afflicted Indigenous people; then and now, cancer occurs more often in old age (Canadian Cancer Society 2020a). Moreover, Indigenous people then would not have been exposed to the environmental and lifestyle factors that are associated with cancer today.

Although there may have been some sex differences in life expectancy among Indigenous peoples, the majority of deaths for both sexes would have occurred before old age. Death from injury sustained in the course of hunting or war-related activities would have been common, with boys and younger men most prone to such injuries. Men were sometimes tortured to death following capture by an enemy group (Dickason 1984), although it is not known how often death occurred under such circumstances. Captured women and children were typically not killed in inter-tribal conflict; instead, they were usually kept to perform necessary functions within the adopting tribe (Dickason 1984).

Some Indigenous women would have died in childbirth. They may also have been more vulnerable than men during times of food shortages. Hunters, who were primarily male (Kelm and Townsend 2006), may have survived when those dependent on them for sustenance did not. Hunters had more immediate access to mobile food sources than women or children; moreover, hunters may have been given preferential access to food when it was in short supply. According to Bryce (1902, 103), one fur trader was told by an Indigenous chief that, on fur-trade expeditions, women "are maintained at a trifling expense, for as they always stand while cooking, the very licking of their fingers in scarce times is sufficient for their subsistence."

Children, too, would have been vulnerable in times of food shortages. Children, both then and now, are particularly susceptible to insults on their health. Starvation has a more serious impact on younger children than older children and adults, either through loss of life or permanent damage to growing organs, muscles, and bones. Infanticide was practised by some Indigenous groups in response to unwanted children, multiple births, and "in defence against privation and hunger" (Brown 1980, 150). There is no evidence to suggest that male children were favoured during times of food shortages or that female children were more deliberately euthanized. Generally, children of both sexes were highly valued and considered necessary to ensure the continuance of their group and to assist their elders (Morton 2006). Nonetheless, it is likely that Indigenous children had a high death rate.

As a consequence of a much higher death rate than today and the greater visibility of dying and dead people in smaller, more intimate communities, dying and death would have been a relatively common life circumstance for Indigenous peoples. There is no evidence that dying people or dead bodies were shunned. Other evidence suggests an acceptance of, if not reverence for, the dead. For instance, Dickason (1984, 115) indicated that "burial customs formed the most distinctive aspect of Huron culture." Whenever a Huron village moved, the bones of deceased individuals were exhumed, cleaned, wrapped, and reburied in a common grave during a 10-day ceremony. An **ossuary** (a burial mound for the bones of the dead) could hold 800 to 4,000 skeletons (Carter 1973).

Carter (1973), who studied the burial customs of Indigenous peoples across Canada, indicated that many tribes regularly revisited their dead every 8 to 12 years in a "Feast of the Dead." He relates an eyewitness account of an Indigenous woman caressing the bones of her children and father. This revisiting was made possible by careful storage of the body, which was prepared

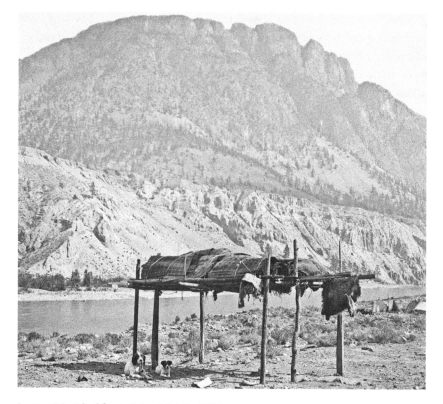

Image 1.2. Blackfoot air burial, late 1800s
Source: Library and Archives Canada/PA 066552.

so that the bones, and at times skin or hair, would be preserved. It was apparently common for the deceased to be bound tightly together by straps so that the knees were touching the chest, although at times the body was wrapped in a prone position. Women often prepared the bodies for burial and in some cases performed the burial unaided by men (Carter 1973).

Indigenous burial customs varied across Canada and included cremation, mummification (mummies consisting of skin wrapped around bones after the flesh was removed have been found on the West Coast), grave burials, surface or mound burials (using dirt, stones, furs, and/or wood to cover the body), tree or scaffold burials, urn burials of cremated remains or bones, and ossuarial (group) burials (Carter 1973). According to Carter (1973), a common type of burial involved a round grave dug approximately five feet deep with the tightly bound body placed to rest sitting on its heels and facing east. Bark and furs were used to keep the earth from touching the body, and various articles were placed next to it. Loud wailing and other displays of grief continued for approximately 10 days after the rapid burial (within one day of death) had taken place. Mourning continued for one year, during which time remarriages did not occur, in part, perhaps, because isolation of the bereaved was common.

Dying Indigenous people frequently participated in preparing for their own death by praying, calling their family together, and making other arrangements. If unable to effect a cure, then the healer's role was to call upon the spirits to help the dying person and to assist the soul on its journey into the afterlife (Carter 1973).

It is likely that dying was considered a normal life process among Indigenous peoples. The folklore surrounding elderly, disabled, or starving Inuit, and their apparent willingness to sacrifice their own life for the good of the family or community, is but one example (Burch 1988). Indeed, death may have been welcomed at times if it occurred during a battle to defend territory or kinfolk, during a hunt to test manhood, or as an end to suffering (Carter 1973; Heagerty 1928). Folklore about ancestral souls revisiting earth provides another example of how death was perceived (Burch 1988). If Indigenous peoples considered death to be a part of the natural cycle of life, just as the seasons ebb and flow, then it may not have been as unexpected or as unacceptable as it is for most Canadians today. Morton (2006) made the point that Indigenous peoples saw themselves as one with nature, not masters of nature. While death would have precipitated grief, it nevertheless could have been perceived as more of a practical issue: a loss of hunters, gatherers, or defenders would threaten the lives and well-being of others in a community, while the loss of women and children would threaten its continuity.

In summary, for Indigenous peoples across Canada during the pre-contact era, death often came early in life. Nevertheless, some individuals survived to old age. Dying and death were familiar in early Indigenous societies because death was a common, anticipated, and visible occurrence shared by members of the community.

DYING AND DEATH ACROSS CANADA FOLLOWING THE ARRIVAL OF THE EUROPEANS

Associations between Indigenous peoples and European newcomers were initially sporadic, later followed by more sustained relations between various Indigenous groups and European explorers, fur traders, missionaries, and then farmers and other settlers. Indigenous camps were often established close to missions and fur-trading posts. Both the missions and trading posts had an enormous impact not only on Indigenous ways of life but also on ways of dying and death.

It is estimated that, in the 1500s, the Indigenous population across Canada numbered 350,000 to 500,000, but possibly as high as 2 million, with the majority living in Central and Eastern Canada (Aylsworth and Trovato 2015). By 1867, only 100,000 to 125,000 First Nations people, 10,000 Métis (in Manitoba mainly), and 20,000 Inuit in the Arctic were left (Aylsworth and Trovato 2015). What had happened to so drastically reduce the Indigenous population?

The most important factor was death from infectious diseases, although starvation and warfare stemming from European interests were also significant (Aylsworth and Trovato 2015). Contact with Europeans brought exposure to infectious pathogens to which Indigenous peoples had little or no natural resistance (Decker 1991). Because the first contacts occurred in Eastern and Central Canada, a rise in the death rate for Indigenous peoples started in these areas and then spread to the north and west. Trading posts that opened following the formation of the Hudson's Bay Company in 1670 served to widen contact between Europeans and Indigenous groups (Morton 2006; Wilson 1983), and thus to increased exposure to deadly infectious diseases.

Reductions in Indigenous populations were dramatic. Morton (2006) reported that half of the Huron, who lived near the Great Lakes, died of contagious illnesses within the first five years of contact with Europeans. By 1650 the Huron ceased to exist as a nation, victims of disease and starvation. By 1680 their rivals, the Iroquois, were also reeling from the effects of European diseases (Heagerty 1928). Smallpox was the deadliest of the epidemics. The first such epidemic likely occurred in 1627, with recurrences afflicting both Indigenous peoples and Europeans until well after the cowpox inoculation was developed around 1800 (Heagerty 1928). According to Bryce (1902, 98), smallpox blotted out entire Indigenous bands as illustrated by this example: "Of one tribe of four hundred lodges, only 10 persons remained; the poor survivors, in seeking succour from other bands, carried the disease with them."

Epidemics radiated outward as European explorers and traders fanned across the country (Decker 1991). Beginning in the eighteenth century and over the nineteenth century, many of the Indigenous peoples living on the Prairies succumbed to infectious diseases (Young 2015). In the far North, the first epidemic of measles reached the Inuit in 1952; it brought death to 7 in every 100 cases (Coleman 1985).

The ineffectiveness of traditional Indigenous healing methods for treating these new infections is thought to have been a factor in their adoption of European health care measures, although these were no more effective against raging epidemics (Dickason 1984; Heagerty 1940; Stone 1962). An alternative explanation for the adoption of European medicine by Indigenous peoples is that many healers died of infection, perhaps in greater numbers than the general Indigenous population because of their more frequent exposure to the infectious agents. Their store of knowledge, which had been gained over centuries (Erichsen-Brown 1979), would have been lost.

In the days before public health, immunizations, and antibiotics, contagious diseases also took the lives of many Europeans (Rutty and Sullivan 2010). Ewart's (1983) study of the daily records of York Factory, a Hudson's Bay Company fur-trading post in northern Manitoba, reveals a continuously high death rate from infections among the European inhabitants—but higher still among their Indigenous contacts. Not surprisingly, cemeteries grew quite large around fur-trading forts (Brown 1980).

Unquestionably, infectious diseases imported by Europeans was the most important factor in a major reduction in life expectancy among Indigenous populations. Yet this was not the only cause of death that could be traced to the Europeans. Territorial disputes also resulted in Indigenous deaths. Outright wars and ongoing skirmishes between Indigenous and European factions, and between Indigenous groups, continued throughout the colonial period (Morton 2006).

The displacement of Indigenous peoples from their traditional lands by European settlement and the reduction of food sources as a result of the growing European presence in Canada are two additional important reasons for the decline and, in some cases, total destruction of Indigenous populations (Aylsworth and Trovato 2015). The last surviving member of the Beothuk, a nation native to Newfoundland, died in 1829. Although she died of tuberculosis, the disappearance of her nation "was at least partly owing to [its] loss of access to the coast and its food resources" (Dickason 1984, 100); the Beothuk were effectively barred from sea access by European fisheries and, later, settlers. On the Prairies, the destruction of the bison herds by overhunting, with bison nearly extinct by 1850, had a major impact on local First Nations and Métis, depriving them of their primary source of food and trade goods (Wilson 1983).

Thus, the initial and ongoing impact of Europeans on Indigenous peoples was devastating. Infectious diseases previously unknown to First Nations peoples reduced, if not annihilated, whole populations. Armed conflict and the destruction of Indigenous economies, food resources, and ways of life further contributed to high death rates.

Largely as a result of inadequate provisions, misadventure, and infectious diseases, early European settlers in Canada also had high death rates (Morton 2006). The incidence of death would have been much higher initially if Indigenous peoples had not provided direct assistance in the form of food and shared knowledge about survival in the new land (Morton 2006). For example, over the winter of 1535–6, local people showed Cartier how to brew white spruce and hemlock bark to treat scurvy (Roland 1985; Stone 1962). Prior to this, Cartier had resorted to prayer when European medicines failed to prevent death from this disease (Jack 1981). The Indigenous people who demonstrated this rapid and effective cure were annihilated by disease soon after. It would be another 300 years before Europeans began to use Vitamin C food supplements to prevent scurvy (Stone 1962); thus, this disease remained a major cause of death in Canada until the nineteenth century (Heagerty 1928).

The European adoption of the Indigenous treatment of scurvy seems to have been something of an exception. Although folklore hints at the use of some Indigenous medicines by the early Europeans in North America (Dickason 1984), it is not evident that there was much transfer of health care knowledge between them. In general, Europeans neither understood nor valued Indigenous peoples' health care knowledge (Erichsen-Brown 1979; Stone 1962). This is unfortunate, as some Indigenous health care practices, such as suturing, keeping wounds clean, reducing dislocations, splinting fractures, and physiotherapy, were observed by the Europeans to be very effective (Heagerty 1928; Stone 1962).

The harsh climate, tough pioneer existence, low standard of living, and unsanitary habits of settlers contributed to many deaths. One-quarter to one-third of all Europeans who immigrated to Canada before 1891 died of infectious diseases (Marsh 1985). Virtually every ship that arrived from Europe brought a new wave of infection. The death rate on these transatlantic voyages was high; one in three travellers became ill, and one in seven died (Heagerty 1928). To try to protect the settlements from imported diseases, quarantine was established in 1720. Later that century, legislation was passed to authorize quarantine hospitals and screening centres in strategic parts of the country (Amyot 1967). After immigrant-bearing ships introduced cholera to British North America in 1832, a permanent quarantine station was set up on Grosse Île near Quebec City in an ultimately unsuccessful attempt to stop its spread (Heagerty 1940).

The death rate from infections remained high among Europeans (Rutty and Sullivan 2010). Although the existence and significance of germs began to be understood as a result of the development of the microscope by Zacharias Janssen in 1590 and its refinement in the mid-1600s by Antonie van Leeuwenhoek, it was not until much later that knowledge about germ transmission and avoidance (**asepsis**) was applied in society. Although surgeons in Canada were first introduced to the principles of asepsis in the 1890s, the medical profession resisted the introduction of aseptic techniques (Roland 1985). During the First World War, some Canadian physicians were still performing surgery with their bare hands (Agnew 1974).

Inadequate health care was another major contributor to the low life expectancy and high death rate in early Canada (Rutty and Sullivan 2010). From the 1500s through the 1800s, health care was more often a liability than an asset in preserving life (Coleman 1985; Dickason 1984). Although Europeans possessed only rudimentary knowledge of the human body, they were interventionist in their approach to treatment (Bettmann 1956). This was a deadly combination. European health care was based on reducing imbalances in the four humours (blood, phlegm, bile, and lymph) of the body, and treatment usually consisted of bloodletting, enemas to induce the passage of stool, and emetics to induce vomiting (Lessard 1991). Through these and a variety of other questionable health care practices, a well-intentioned healer could weaken a person further and spread an infection from one site of the body to another or from one person to another (Heagerty 1928, 1940).

Moreover, most people could not afford either the expense of a hospital stay or the services of the very small number of doctors in early Canada. Given the primitive state of both medical knowledge and health care technology, this was not entirely to their disadvantage. It is not surprising that the few hospitals existing then were considered places of death (Heagerty 1940; Stone 1962).

Reducing suffering during the dying process does not appear to have been a common focus of care by European healers in early Canada. For many centuries, healers across Europe are thought to have shunned dying people because the death of patients would negatively affect their reputations (Veatch 1989). Palliative knowledge and skills consequently remained undeveloped. Trade with the Far East brought opium to Europe in the 1600s, and that substance is thought to have been one of the few early **analgesics** in Europe (Bettmann 1956). It is not clear how available opium was in early Canada. Instead, alcohol was a common analgesic. Healers in early Canada were thus unlikely to have either the tools or the expertise to effectively reduce pain or other unpleasant symptoms during the dying process. Religious doctrine may also have served to restrict efforts to relieve suffering. Until the eighteenth century, Europeans commonly thought illnesses were a punishment or warning from God, and that suffering was to be accepted (Lessard 1991).

Other factors are also certain to have had an impact on dying and death in early Canada. One was a gender imbalance. Almost all of the early explorers and settlers were men, as were the mainly Scottish fur traders arriving to work in Hudson's Bay Company posts (Brown 1980). These young men had a high risk of death through misadventure and starvation during explorations to map the land and gather furs. Because their travels took them away from population centres where health care was more available (Decker 1997), it is not known how much assistance was provided to them when they were ill or dying. In any case, male gender roles emphasized stoicism. This quality may have been enhanced through contact with Indigenous cultures that typically considered pain and suffering an intrinsic aspect of living and valued courage in the face of such challenges.

The demographic makeup of early Canada changed slowly. Precarious European settlements of men gradually became home to an increasing number of women and children. Fur traders and other men had children with Indigenous women, the outcome of which were **Métis** descendants. French settlement schemes brought unmarried women to New France to promote the development of families. By the early nineteenth century, waves of British immigrants, many of them families with children, arrived to expand or develop new British North American communities.

The increasing presence of European women brought new patterns of dying and death. Maternal and child deaths were frequent, and these deaths served to further reduce the life expectancy of Europeans in early Canada. It was not until 1737 that the Grey Nuns of Montreal began caring for women, a remarkable feat since the General Hospital there only accepted males until 1747, when Saint Marguerite d'Youville was appointed administrator of this bankrupt hospital (Grey Nuns of Montreal 2014).

As the number of European immigrants increased, the cultural values they brought with them also began to change Indigenous meanings attached to life and death. Christian religious views of life and death were in sharp contrast to the values common among Indigenous peoples (Dickason 1984). For Indigenous peoples, death was viewed as a natural or unavoidable part of life, explained by their cosmology and given meaning by their spirituality. Death began to be viewed in the European context of everlasting suffering in hell or eternal reward in heaven. Similarly, new meanings of dying and death were introduced, such as death being a punishment for sin and suffering while dying was a means of securing a place in heaven (Lessard 1991).

In addition to religious values, the new immigrants brought a contemporary European emphasis on the individual (Morton 1997). In traditional Indigenous communities, the loss of an individual, while serious, could be somewhat compensated for by the larger group. The individualism and self-reliance of pioneer life meant that death took on a different meaning, becoming more personally significant. In practical terms, the death of either wife or husband in an isolated pioneer or reserve family could be disastrous for the survivors.

And death did come. The life of pioneer families was extremely difficult. Morton's (1997, 39) account is particularly revealing:

> For pioneers in a harsh and unfamiliar land, survival was a preoccupation, to be achieved only through relentless, back-breaking work. . . . Pioneers were described as being reduced to an unsmiling grimness by loneliness and labour. Women faced the terror of childbirth without even a neighbour to help. A single careless blow with an axe could cripple a man or leave him to die in the stench and agony of gangrene.

Life in early Canada was difficult and dangerous, and the state could do little to make it safer. It was not until the late nineteenth century that public health measures were introduced by various levels of government, reflecting the public health movement that originated in Britain earlier in the century (Rutty and Sullivan 2010). Long before hospitals and medical care became effective at saving lives, public health was rapidly extending life expectancy in Canada, in part by significantly reducing maternal and child death rates (Rutty and Sullivan 2010). Enhanced cleanliness, including sewage management, more effective quarantines, and better-quality water and food, reduced contact with infectious agents and raised the level of health among Canadians. Public health measures reduced the risk of acquiring common infectious diseases such as measles, cholera, scarlet fever, influenza, diphtheria, tetanus, tuberculosis, and typhoid. These illnesses claimed the lives of many people, particularly children. By the turn of the century (late 1800s to early 1900s), campaigns for clean water and pasteurized milk were also beginning to reduce the high death rates among children from gastrointestinal diseases, particularly among the urban poor.

In summary, before the middle of the twentieth century, Europeans in Canada had a low life expectancy, with many dying from infectious diseases. Health care was largely ineffective and public health practices were inadequate, although things were beginning to change. Death came frequently, often claiming young people, and little could be done for the dying. Although health care was practised in various forms in early Canada by both Indigenous and European healers (Heagerty 1940; Scalena 2006), its success in preventing death was limited. Prior to the emergence of modern health care measures, death for both Indigenous and non-Indigenous people was a common outcome of illness or injury. The dying process would have typically been shorter than it is today because a severe illness or injury without specific and effective care often leads quickly to death.

DYING AND DEATH IN CANADA IN THE TWENTIETH AND TWENTY-FIRST CENTURIES

Until the twentieth century, there were no dramatic gains in life expectancy in Canada. From the early 1900s on, gradual changes served to reduce the death rate and enhance the prospect of long life. These changes were mainly caused by improvements in the standard of living and a concerted public health movement. These improvements benefited some Canadians more than others. Indigenous people, for example, continued to suffer from a lower standard of living than their European counterparts (Corlett 1935; Wilson 1983), which then as now increased the incidence of health problems among First Nations individuals and led to a higher death rate and lower life expectancy (Adelson 2005). Chief George Baker recounted how, when he was a child in the early 1900s, every member of a poor Indigenous family he knew died of smallpox, and how during the epidemic no doctor came to the reservation (Wilson 1983). By the 1970s, when health care advances had significantly reduced the incidence of death from acute conditions among the general population, pronounced differences continued to exist between Indigenous and non-Indigenous people in terms of health status, life expectancy, and rates of illnesses and injuries causing sickness and death (Aylsworth and Trovato 2015).

Modern health care treatments provided in hospitals by doctors and nurses, and the 1957 federal Hospital Insurance and Diagnostic Services Act, which initiated a universal health care system to serve Canadians, are commonly believed to be the most important factors explaining the dramatic increase in life expectancy in Canada in the latter half of the twentieth century. However, most of the reductions in the death rate and the resulting increases in life expectancy occurred before both the development of the Canadian health care system and the availability of the surgical and medical treatments that began to save people. In 1770, the death rate in Canada was 37 per 1,000 persons, but this increased to more than 50 per 1,000 during epidemics (Heagerty 1940). By 1926, the death rate had decreased to 13.5 deaths per 1,000, and by 1939 it had dropped to 10.4 per 1,000 (Heagerty 1940). The rate in 2018 was 7.7 deaths per 1,000 persons (Statistics Canada 2020b). This early twentieth-century decline in mortality rate is attributable largely to the public health movement's impact on life expectancy through disease prevention (Rutty and Sullivan 2010).

Public health measures had the effect of reducing the incidence of most types of illnesses, infections, and other types of health problems. Millar (1995, 25) credits public health for improvements in longevity through "public health programs in the areas of infectious disease control, maternal and child health, chronic disease prevention, environmental health, nutrition education, and injury prevention." Major public health measures at the beginning of the twentieth century included sewage management, milk pasteurization, and the sanitation of drinking water (McGinnis 1985). Other public health initiatives included the promotion of cleanliness in the home and community, and the enactment of legislation to ensure the safety of food, drugs, and health products. This public health movement led to increased community and personal standards for cleanliness and health.

In addition to continuing efforts to improve sanitation, hygiene, and food safety, public health efforts after the First World War began to include **immunization** programs to create resistance to infectious pathogens. In the past, resistance usually developed through surviving an infection, but many did not survive serious illnesses such as smallpox or diphtheria. Mass immunizations greatly reduced the death rate from infectious diseases (Harding le Riche 1979). For instance, diphtheria was one of the leading causes of childhood death until its vaccine became available in 1930. Mass immunizations for diphtheria, as well as smallpox, whooping cough, and tetanus, were administered in Canada in the 1940s (Grant 1946). Some significant vaccines were developed more recently, such as those in the 1950s to prevent poliomyelitis (polio), the human papilloma virus (HPV) vaccine that became available in Canada in 2006, and the coronavirus (COVID-19) vaccines that became available in early 2021.

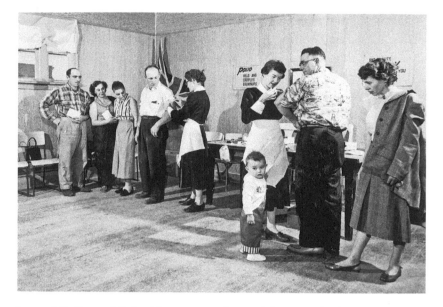

Image 1.3. Two public health nurses vaccinate adults at a polio clinic in Southey, Saskatchewan, 1960
Source: Canadian Nurses Association/Library and Archives Canada/e002504596.

Regardless, epidemics and even pandemics occurred during and after what could be considered the heyday of public health—that is, the period immediately preceding the introduction and subsequent widespread use of antibiotics in the 1940s. The worldwide influenza pandemic of 1918–20, the polio epidemic in the 1950s, the HIV/AIDS pandemic starting in 1981, and other less-well-known infectious episodes claimed tens of thousands of lives in Canada (Hammond 2020). Indeed, the influenza pandemic following the First World War killed 50,000 to 70,000 Canadians (Buckley 1988; MacDougall 1994). The federal Department of Health was established in 1919 as a direct result of this pandemic (McGinnis 1985). One reason why this infection was studied, reported on, and acted on was the fear that it induced. Death was particularly gruesome—the victim drowned slowly from fluid buildup in the lungs. It also tended to strike young adults in the prime of life.

Marion and Scanlon (2011) examined the 1918–20 influenza pandemic as it impacted Kenora, Ontario. At the time, Kenora (including neighbouring Keewatin) had a population of about 4,700. Deaths of young men who left Kenora for the war overseas (the First World War) had averaged about three per month from 1915 to 1918, totalling 130. As the war ended, influenza came to Kenora. In November 1918, 36 people died. In total, 66 died in Kenora in five months beginning in October 1918. All but four were under 40 years of age. Thousands became ill. Schools were closed, as were churches and all other public places. There were no funeral services, and bodies were buried within 36 hours despite winter conditions. Volunteers were organized to deliver food to afflicted families. The library was converted into a hospital to supplement the two overloaded town hospitals. This story was repeated across Canada as every community, small and large, was afflicted.

Changes in the historical rate of death from tuberculosis (TB) present a positive assessment of the impact of public health measures across Canada. In the late 1800s, TB had become the most common cause of death in Canada, and it was particularly severe among Indigenous peoples across Western Canada, who until 1870 were free of it (Daschuk, Hackett, and MacNeil 2006). Its incidence was reduced by the 1920s through public health measures. This abatement occurred fully 20 years before antibiotics began to be used widely to treat infections, including TB (Zilm and Warbinek 1995).

As early as the 1930s, immunizations and other public health measures had reduced infectious diseases to the point where they were no longer the leading cause of death in Canada. The leading cause of death shifted from infections to **chronic illnesses**—that is, to conditions that are incurable and typically progressive, usually with increasingly debilitating effects (World Health Organization 2020).

Health care did not become effective at saving people until after the Second World War. For instance, although Canadians Frederick Banting and Charles Best developed insulin in the 1920s, its successful use in conjunction with dietary and exercise regimens for the treatment of diabetes was not perfected until after the 1940s (Winterfeldt 1991). Antibiotics such as penicillin and the sulfonamides were also not in widespread use until after the Second World War. Furthermore, even though the X-ray machine and laboratory testing of blood and other bodily materials were developed around the beginning of the twentieth century, these advancements in diagnostic capacity did not immediately lead to improvements in health. Most parts of Canada had neither a reliable laboratory nor an X-ray machine until after the 1940s, when the federal government began to directly fund hospital construction and modernization (Agnew 1974). Major surgery such as heart surgery, vascular surgery, and kidney transplants did not begin in Canada until the 1960s (Audette 1964; Hayter 1968). The modern method of closed-chest cardiopulmonary resuscitation (CPR) was developed in 1960 (Kouwenhoven,

Jude, and Knickerbocker 1960). Intensive care units and coronary care units, along with the drugs and other technologies for them, did not become available across Canada until after 1960.

Ongoing breakthroughs after the Second World War in health care knowledge and subsequent progress in diagnostic capacity and in surgical and non-surgical procedures for treating illnesses had a marked effect on society. Faith in health care and physicians increased rapidly, justified to a degree as the efficacy of health care grew quickly and substantially. These developments overshadowed the earlier and still ongoing successes of public health. In comparison to public health programs, which promote population health and seek to prevent the development of illnesses that cause widespread disability and death, modern health care comprised an immediate and dramatic way of saving lives. An illness-based and cure-oriented care perspective quickly began to prevail in the Canadian health care system (Ajemian 1992). Treating illnesses and preventing death became the focus rather than preventing illnesses or providing hospice/palliative care to the terminally ill and dying.

This shift from prevention to treatment was reinforced by hospital developments (Ajemian 1992). Until the 1940s, health promotion and health care were most often carried out at home by family members, assisted at times by visiting nurses or physicians. Thereafter, health care shifted increasingly to hospitals and the professionals there (Bradley 1958; McPherson 1996; Wilinsky 1943).

This was a remarkable shift, as early hospitals had been thought of as places of death and were often shunned. Throughout the twentieth century, however, as the number of hospitals grew, the care of dying persons began to shift there (Wilson, Northcott, et al. 2001; Wilson, Smith, et al. 2002). For instance, in 1930, 39 per cent of deaths in Alberta occurred in hospital (Wilson, Northcott, et al. 2001). By 1953, four years before publicly funded hospital care was guaranteed to Canadians by federal law, half of all deaths were taking place in hospitals. In 1994, three-quarters of all deaths in Canada were recorded as occurring in hospitals, although this rate has since declined substantially (Wilson, Northcott, et al. 2001; Wilson, Smith, et al. 2002).

Not only did the location of death change, but also its causes. The shift over the last half century from acute to chronic illnesses has had a remarkable, although largely untold, effect on society. One overlooked consequence is that Canadians lost their fear of sudden and **premature deaths**. For example, pneumonia used to be a common illness that could bring a relatively quick death at any age. It could strike any person, and without good nursing care, or even despite good nursing care, death frequently occurred. After antibiotics became available, pneumonia quickly became an almost unheard-of cause of death, except in old age or cases of considerable disability.

The shift from acute to chronic illnesses also impacted nurses and physicians. Although the sick and dying have been nursed for centuries, the years from 1890 to 1940 are significant in that many nursing schools and medical schools opened across Canada to ensure enough well-educated nurses and physicians for public demand (McPherson 1996). Licensure that restricted the practice of health care to educated physicians and nurses was enacted during this time (Scalena 2006). Although medical schools were university based, most early nursing schools were hospital based, with student nurses a source of reliable, high-quality, as well as cheap labour. Upon graduation, nurses typically provided private care in the home (McPherson 1996). Often, they cared for the chronically ill and the dying.

By 1943, however, only 2,000 of all 16,000 registered nurses in Canada were working in private practice (Clamageran 1964). Dire working conditions and either unemployment or underemployment forced nurses to seek more secure and also more familiar work in hospitals (McPherson 1996). Almost every town and city across Canada had a hospital by the 1920s (Agnew 1974). Ongoing demand for skilled nursing care in hospitals and the need to keep pace with rapid hospital-based developments continued to impact nursing throughout much of the twentieth century. In 2019, over half of all nurses were employed in hospitals (58.5 per cent), while the remainder worked primarily in community-based settings such as community health (15.6 per cent) or nursing homes/long-term care (15.5 per cent) (Canadian Nurses Association 2020; Canadian Institute for Health Information 2020a).

It is important to note that nursing the dying became less significant in the excitement generated by health care developments during the latter half of the twentieth century (Langham and Flagel 1991). Furthermore, with nursing and medicine both shifting their focus to preserving life, it is not surprising that there was little progress made in the area of hospice/palliative care. **Hospice/palliative care**—the art and science of caring for and comforting the dying—was not present in Canada until 1975, when two Canadian hospitals opened inpatient units dedicated to the noncurative care of dying persons (Ajemian 1990).

Although dying and death were frequent topics in the health literature until the 1940s, there was little mention of either in the health literature from 1950 to 1990, and there was very little discussion about providing supportive care to dying persons (Wilson, Northcott, et al. 2001; Wilson, Smith, et al.

2002). One issue that did generate concern during those years was aging. Starting in the mid-1940s, numerous reports highlighted the growing number and challenges of older individuals in Canada (Clamageran 1964; Hall 1947; Miller 1960).

Most chronic illnesses, although they usually have their origins in early or mid-life, typically do not become symptomatic until later life (World Health Organization 2020). Most of these worsen with aging. Heart and lung diseases, for instance, are often progressively debilitating in nature and not amenable to a complete cure. Lungs, once scarred from smoking or lung infections, cannot be regenerated. Furthermore, atherosclerosis—hardening of the arteries—develops over many years and it is not fully dissipated by life-saving surgery, which (sometimes temporarily) opens blocked arteries in the heart, neck, legs, or elsewhere. Although surgery, drug therapies, and other treatments have proven to be very successful at saving lives, they have also extended the length of many terminal illnesses and the final or end-stage dying process (Millar and Hill 1995). In the second half of the twentieth century, death shifted from being an inevitable and generally quick event to a much less certain outcome of therapeutic treatment. In short, death began to be delayed through health care, even though the underlying illness remained.

In the mid-1970s, a concerted attempt to reduce the impact of unhealthy lifestyles began, as it had become evident that inactivity, obesity, unhealthy dietary habits, unrelieved stress, and the use of tobacco products and excessive alcohol consumption led to serious health problems (Lalonde 1978). The wellness or health promotion movement has since helped reduce the incidence of illness and death from accidents and acquired illnesses (Rutty and Sullivan 2010). For instance, seat belt legislation in the 1970s and 1980s greatly reduced the incidence of vehicular deaths (Hauser 1974; MacKillop 1978). More recently, the environmental movement is drawing attention to the unhealthy consequences of pollution and mismanagement of the environment in which we live. The implications of global climate change are becoming increasingly apparent. While health care may be needed for the illnesses that occur as a result of global warming, the solutions to climate change are not within its realm.

Public perceptions of health care, despite being bolstered considerably in the middle of the twentieth century by many significant diagnostic and treatment advances, began to change as the end of the twentieth century neared. Not only did the irreversibility of aging effects, particularly in light of an aging Canadian population, become more evident, so too did the limitations of modern health care treatments (Millar and Hill 1995). For all our progress, human beings have escaped neither death nor disability.

The optimism generated by the wonder of modern scientific health care has dissipated considerably. Canadians once again are more conscious of the inevitability of death. The Supreme Court of Canada's ruling on 6 February 2015 to decriminalize assisted death so that some dying people can get help to end their life early was a major indication of how far this shift has gone. Hospice/palliative care is an expected duty of all health care professionals now, and it is a respected specialization for those who dedicate themselves to the compassionate care of the dying.

SUMMARY

For Indigenous peoples in Canada before the arrival of Europeans, death was common, visible, often came early in life, and was thus a familiar circumstance. Life expectancy was modest, although some Indigenous persons reached advanced old age. Death followed a similar pattern for the Europeans who came to Canada from 1500 to 1900. However, the consequences of the European presence were disastrous for Indigenous peoples, who were devastated by epidemics and by the destruction of their economies, food sources, and ways of life. By the end of the nineteenth century, the public health movement was benefiting European immigrants in Canada. As a consequence, death rates declined and life expectancy increased.

Throughout the twentieth century, the public health movement continued to produce significant gains in health. The development of health care knowledge and technologies, coupled with universal access to hospitals and medical care for Canadians, led to further, often spectacular gains in the saving of lives. The welcome and continuing successes of modern health care substantially eclipsed the public health movement in public consciousness. In the twentieth century, the causes of death shifted from infectious diseases and other acute conditions to chronic illnesses. The timing of death also shifted increasingly to later life. Care of the dying was transferred from family members to health care providers, with dying and death largely moved from the family home to the hospital or nursing home. Death, which had been common and familiar for centuries, became unfamiliar, remote, invisible, and expected only in old age.

QUESTIONS FOR REVIEW

1. Describe the experience of dying and death for Indigenous peoples in the pre-contact era (before the Europeans arrived), and later for Indigenous peoples and Europeans in Canada during the early contact era.
2. Discuss the historical and current significance of epidemics and pandemics in Canada. Consider infectious diseases such as smallpox, cholera, measles, tuberculosis, the influenza pandemic of 1918–20, polio in the 1950s, HIV/AIDS beginning in the 1980s, and the recent COVID-19 pandemic. What have been the social and economic impacts of these events? What have been the consequences of epidemics and pandemics for anticipating and accepting dying and death?
3. How do dying, death, and bereavement reflect the society in which we live our lives? That is, discuss the notion that how we live influences how, when, and where we die.
4. What have been the consequences of the public health movement, the rise of modern health care, and the evolution of the hospital for the life expectancy of Canadians? How has the expectation of a lengthy life impacted views of dying and death?

KEY TERMS

analgesic – A substance used to reduce pain. (p. 15)
asepsis – Keeping a clean, germ-free environment. (p. 15)
chronic illness – Illnesses that are incurable and typically progressive. (p. 21)
hospice/palliative care – End-of-life care designed to relieve suffering and improve the quality of life for persons who are dying and their family members. (p. 23)
immunization – Injection of substances that create resistance to infectious pathogens. (p. 19)
Métis – The descendants of European fur traders and their Indigenous wives. (p. 16)
ossuary – A container or burial site for the bones of the dead. (p. 9)
premature death – Death before the age of 75. (p. 22)
shaman – An Indigenous healer. (p. 7)
taboo – A widely and strongly held social rule that results in social sanctioning (punishment) when broken. (p. 5)

CHAPTER TWO

Dying and Death in Canada Today

This chapter examines contemporary patterns of dying and death in Canada. The chapter starts with a discussion of mortality rates and the number of deaths in Canada, and then explores who experiences what terminal conditions, when, and under what circumstances, including the length and course of the dying process and the timing and location of death. The chapter includes a discussion of current causes of death and examines death by age, sex, and other significant factors.

MORTALITY RATES

Every year, an increasing number of deaths are occurring in Canada, largely because of population growth and population aging. In 2018, records show that 283,706 Canadians died, as compared to 258,821 in 2014; a 10 per cent increase in only four years (Statistics Canada 2020b). Population aging has impacted the death rate, which has been rising steadily over the past decade after years of decline. In 2011, Canada's death rate was 7 per 1,000 persons; it has since risen to 7.7 in 2018 (Statistics Canada 2020b). This is still a low rate comparatively; most developing countries have higher rates. Some developed countries also have a higher rate than Canada's, including the United States and the United Kingdom, both at 9 per 1,000 persons (World Bank 2020). Bulgaria and Latvia have the highest recorded death rates among developed countries at 15 per 1,000 persons each (World Bank 2020). In addition to long-term trends that influence mortality rates, temporary events such as hurricanes, tsunamis, and pandemics can suddenly affect mortality rates. The COVID-19 pandemic that started in Canada in 2020 became the most deadly pandemic since the influenza pandemic a century earlier.

CAUSES OF DEATH IN CANADA

Table 2.1 reveals that over half of all deaths in Canada in 2018 were from only two causes (Statistics Canada 2020c): cancer (28 per cent of the total) and circulatory (e.g., heart and cardiovascular) diseases (23.5 per cent of the total). Three less common causes of death in 2018, each with under 5 per cent of deaths, were accidents or unintentional injuries, chronic lower respiratory diseases, and influenza and pneumonia. Four additional causes of death are also notable for their top-10 frequency: diabetes mellitus, Alzheimer's disease, suicide, and kidney diseases. Most developed countries have similar causes of death associated with the predominance of chronic illnesses, while less developed countries still have acute illnesses, accidents, and other sudden and serious health conditions resulting in more deaths at younger ages (World Bank 2020). Unfortunately, although aging has many impacts on health, old age is not listed as a cause of death in Canada or elsewhere. Moreover, from 16 March 2020 to 16 March 2021, over 22,500 persons died of the COVID-19 pandemic in Canada, which ranked it as the third leading cause of death in 2020.

One of the most concerning issues about death reporting is determining the primary or most important cause of death. Autopsies are infrequently done to verify cause of death; they are carried out only if foul play is suspected or if a patient dies soon after a surgical or diagnostic procedure. In 2018, only 15,803 (5.6 per cent) decedents in Canada were autopsied (Statistics Canada 2020d). It is therefore not possible to say with complete accuracy what the main cause of death was for every decedent in Canada. For instance, someone who is well and dies suddenly could have died from a heart attack, a heart rhythm disturbance (arrhythmia), a stroke (brain bleed), a pulmonary embolus (a blood clot travelled to the lungs), or other less common causes. Most of these causes are vascular in nature, and it is not unusual for the most probable circulatory disorder to be listed as the primary cause of death. Indeed, it is often said that circulatory diseases are assigned by "default" when there is uncertainty about the cause of death. Another issue is illustrated by the case

Table 2.1. Leading causes of death in Canada in 2018 (sexes combined)

	Rank	Number	%
Total, all causes of death		283,706	100.0
Malignant neoplasms (cancer)	1	79,536	28.0
Diseases of the heart and cerebrovascular diseases (including stroke)	2	66,614	23.5
Accidents (unintentional injuries)	3	13,290	4.7
Chronic lower respiratory diseases	4	12,998	4.6
Influenza and pneumonia	5	8,511	3.0
Diabetes mellitus	6	6,794	2.4
Alzheimer's disease	7	6,429	2.3
Intentional self-harm (suicide)	8	3,811	1.3
Nephritis, nephrotic syndrome, and nephrosis (kidney disease)	9	3,615	1.3
All other causes combined	–	82,108	28.9

Source: Statistics Canada 2020c. Table 13-10-0394-01.

of a person who has cancer slowed by treatment. If this person dies suddenly from a heart attack, a reaction to a drug, or a fall, what should be listed as the primary cause of death? In this case, according to both Statistics Canada and the criteria set out under the International Classification of Diseases, cancer should be listed as the cause of death since it is the condition that primarily contributed to death or to conditions favourable for death. Given these issues, it is unlikely that all physicians, nurses, and other people who are authorized to complete death certificates in Canada will list the correct primary cause of death.

Selecting and recording a correct primary cause of death is important. The reported incidence of a disorder, particularly if it causes illness, hospital utilization, disability, or premature death, is a significant indicator of the level of effort and resources that will be devoted to combat it. It is said that more money has been devoted to researching the treatment of heart disease and cancer than has been committed to all other illnesses combined. Tremendous advancements in care have resulted. These advancements have helped reduce suffering and death; indeed, heart attack deaths have become less common, and 2018 marks the first reduction in annual cancer deaths (Statistics Canada 2020c).

Regardless, heart attack (death of heart tissue from blocked arteries feeding the heart muscle) continues to be one of the most common sudden lethal diseases, along with arrhythmias that reduce heart functioning from heartbeat irregularities. Strokes and accidents are two additional common causes of sudden death. Sudden deaths are more difficult for families and friends, who have no opportunity to have the meaningful last conversations that can and do take place in less rapid dying processes. Moreover, most deaths from circulatory diseases occur in mid- to late life. They are usually progressive in nature, with few symptoms showing until the disease is advanced. At this stage, they are incurable and thus "chronic." This is not to say that they are untreatable, but most cannot be eliminated once they are symptomatic. Furthermore, the risk factors for acquiring cardiovascular diseases (such as smoking, inactivity, obesity, and a diet high in saturated or trans fats) are often associated with long-standing personal habits.

Cancer also tends to be diagnosed in mid- to later life. There are many different types and sites of cancer, and they are often sex specific. Breast cancer is the most commonly diagnosed cancer for females, followed by lung, colorectal, and uterine cancers. Prostate cancer is the most commonly diagnosed cancer for males, followed by lung, colorectal, and bladder cancers (Canadian Cancer Society 2020a). Although lung cancer continues to be the most lethal type of cancer resulting in death, 63 per cent of Canadians diagnosed with cancer will live five or more years. This is remarkable, as the five-year survival rate was only 25 per cent in the 1940s (Canadian Cancer Society 2020a). Although cancer can cause death quickly, it is considered a chronic illness because its cause, impact, progression, and treatment are usually long term.

THE COURSE OF THE DYING PROCESS

The course or process of dying, including symptoms of illness and the speed at which death occurs, varies considerably. A terminal illness may progress rapidly to death, or it may be present for weeks, months, or even years, during which time it may abate but eventually worsen. Dying processes are also influenced by a person's age; the number and type of concurrent health problems (or co-morbidities) they have; their willpower, personal strength, and support network; and the treatments used to combat the disease or manage the symptoms arising from it.

Heart diseases have highly variable dying processes. A person who experiences a heart attack or arrhythmia, for instance, may die immediately, with little or no warning. It is also possible that a person may be resuscitated from cardiac arrest. If resuscitated quickly, he or she may experience few, if any, lasting effects. On the other hand, the survivor may remain critically ill, needing a mechanical ventilator to breathe and sustain life. During this illness episode, the person may or may not be conscious. Numerous medications will be needed to sustain life, along with the many other technologies that are available in hospital intensive care or coronary care units. Complete recovery or partial recovery can result from aggressive treatment, but death may also occur in one or more days. Death is almost inevitable if a critical mass (40 per cent or more) of heart tissue has been irrevocably damaged (and no heart transplant occurs), or if the brain and other vital organs have been damaged by a lack of oxygen during an episode of interrupted blood flow.

Heart failure provides another example of a variable dying process (Heart and Stroke Foundation of Canada n.d.). Most people who survive heart attacks will develop heart failure because the heart has been affected by the death of tissue. Everyone diagnosed with heart failure lives with a weaker heart. New drug therapies are extending life expectancy and wellness for people living with heart failure, but only half live as long as five years. Sudden death, if it occurs, generally comes as a result of a fatal disturbance in the heart rhythm. The dying process, however, is usually gradual. Signs of heart failure are present when the heart is not strong enough to pump blood to other organs, resulting in their reduced functioning and also generalized weakness. A backlog of blood in the lungs and other parts of the body that deliver blood to a heart that can no longer pump all of it onward creates additional symptoms. This backlog causes foot and lower leg swelling (i.e., peripheral edema, or "fat" ankles) and shortness of breath from lung congestion (i.e., pulmonary edema). Acute air hunger can also result, which presents as restlessness or agitation and blue or unoxygenated skin. People suffering from end-stage heart failure may or may not be conscious during the final hours or days of life. The mental and physical states of these individuals, as well as the length of each dying process, are partly dependent on the treatments employed to extend life. Oxygen is commonly used during acute episodes of heart failure to reduce the work of breathing and raise the oxygen level in the bloodstream, thereby improving the condition of the heart and other tissues. If the heart continues to fail, however, and oxygen is used until death, then the dying process can be lengthened by a few hours or even days. Heart failure was the third most common reason for hospital admission in Canada in 2018–19, although only 2.3 per cent of all hospitalizations were due to heart failure that year (Canadian Institute for Health Information 2020b).

The dying process also varies in cancer deaths, but sudden death from cancer is rare. Although death may occur quickly over a few weeks, it normally does not come for a few months, if not years, after a diagnosis is made (Canadian Cancer Society 2020b). Over that time, the diagnosed person is likely to experience varying states of health, ranging from good to poor. Today, with health care advances allowing most diagnostic tests and health care treatments to be conducted on an ambulatory or outpatient (not inpatient) basis, people diagnosed with cancer and other chronic diseases are much less frequently hospitalized than they were in the 1990s (Canadian Institute for Health Information 2020c). Patient visits lasting only a few hours to hospitals, community clinics, or physician and nurse practitioner offices are now the norm. Much of the ongoing supportive care that cancer victims receive is provided at home, with family and friends often responsible for the transportation and other needs that arise throughout six-month or longer treatment regimens. Home-based care may continue over the end-stage dying process as well, as terminally ill people typically want to die at home (Wilson, Cohen, et al. 2013). The suffering associated with cancer both during the treatment and end-stage dying processes is often considerable. As a result, people dying of cancer are the most common users of specialized hospice/palliative care services (Canadian Institute for Health Information 2018). This suffering, coupled with other factors such as not having a healthy family member living nearby, can make it difficult, if not impossible, to die at home.

Symptoms during the dying process depend a great deal on the location and type of cancer. Symptoms are associated with the specific organs and bodily processes that are affected by the cancerous growths, with symptoms tending to appear and worsen as death nears. Some symptoms are partially or entirely caused by the treatments used to cure or slow cancer. Chemotherapy, surgery, and radiation are the most common cancer treatments. They may be undertaken early in the course of an illness to eradicate cancer or to slow cancer growth, or later, even when it is evident that an end-stage dying process has begun. Treatment may be simply aimed at reducing the size of a tumour to lessen the symptoms that result from blocked blood or lymph flow, or from pressure on surrounding tissues and nerves. Analgesics used to combat pain can cause constipation and other unwelcome side effects such as sedation or sleepiness. Symptoms arising from cancer care may be mistaken for symptoms of the disease.

CAUSES OF DEATH BY AGE

The most common causes of death vary considerably by age (see table 2.2). Canadian mortality data from 2018 (Statistics Canada 2020c) reveal that the leading cause of death for infants younger than one year of age is congenital malformations, deformations, or chromosomal abnormalities (23.5 per cent). In contrast, accidents are the most common cause of death for youths aged 1–19 (25 per cent) and also for adults aged 20–44 (26.7 per cent). Cancer is the leading cause of death for adults aged 45–64 (39.7 per cent) and for those aged 65–84 (36.6 per cent). For people aged 85 and older, heart diseases comprise the most common cause of death (23 per cent) (Statistics Canada 2020b, 2020c). Age has similarly been identified in other countries as linked with specific causes of death (United Nations 2020).

It is also important to recognize relationships between age, cause of death, and number of deaths. In 2018, there were only 1,750 deaths of infants under one year of age and 1,342 deaths involving youths aged 1–19, as compared to, for example, 106,525 deaths of adults aged 85 or older (Statistics Canada 2020b). The number of people aged 85 or older who die of Alzheimer's disease alone (n = 4,384) is more than double the number of deaths of infants (Statistics Canada 2020c). Regardless of the fact that decedents are most likely older, some infants do die, but one-quarter of those deaths are due to a condition the infants were born with that is incompatible with life.

Focusing only on the primary or main causes of death tends to overshadow a number of serious disorders that, although common, are uncommon causes of death at any age. One relatively well-known disorder is diabetes mellitus, currently the fifth most common cause of death among adults aged 65–84. Technological advances that allow rapid, direct blood glucose testing have almost eliminated death from diabetic coma (too much sugar in the blood) and insulin reaction (too little sugar in the blood). Nevertheless, diabetes is still a major contributor to high blood pressure (hypertension), heart disease and heart attack, stroke, kidney failure, blindness, and other illnesses. These illnesses are more life threatening than the original disease of diabetes mellitus. Advanced-age frailty is another disorder that is not yet recognized as a major contributor to death in Canada (Canadian Frailty Network, n.d.). However, as more people are living to be very old, weight loss and other features of frailty have made it a marker for increased vulnerability to falls, pneumonia, other illnesses, and death.

Table 2.2. Causes of death by age group in 2018 (283,706 deaths in total)

	Age at Death					
	Under 1 Year N = 1,750 n/%	1–19 Years N = 1,342 n/%	20–44 Years N = 10,669 n/%	45–64 Years N = 41,970 n/%	65–84 Years N = 121,450 n/%	85+ Years N = 106,525 n/%
Most common primary cause of death	Congenital malformations, deformations, and chromosomal abnormalities 412/23.5	Accidents 336/25.0	Accidents 2,848/26.7	Cancer 16,654/39.7	Cancer 44,447/36.6	Heart diseases 24,505/23.0
Second most common primary cause of death	Disorders related to short gestation and low birth weight, not elsewhere classified 171/9.8	Suicide 249/18.6	Suicide 1,499/14.1	Heart diseases 6,365/15.2	Heart diseases 21,643/17.8	Cancer 16,782/15.8
Third most common primary cause of death	Newborn affected by maternal complications of pregnancy 167/9.5	Cancer 161/12.0	Cancer 1,487/13.9	Accidents 2,666/6.4	Chronic lower lung diseases 7,209/5.9	Cerebrovascular diseases 6,727/6.3
Fourth most common primary cause of death	Newborn affected by complications of placenta, cord, and membranes 93/5.3	Assault 34/2.5	Heart diseases 581/5.4	Liver failure 1,494/3.6	Cerebrovascular diseases 5,499/4.5	Influenza and pneumonia 5,047/4.7
Fifth most common primary cause of death	Newborn affected by complications of labour or delivery 65/3.7	Influenza and pneumonia 28/2.1	Liver failure 245/2.3	Suicide 1,472/3.5	Diabetes mellitus 3,443/2.8	Chronic lower lung diseases 4,528/4.3

Source: Statistics Canada 2020b, 2020c, and 2020e. Tables 13-10-0710-01, 13-10-0394-01, and 13-10-0395-01.

It is also important to recognize that most deaths today do not result from a single cause. Instead, the majority of deaths result from a combination of the accumulated impact of various health conditions that have occurred throughout the years, the direct and indirect effects of more than one illness or disease, and—to a major degree—the effects of aging (Betancourt et al. 2014). As such, focusing only on the primary cause of death does not provide much insight into the more normal consortium of death causes, nor does it indicate much about the dying process.

THE LENGTH OF THE DYING PROCESS

Most terminal or life-limiting conditions now do not result in death immediately after diagnosis or after a life-threatening episode of acute illness. Instead, a period of decline or even improvement in health follows. This trajectory of life is dependent on many factors, one of which is the availability of effective health care treatments. Most diseases, once correctly diagnosed, can be managed or stabilized through medication, surgery, or a change of living and eating habits. It is not surprising, then, that terminal illnesses can last for many years. Whereas a quick death often occurred in the past, a much longer end-of-life phase is now possible. During a long illness, a person is likely to come to consider themself to be dying; yet others, including family and health care providers, may not think of the person as dying, or even as gravely or terminally ill. This dichotomy in perceptions can bring about some difficult decision making. The location of death and thus also the final place of end-of-life care is dependent on the decisions that typically are made during a terminal illness. Many such decisions now favour a home death, with this responsible for a major shift of dying and death out of hospital since 1994 (Wilson, Hewitt, et al. 2014).

During a terminal illness, a person's health may be relatively stable with only a slow decline over time. The term "holding their own" is often used in response to queries about their health. Another trajectory that is common, particularly among people with dementia and those at an advanced age, is that of a progressive "dwindling" (Cable-Williams and Wilson 2014; Cable-Williams, Wilson, and Keating 2014). This decline is marked at times by sudden illness episodes during which death may occur, but often with a recovery that does not return the individual to their pre-crisis health state. For this reason, this trajectory has also been characterized as "bouncing on the bottom." Many of these terminal illness trajectories are lengthy. Work has gone into estimating the length of life remaining for terminally ill individuals because it can be important to have an idea of when death will occur; consequently, some reasonably useful prognostication tools are now available, although mainly for cancer (Sax Institute 2017).

In contrast to highly variable terminal illnesses, the final end-stage process—when death becomes immediate and inevitable—typically proceeds quickly and with more certainty, with death occurring in minutes or at most a few days. This shift to an **active dying** process generally results from a major irreversible change in health. With 80 per cent of terminally ill people able to walk until the last few hours or days of life, the change to becoming bedridden is significant (Wilson 2002). Most final dying processes are recognized by close family members and friends, as they see a critical change in the condition of the terminally ill person (Cable-Williams and Wilson 2014). Health care workers, particularly those who have come to know the dying person and those who have witnessed numerous deaths, are also likely to recognize impending death (Cable-Williams, Wilson, and Keating 2014). Unconsciousness may be the most commonly recognized signal of impending death, but becoming bedridden or refusing to eat also indicate that death is approaching (Sax Institute 2017). Impending death tends to be accepted now, with more home and nursing home deaths, and fewer hospital deaths as a result (Cable-Williams, Wilson, and Keating 2014; Wilson, Hewitt, et al. 2014).

Death is commonly considered the end of cognitive (brain) and physical (heart and respiratory) functioning; it is also considered the culmination of all dying processes. For example, a massive head injury or major stroke can result in almost instantaneous death. A heart attack that stops the heart from beating can cause death in as few as 10 minutes. A more typical death takes place now after an end-stage dying process that lasts one to four days, with unconsciousness and irregular, laboured breathing signalling an irreversible decline before the cessation of heart, lung, and brain functioning (Wilson 2002).

FACTORS AFFECTING THE DYING PROCESS

Countless factors can affect the dying process. Around 40 per cent of deaths in Canada take place in hospital now (Wilson, Shen, and Birch 2017)—a location where oxygen, intravenous fluids, and other life-saving or life-prolonging technologies are readily available for use. A Canadian study of deaths in hospital found that 95 per cent of the patients who died had at least one continuous life-saving technology in use at the time of death (Thurston, Wilson, and Hewitt 2012). Deaths in nursing homes are increasing because of an aging population and a greater number of older people living alone and needing help from formal rather than family sources (Cable-Williams and Wilson 2014; Cable-Williams, Wilson, and Keating 2014). Many of the same technologies that exist in hospitals to save or extend lives can be found in nursing homes. There is considerable ongoing controversy over the use of these technologies near death, although terminal sedation has come to be an accepted technology that allows for a peaceful death. Each dying process should be considered unique and, therefore, one in which the benefits and drawbacks of each technology should be considered. The issue of how best to comfort dying people is not confined to hospitals and nursing homes; these same technologies can be transported to the home, which means that the final dying process can be extended in any setting.

As mentioned previously, there is often considerable uncertainty about the primary or main cause of death. Furthermore, death is often the outcome of several concurrent illnesses or health conditions, usually coupled with the influence of aging. Thus, the practice of recording a single disease as the cause of death means that some illnesses, most often those involving the heart, appear to be more prevalent and more serious than they really are, while other illnesses do not appear to be as significant as they truly are. The consequence of this practice is significant. If the method of assigning a single cause of death is not considered when population mortality data are examined, then faulty health care and social sector planning follow.

Of considerable concern is that efforts and funds are spent primarily on curing diseases as opposed to developing and providing support for dying persons and their families. Indeed, minimal assistance is currently available in Canada for families, although they provide the majority of the end-of-life care needed by dying family members. An Alberta study found only 20 per cent of all decedents had received any formal home care services in the last year of life (Wilson, Truman, et al. 2005, 2007). Other current forms of assistance, such as paid leave from work, are growing but still minimal. The Employment Insurance Compassionate Care Benefits program, first initiated in January 2004, was expanded in January 2016 to 26 weeks of coverage during the last 52 estimated weeks of life, with this benefit able to be shared between family members. In February 2020, there were 1,590 persons receiving this benefit, which is less than 0.2 per cent of the total 864,350 Canadians receiving employment insurance benefits (Statistics Canada 2020f). Providing end-of-life care to a loved one at home is challenging, in part because the primary caregiver gets so little support. As such, considerable concern exists over fostering and ensuring a "good" death where the dying process is as optimal as possible for all involved (Wilson, Fillion, et al. 2009).

Despite advances in determining the length of life remaining for people who are terminally ill from cancer, it can be difficult to determine when a person is in their last days of life since chronic health conditions that threaten life may exist for years before death. Nearly half (44 per cent) of all adult Canadians report at least one chronic health condition, with more than one condition common among older individuals (Public Health Agency of Canada 2019). The most frequent chronic health problems are (in this order) hypertension, osteoarthritis, mood and/or anxiety disorders, osteoporosis, diabetes, asthma, chronic obstructive lung disease, ischemic heart disease, cancer, and dementia (Public Health Agency of Canada 2019). The incidence and severity of both chronic and acute health problems tends to vary considerably among mid-life and older individuals; some are much healthier than others. It is also important to remember that other factors impact health, as well as perceptions of one's own health, such as income adequacy, highest level of education achieved (Canadian Institute for Health Information 2016), deafness, needing to wear glasses, and waiting for cataract removal surgery.

Not surprisingly, the prevalence of health problems among institutionalized older individuals is high. Advanced Alzheimer's disease and other dementias causing both confusion and physical disability are common reasons today for the institutionalization of older people. In 2013, 60 per cent of Canada's nursing home residents lived with dementia, with 95 per cent needing help with activities of daily living (e.g., bathing, dressing, eating), and 80 per cent needing extensive assistance (Canadian Institute for Health Information, n.d.).

Chronic health conditions indirectly influence both dying and death. For instance, arthritis and many other health limitations that older people experience serve to impede their mobility. Several problems can result from limited mobility, which can reduce not only physical activity and exercise tolerance but also the ability to obtain and prepare food and engage in social activities. However, in cases such as these, in the end, heart disease will be the most likely primary cause of death listed on the death certificate, particularly if the deceased was obese. This situation raises the proverbial "chicken or egg" argument of what came first. Death certificates and other health records generally emphasize what came last and fail to recognize the range of factors that contribute to death and that impact the dying process.

Hospital utilization is at times used to describe the prevalence and seriousness of health problems, both chronic and acute, with utilization rates and figures often related to age. For instance, in the 2018–19 fiscal year, acute respiratory infections (e.g., acute bronchiolitis) comprised the most common cause of hospitalization for children up to five years of age, compared to several mental health (not mood or anxiety) disorders for children aged 5–17, giving birth for women during their reproductive years, and chronic obstructive pulmonary diseases (including bronchitis) for people aged 65 and older (Canadian Institute for Health Information 2020c). Older people tend to have longer hospital stays than younger people because they are more likely to have serious life-threatening disorders combined with other co-morbidities (illnesses) and limiting social factors such as not having someone at home who can provide assistance if discharged early (Canadian Institute for Health Information 2020b). It must also be recognized that longer hospital stays may include the care of those who are actively dying and, for compassionate reasons, are kept in hospital until that process is complete.

AGE AT DEATH

As figure 2.1 illustrates, the vast majority of deaths in Canada occur in old age. More specifically, in the year 2018, 80.4 per cent of all Canadians who died were 65 years of age or older. The fact that death in Canada now typically comes in old age is also illustrated by the finding that individuals aged 85 and older compose 37.5 per cent of the total number of deaths. It is also remarkable that 60,402 decedents were aged 90 or older, while only 55,731 were aged 0 to 64. As was discussed in chapter 1, childhood deaths have become increasingly uncommon, as have premature deaths in the adult years. Death has clearly shifted to advanced old age.

Age at death has a major impact on how death is perceived. If a young person dies, it is often unexpected and normally considered tragic. In contrast, the death of an old person, particularly someone very old, is much more common and also more likely to be expected and accepted, or at least anticipated to some degree. This does not mean that the death of an older person is not

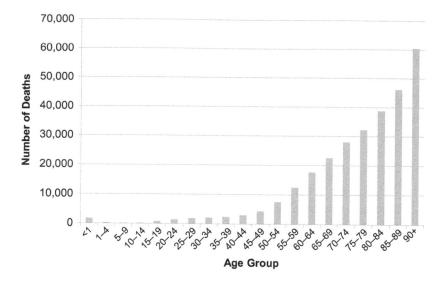

Figure 2.1. Age at death in Canada, 2018
Source: Statistics Canada 2020b. Deaths and mortality rates, by age group. Table 13-10-0710-01.

mourned; it simply means that death at an advanced age is a more normal and expected occurrence now than death at younger ages.

It is also remarkable that in 2019 a total of 10,795 Canadians were 100 years of age or older, a number almost two times greater than a decade ago (Statistics Canada 2020g). These 10,795 individuals overcame many barriers to a long life and as such could be considered "hardy" survivors. Ongoing public health improvements, continuing social and economic progress, and advances in health care are likely to continue to reduce barriers to a long life. Barring a world war, global economic or environmental collapse, or the emergence of new untreatable illnesses including unchecked pandemics, it is likely that more and more Canadians in the near future will reach the advanced age of 85 or 100 or even older. However, there is less certainty about the life expectancy of today's younger people, as the majority of young adults and one in five children in Canada and other developed countries are either overweight or morbidly obese (Organisation for Economic Co-operation and Development [OECD] 2014).

Population aging has led to some interesting conjectures on life expectancy. Some experts have long believed there is a biological limit to life—that humans have a fixed lifespan (of perhaps 120 years) beyond which life cannot be extended (Fries 1980). Others argue that the human lifespan is not fixed. In either case, human life expectancy increased markedly throughout the twentieth century, meaning that a much higher proportion of people lived into advanced old age. This trend is expected to become even more pronounced as the baby boom generation ages. This large and influential cohort, born in the years 1946 through 1966, began to reach the age of 65 in 2011 and will contribute significantly to the pattern of dying and death in Canada—an influence that will extend well into the twenty-first century. The baby boom generation has benefited from many social and health care advances throughout their lifetimes, so their deaths are expected to further emphasize the century-long trend toward death at old and very old ages.

Senescence is the term used to refer to the "wearing out" of body parts as a result of aging, with G. Stanley Hall reporting in 1922 that senescence occurred over the last half of one's life. More recent information shows senescence begins early in life and progresses with aging. With more people reaching advanced ages, senescence has become a major factor in both the quality and quantity of life today. Senescence tends to be overlooked, though, as a "cause" of death, or even as a cause of the many health limitations that can lead to death. For instance, when a **centenarian** dies, a disease or illness—not senescence or "old age"—is registered on their death certificate as the cause of death. Chappell (1992) referred to this phenomenon as the **"medicalization"** of death. Chappell considers dying to be a normal physiological event at the end of a long life. As we have argued, the practice of labelling every death as an outcome of a potentially treatable disease is problematic. If it appears that people are dying from unsuccessfully treated illnesses, then it is much more likely that health care efforts will focus on finding cures than on finding ways to make dying people more comfortable. This issue is increasingly a concern now that more and more people are living into their eighties and beyond.

By the age of 85, or increasingly by age 90, considerable senescence in the form of physical frailty is usually clearly evident (Lindsay 1999; Rosenberg and Moore 1997). For this reason, persons aged 85 and older are often referred to as the "oldest old" and the **"frail elderly."** This population group is one of the fastest-growing segments of the Canadian population. This aging trend is significant. Despite being survivors, the frail elderly tend to become very ill if they experience a common cold, flu, or another illness that would not be life threatening at an earlier age. In 1989, the World Health Organization recognized this health state as a loss of physiological adaptability with aging.

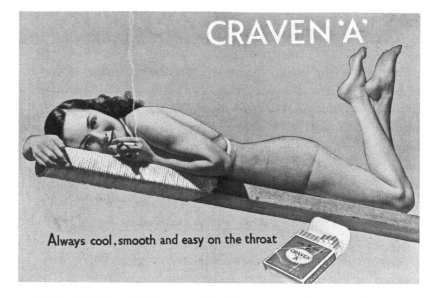

Image 2.1. Cigarette advertisements, like this one, were often targeted specifically at women during the twentieth century. As more women took up smoking, an increase in the number of smoking-related illnesses has led to a narrowing of the sex differential in life expectancy between women and men. Source: Popperfoto/Getty Images.

While Canadians in general are living longer than past generations, females typically live longer than males at most age groups. For instance, until the age of 84, more male than female deaths occur each year. This difference is most stark for individuals between 25 and 29 years of age; males comprised 69.5 per cent of all deaths in Canada in 2018 for that age group. Females, however, comprised 66.5 per cent of all deaths in Canada among adults aged 90 and older, and 52.9 per cent among those aged 85–9 (Statistics Canada 2020b).

This sex difference in life expectancy has been clearly evident for some time (Millar 1995); consequently, it is important to calculate life expectancy separately for males and females. According to Statistics Canada (2020h), the life expectancy for girl babies born in 2016 to 2018 is 84.1 years and for boy babies is 79.9 years. The sex differential in life expectancy is not static, and while it grew over the past 100 years, this gap is now closing. This narrowing of the sex differential in life expectancy may be the result of current and past factors negatively affecting the health of women, such as increased smoking and alcohol use rates (Bushnik 2016).

Table 2.3. Causes of death by sex in 2018 (283,706 deaths in total)

Causes of death	Male decedents (N = 144,483) % (Rank)		Female decedents (N = 139,223) % (Rank)	
Cancer	29.1	(1)	26.9	(1)
Circulatory	23.8	(2)	23.1	(2)
Accidents	5.3	(3)	4.0	(4)
Chronic lower respiratory	4.5	(4)	4.7	(3)
Influenza and pneumonia	2.7	(5)	3.3	(5)
Diabetes mellitus	2.6	(6)	2.2	(7)
Suicide	2.0	(7)	0.7	(10)
Chronic liver failure	1.5	(8)	0.9	(9)
Alzheimer's disease	1.5	(9)	3.1	(6)
Kidney diseases	1.2	(10)	1.4	(8)
Assault (homicide)	0.19	(11)	0.07	(11)

Source: Statistics Canada 2020c. Table 13-10-0394-01.

There is some ongoing speculation, however, about why females typically live longer than males and why males have higher numbers of death than females until the age of 85. Clearly, women outnumber men in the oldest age groups because of their higher rates of survival in earlier years, but there are, in fact, several ways in which sex influences age at death and thus all aspects of dying and death.

Not only are males more likely to die at younger ages than females, but as table 2.3 shows, the causes of death also differ between the two sexes. In 2018, males and females died most often of cancer and circulatory diseases, although small sex-based differences in these proportions are apparent. Differences in causes of death are more apparent when the less common causes of death are compared. In particular, males are more likely to die from accidents and are more than twice as likely as females to die by suicide and assault (homicide). In contrast, females die more often of Alzheimer's disease, influenza and pneumonia, and chronic lower lung diseases than males do. These disorders largely reflect the greater age of females at death.

PREMATURE DYING AND DEATH

Deaths are considered "premature" if they occur before the age of 70 (Canadian Institute for Health Information 2016). This age is a measure of "unfulfilled" life expectancy and is used to calculate **potential years of life lost (PYLL),** an estimation of the additional years a person might have lived had premature death not intervened. For example, if a person died at the age of 60, they would have a PYLL of 10 (70-60). If a child died at 10 years of age, then PYLL would equal 60 (70-10). While premature mortality has declined greatly over the last century, over one-quarter of all deaths in the 38 OECD (Organisation for Economic Co-operation and Development) countries that have more developed economies are still premature, and there is concern now over stagnant or even rising rates (OECD 2019). For instance, in 2015, many OECD countries had a reduction in their life expectancy because a severe influenza killed many people (OECD 2019). Cancer and circulatory deaths have long been identified as causing premature deaths, but the OECD (2019) noted that other illnesses such as diabetes, pneumonia, and asthma are increasingly causing premature deaths. Moreover, road and other accidents, suicide, obesity, air pollution and global climate change, and alcohol, tobacco, and drug-related deaths (opioids in particular) are increasingly of concern for their high PYLL (OECD 2019). Although premature death may seem an unimportant consideration, treatment decisions are often based on age. If a person is thought to be dying prematurely, then aggressive, cure-oriented treatment is more likely to occur.

Using a set age as a benchmark for premature death disregards sex and other more individualized factors. For instance, males in Canada have 90 per cent more preventable deaths than females do (Canadian Institute for Health Information 2016). Most premature deaths are lifestyle related (OECD 2019), but some people are born with life-threatening conditions, such as cystic fibrosis. Health care has done much to improve and extend life for people with cystic fibrosis, but few if any individuals living with this disease can expect to reach age 75. In the 1940s, most individuals with cystic fibrosis died in infancy. By the 1970s, with health care advances and a publicly funded health care system providing assured access to health care, the majority could expect to live into their twenties. Even today, death from cystic fibrosis comes early—the median age of survival in Canada currently is around 50 years (Cystic Fibrosis Canada 2018).

In summary, most deaths occur in old age, and increasingly at very old ages. Deaths in childhood and even in middle age are uncommon. Deaths occurring before age 70 are characterized as premature, although there are some issues with this definition. It follows that death is now expected only in very advanced old age.

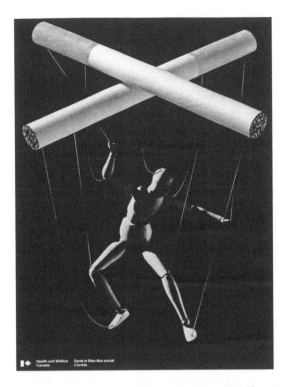

Image 2.2. Cigarettes Control You: An ad from Health and Welfare Canada. Just as tobacco companies used ads to promote smoking, the government has used ads to warn the public about the risks of smoking.
Source: Library and Archives Canada, Acc. No. 1978-29-255; Health and Welfare Canada.

OTHER INFLUENCES ON DYING AND DEATH IN CANADA

Indicators of social class such as income, education, housing, and where one lives have clearly and repeatedly been associated with premature death and therefore life expectancy (Canadian Institute for Health Information 2016). For instance, not only are more health problems evident in rural and remote areas of Canada, but a lack of health care access and thus early attention to health problems means more life-threatening conditions need hospital-based interventions and unfortunately result in higher rates of avoidable death (Subedi, Greenberg, and Roshanafshar 2019). Many factors noted for premature deaths are interlinked. Income level is often directly linked with education level, and higher incomes and more income security are associated with better health (Canadian Institute for Health Information 2016). Occupation is another related factor. Workplace injuries, exposure to toxic chemicals, toxic work environments, and workplace deaths are under-recognized issues in Canada (Tucker and Keefe 2019).

Ethnicity, race, and culture are additional factors that can contribute to longer or shorter life expectancies, and therefore to premature deaths. A prime example is the continuing lower life expectancy among First Nations, Métis, and Inuit populations. Not only is this a result of lower social determinants of health such as income, education, and occupation, but it is also a consequence of colonization and racism (Tjepkema, Bushnik, and Bougie 2019). The lower life expectancy and considerable burden of illness among Indigenous peoples was the impetus for the establishment in June 2000 of an Institute of Aboriginal Peoples' Health under the Canadian Institutes of Health Research. This Institute (now called the Institute of Indigenous Peoples' Health) was formed to foster a research agenda in the area of Indigenous health and to promote innovative research to improve the health of Indigenous people across Canada.

The "**healthy immigrant effect**," where most immigrants are healthy young adults, is another consideration (Lu and Ng 2019). Although the health status of immigrants may be superior to Canadians on arrival, this advantage is often lost over time when language barriers, reduced access to health care services, and underemployment exist (Lu and Ng 2019). This is not an inconsequential concern, as 21.9 per cent of Canadian citizens in 2016 were identified as having been born in another country, and another 17.7 per cent had parents who immigrated to Canada. Moreover, immigrants to Canada are increasingly members of "visible" minorities, as people from India, China, the Philippines, and a number of African countries are the most common immigrants to Canada now (Statistics Canada 2017a). Visible minorities often experience occupational and socioeconomic disadvantages (Trovato 2015), which have implications for health and life expectancy.

The climatic variation in Canada, with extremes of hot and cold weather occurring throughout the year, is another factor to consider. More deaths occur in Canada in the winter months than the summer months (Statistics Canada 2020i), although days of extreme heat and humidity are associated with increased deaths, especially for the socially vulnerable (Ho et al. 2017). A seasonal incidence of hospitalizations, particularly for chronic illnesses, is also notable for Canada. There are several possible explanations for this seasonal variation in death rates and hospitalization rates, such as different patterns of exercise and socialization, as well as an increased incidence in the winter of influenza, colds, and pneumonia; falls on ice; and road accidents. In short, the weather affects our health and our death rates.

LOCATION OF DEATH

As outlined in chapter 1, there was a pronounced trend toward the hospitalization of death from the middle to near the end of the twentieth century. The percentage of deaths occurring across Canada in hospital reached a peak in 1994 and then began to decline (Wilson, Anderson, et al. 1998; Wilson, Hewitt, et al. 2014; Wilson, Truman, et al. 2009). It is becoming evident, now with only around 40 per cent of deaths taking place in hospital (Wilson, Shen, and Birch 2017), that the final days of life are increasingly occurring either at home or in a nursing home (i.e., a long-term or continuing care facility). The COVID-19 pandemic, where 81 per cent of all related deaths in Canada occurred among nursing home residents in the first half of 2020 (Estabrooks et al. 2020), should be recognized not just for illustrating the vulnerability of nursing home residents to death from infections, but also for having increased the profile of nursing homes as places were dying and death occur. Other places are also becoming noted for providing end-stage end-of-life care, including hospices, jails, retirement homes, and assisted living facilities.

The actual location of death and also the location (or locations) of end-of-life care are affected by many factors, one of which is the type of dying process. Persons experiencing long, drawn-out dying processes and who have developed considerable dependency are more likely to be living in a nursing home or another type of care facility before their death in those places. Other persons with a relatively short dying process are more likely to live at home before death either at home or in hospital.

While dying at home has its appeal, it also raises certain issues. One major problem, given limited formal home care support (Gilmour 2018), is that there must be one or more family members willing and able to care for the dying person in the home. This informal care tends to fall disproportionately on female family members, generally the spouse or a daughter (Gilmour 2018). This work often involves a great deal of physical and emotional labour over long hours with potentially negative effects on the health of these caregivers (Gilmour 2018).

Much concern has been raised about this informal caregiver burden, and it is important to point out that more formal home care is needed to support dying and death in the home, as well as for the ongoing care of terminally ill people at home. At the same time, it is unfortunate that the many benefits of informal family caregiving have been overlooked. There is often tremendous benefit to all people involved in the shared caring that occurs between caregivers and care recipients (Canadian Institute for Health Information 2018). When these benefits occur over the final days of life, this is a unique and special time for dying people and their families. However, more care must be taken to mitigate or prevent intra-family end-of-life conflict that is common given the many possible stressors associated with caring for the dying (Wilson, Anafi, et al. 2020).

It is now believed that most, if not all, of the care needs of dying individuals can be managed outside of hospitals. While a small proportion of people (5–10 per cent) experience difficult dying processes such that they require specialized hospice/palliative care (Canadian Institute for Health Information 2018), most people have a relatively short phase of dependency near death and fairly basic care needs near the end of life (Wilson 2002).

Although much dialogue is occurring about dying and death in the home, a considerable number of deaths take place in nursing homes and other long-term or continuing care facilities. In the 2018–19 year, there were 191,835 continuing care residents across Canada, with 61.8 per cent of all those residents who died staying onsite for their end-of-life care (Canadian Institute for Health Information 2018–19). Many more retirement home and assisted living beds exist for people who have lower needs for assistance or support with activities of daily living. With chronically long wait lists to get into nursing homes (Garner et al. 2018) and declines in the number of deaths taking place in hospital (Wilson, Shen, and Birch 2017), an increasing number of deaths in retirement homes and assisted living facilities is likely occurring.

This obvious and pronounced shift of dying and death from hospitals to patients' homes, nursing homes, and other non-hospital places is presenting many opportunities for end-of-life care capacity development. Indeed, nursing homes and other care facilities have considerable expertise in the care of dependent older adults, and some are recognized for their provision of specialized hospice/palliative care. Transferring a dying person from a long-term care facility to receive end-of-life care in hospital is rarely required. Furthermore, sending a dying resident of a nursing home to hospital means this person moves from a familiar environment and familiar caregivers to an unfamiliar environment that is primarily concerned with providing acute, cure-oriented care. Considerable discomfort during and after this move is of concern. Another hazard is that the peace and reflection that normally occurs at the deathbed vigil during the final hours or days of life is lost in the rush to transfer and treat what may appear to new and unfamiliar health care professionals as a potentially reversible trajectory.

Some other factors affect the chances of dying in hospital. Deaths from accidents, injury, and suicide are much less likely to occur in hospitals, as there is no longer a requirement that all dead people be sent to a hospital for an autopsy or death certification. In contrast, babies who are born with a congenital disorder are highly likely to die in hospital, either soon after birth there or in the first year of life.

When hospitalized, the time that dying people spend in the hospital varies, but hospitalizations that end in death tend to be lengthy. This end-stage stay is declining in length, however, for many different reasons. One of the most important is that relatively few hospital beds exist in Canada and they are often full, creating pressure to discharge patients from the hospital (Wilson, Brow, et al. 2018). Consequently, hospital patients who are discharged alive are usually under the age of 65 rather than the frail elderly (Wilson, Shen, and Birch 2019).

Although a lack of home-based family or formal caregivers could be a factor contributing to dying and death in the hospital (Canadian Institute for Health Information 2018), it is more likely that death occurs in hospital now after someone suffering an acute illness or injury has not responded to treatment. One notable exception is Medical Assistance in Dying, which has been legal in Canada since June 2016. Although less than 2 per cent of deaths in Canada were medically assisted in the first three and a half years since implementation (up to December 2019), over one-third (36 per cent) of these deaths took place in hospitals, over one-third (35 per cent) occurred in the patients' homes, and the remainder took place in nursing homes, hospices, and other locations (Government of Canada 2020b).

SUMMARY

Today, dying and death in Canada typically occur in old age and usually are the result of chronic health problems such as cancer or circulatory disease. Death is not expected early in life, and deaths before the age of 70 are considered premature. However, the process of dying and the event of death typically come later in life for females than males. This sex differential in life expectancy is not fixed and has been converging for some time. There also continues to be a differential in the health status and life expectancy among Canada's social classes and ethnocultural groups, with the poor and less educated being at greatest risk for poor health and premature death. Finally, although many deaths still take place in hospital, it is becoming evident that hospitals are not the preferred place for end-of-life care, nor should they be. What is certain, as a consequence of both a growing and aging population and the aging of the baby boom cohort, is that an increasing number of Canadian deaths can be expected each year. The challenge is to provide the best possible end-of-life care in settings that improve the experience of dying and death for those who are dying and their families.

QUESTIONS FOR REVIEW

1. Describe the problems involved in recording cause of death in Canada. What are the implications of these problems?
2. How do the causes of death vary by age in Canada? How has this changed over the past century? What is the likelihood that these patterns will continue in the future?
3. Discuss the social pattern of death due to COVID-19 infections focusing on age, sex, residency in a long-term care home, social status, occupation, and other such variables. Compare this new pattern of death to the other established causes of death such as cancer, heart disease, diabetes, and Alzheimer's disease.
4. How does life expectancy vary for males and females in Canada? Discuss trends in sex differences in life expectancy in the twentieth and early twenty-first centuries.
5. Identify and discuss changes in the location of death in the twentieth and early twenty-first centuries in Canada. Consider the impacts of these changes on dying people.
6. Discuss future implications of Medical Assistance in Dying (MAID), such as effects on where and when Canadians will die.

KEY TERMS

active dying – The process of dying leading to immediate and inevitable death. (p. 36) centenarian – A person who is 100 years of age or older. (p. 41)

frail elderly – Individuals in general poor health due to advanced age. Usually aged 85 and older. (p. 41)

healthy immigrant effect – Immigrants who come to Canada often have better health than native-born Canadians because people in ill health are less likely to immigrate. (p. 46)

medicalization – The process of defining and treating phenomena as medical pathology. Medicalized constructions contrast other possible constructions, such as criminalization, immorality, and normalization. (p. 41)

potential years of life lost (PYLL) – An estimate of the additional years a person might have lived had premature death not intervened or if a particular cause of death was eliminated. (p. 44)

senescence – The wearing out of the body as a result of aging. (p. 41)

PART TWO

The Social and Cultural Response to Dying and Death

CHAPTER THREE

Dying and Death in the Context of Canadian Social Institutions

Death is a normal event that occurs at the end of every life. Death in contemporary society is typically something that can be anticipated, expected, and even managed. Dying and death have many different meanings and implications for individuals, families, and Canadian society as a whole. Current views of dying and death, along with existing related practices, are influenced by cultural orientations and by the social institutions of family, religion, the legal system, the health care system, and the death care industry. Although each has developed over many years, these systems are undergoing changes that have consequences for dying and death. This chapter provides an overview of how they affect dying and death in Canada.

CULTURAL INFLUENCES

Cultural backgrounds, expectations, practices, and traditions influence how people view and respond to illness, health care treatments, end-of-life care, dying, death, grief, and after death rituals. It is also important to note that cultural traditions change over time. For instance, second-generation immigrants (the children of immigrants) to Canada often do not hold to the practices that are still common in their parents' home country. On the other hand, immigrants may hold to customs that were present at the time they left their home country even though these customs have since changed. One illustration of this is a reluctance among older Chinese immigrants to die at home, with a preference for dying in the hospital. Chinese families often lacked the resources to care for the dying at home, and death was considered bad luck and a stigma (Hsu, O'Conner, and Lee 2009). Nevertheless, home deaths are common across China now (Dong et al. 2019). Canada is a multicultural country, where many cultural backgrounds influence the experience of dying, death, and other related components such as bereavement. At the same time, seasonal weather, the high cost of funerals, and dominant Canadian norms are also influential.

Cultural norms provide much stability, assistance, and guidance for survivors. These norms are important as experience with dying and death is uncommon now in Canada. The need for family supports and traditions, religion, the legal system, the health care system, and the death care industry is subsequently much greater as people grapple, often for the first time, with dying, death, and bereavement.

THE FAMILY

Family life provides many of the experiences and contexts that shape our personal understandings of dying, death, and bereavement. Although any death can be distressing, the death of a close family member is a major life event. Each surviving individual is likely to be affected differently, however, as the circumstances of family relationships and the dying and death process vary considerably. One such circumstance is when an illness changes the dying person. For example, deaths due to Alzheimer's disease often represent two deaths: (1) the death of the person as previously known and (2) the death of the physical body.

Much of what we understand and come to expect about dying, death, and bereavement is gained during our formative years. Although television and movie deaths or video game deaths may be the closest exposure to death for many children now, the reactions of family members to these deaths and to actual deaths, such as the deaths of grandparents, other relatives, friends, or even family pets teach young people about dying and death. In some families, children are deliberately excluded from discussions about dying or death, visits to dying people, and attendance at funeral or memorial services. These children may learn to respond to dying and death with avoidance, revulsion, despair, anger, or fear (Macy 2013). Death anxiety

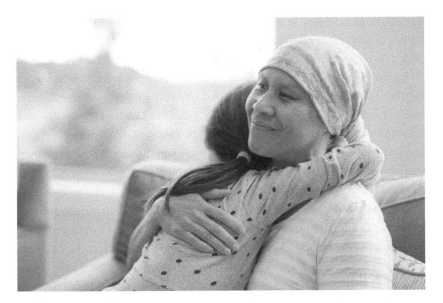

Image 3.1. When children are included in the dying process and death experience, they are more likely to develop positive perspectives and coping skills.
Source: FatCamera/iStock.com.

may result and there are now several measurement tools in existence to determine the extent of personal apprehension over dying and death (Lehto and Stein 2009). In other cases, where children are involved in dying and death experiences or have been exposed to books written specifically to teach children about dying and death, they are more likely to develop positive perspectives and coping skills (Bonoti, Leondari, and Mastora 2013; Malcom 2010–11).

When required, family members typically provide support to dying and surviving family members (Statistics Canada 2014a). Yet not all families are able to help dying or bereaved family members. Dying and death experiences are often stressful and can strain family relationships (Wilson et al. 2020). In some cases, these relationships are already compromised, with dying and death bringing difficult memories forward and bringing together family members who have perhaps not met by mutual consent for years. Families tend to be widely scattered now, with travel distances reducing the possibility of direct support (Statistics Canada 2020j). Moreover, smaller nuclear families and increased longevity have reduced the number of deaths that individual

Canadians experience. In the 1960s and 1970s, Canadian families used to bury a family member every 8 to 10 years on average; by the 1990s, it was once every 15 to 18 years (Flynn 1993). This trend has continued.

Reduced experience with dying and death has made it more difficult for families to develop collective stances, positive role models, and comfortable traditions (Bonoti, Leondari, and Mastora 2013). Deaths in hospitals and nursing homes, and thus outside the home, as well as lack of contact between family members because of physical or emotional distance have contributed to dying and death becoming unfamiliar. In this context, Webb (1997, xvii) reported that "most of adulthood passes without personal contact with dying." Anderson (1980) was among the first to point out that it is in middle age that children usually have to come to terms with the "finitude" of their parents. He coined the term "middle-aged orphan" to indicate the significance of parents passing away. Their passage is a potential personal crisis for the middle-aged, as death seems closer now that their buffer (i.e., their parents) to old age and eventual death is gone. As the first author's distressed middle-aged father-in-law said in the cemetery after burying his last parent: "This is hard. This means that I am next." And indeed he was, dying just a few years later.

The shift of dying and death out of hospital in recent decades is raising the profile of family members as end-of-life care providers and death wish granters, as most dying people now express a wish to die at home (Wilson, Cohen, et al. 2013). Although the traditional view of the family as a married mother and father and one or more children has changed, families in various forms are present and influential in Canadian society. Mirabelli (2018) defines a family as

> any combination of two or more persons who are bound together over time by ties of mutual consent, birth and/or adoption or placement and who, together, assume responsibilities for variant combinations of some of the following: physical maintenance and care of group members; addition of new members through procreation or adoption; socialization of children; social control of members; production, consumption, distribution of goods and services; and affective nurturance—love.

Despite continuing high levels of divorce and an increasing incidence of single or never-married people in Canada, remarriages, common-law marriages, and LGBTQIA2S+ (lesbian, gay, bisexual, transgender, queer/questioning, intersex, asexual, and two-spirit) marriages either sanctioned by the state or not are continuing to ensure that most individuals are part of a family. Long-term friendships, particularly among people who never married, can also constitute a family. In some cases, this means individuals have larger extended families, as may be the case for children whose parents have divorced and remarried. A child could have four people now who fulfill the role of parent, as well as eight whom they consider as grandparents and many additional aunts, uncles, and cousins.

Few Canadians, however, have much experience in providing hands-on care to ill or dying family members. The 2018 General Social Survey on Caregiving and Care Receiving revealed only 25 per cent of Canadians aged 15 and older provided for or helped another person who needed assistance in the last year (Statistics Canada 2020j). This represents a decline from 28 per cent in 2012 (Statistics Canada 2014a). The reasons for this are varied but include geographic mobility and physical distance between family members; elderly parents and their children living separately; people usually being healthy and able to care for themselves most of their adult lives; and two of every three deaths taking place in hospitals or nursing homes (Statistics Canada 2014b; Wilson, Anderson, et al. 1998). Hospitalization is a reality during most bouts of serious illness, and institutionalization in a long-term care facility is common whenever there is a long decline leading to death (Cable-Williams, Wilson, and Keating 2014). In these settings, nurses have taken on many of the responsibilities that family members and friends used to have when home deaths were the norm (Wilson, Anderson, et al. 1998). Even if dying and death take place at home, palliative home care nursing and information on how to care for a dying person are often needed (Stajduhar, Funk, and Outcalt 2013).

The decline in hospital deaths, discussed in chapter 2, is linked with an increased number of deaths at home (Wilson, Hewitt, et al. 2014). Around one in every three deaths take place at home now. This increase in home deaths was forecast in 1994 by McWhinney and Stewart (1994, 240), who said that "during the next few decades, the increasing prevalence of cancer and other chronic disease and the reduced number of [hospital] beds are likely to increase the number of home deaths. Even when patients die in hospital, their length of stay is likely to be reduced, so that a longer portion of their terminal illness will be spent at home."

The main impetus for home deaths is to enable a "good death." **Good deaths** are often thought of as natural dying processes that are not interrupted by life-supporting technologies or other medical interventions (Wilson, Fillion, et al. 2009). However, good deaths are also those where dying people and their families are ready for and accept death (Wilson and Woytowich 2014). Good deaths also avoid bad ones, where pain and other symptoms are not successfully addressed (Wilson and Hewitt 2018).

The shift of dying and death out of hospital is also due to death occurring most often now at an advanced age, with older and possibly retired adult children tending to have the time, emotional maturity, and physical capacity to assist parents through their dying days. This assistance continues even if hospitalization or institutionalization in a nursing home occurs. As a consequence of these changes, dying and death is increasingly "up close and personal" instead of something completely delegated to health care professionals (Donnelly, Michael, and Donnelly 2006).

Regardless, few families plan for a home death or home-based end-of-life care. Another problem is that it is difficult to forecast the time to provide for supportive end-of-life care, so family members may not be present in the home, hospital, or nursing home when needed (Cable-Williams, Wilson, and Keating 2014). As a result, many Canadians have never actually witnessed a death. Contact with death is often limited to attending a funeral or memorial service. In some cases, the casket is closed or the increasing practice of cremation and other constraints such as short viewing hours mean there is limited opportunity to see the deceased person. Today, people other than family members normally care for the body after death (Waugh 2013). In short, few families perform the required duties that arise before or after death.

In a few cases, decisions are made at or near the time of death to enable organ or tissue donation. In 2018, 2,782 organ transplants were undertaken in Canada, using tissue from 762 deceased and 555 living persons (Canadian Institute for Health Information 2019). Although individual Canadians can arrange before death to donate all or selected organs and tissues through registering their intention provincially, families of the deceased usually have the right to determine if this harvesting will occur. Many different body organs and tissues, including skin and bone, can be harvested. Decisions about organ and tissue donation, as well as the rituals, ceremonies, and customs that follow death vary depending on the cultural origins of the family of the deceased person, the relationship of the deceased person to other members of the family, and changing social concepts of what is deemed acceptable. With the advanced age of many deceased persons now and other factors limiting the number of organs and tissues that can be harvested, the families of younger individuals who have suddenly died are typically the ones making decisions about donation. Although this decision comes at a difficult time, donor families are often comforted by the knowledge that their loved one's death was not in vain. Regardless, sudden deaths are normally the most difficult in terms of bereavement impact (Bolton et al. 2013).

Following death, a funeral home is usually given the responsibility of taking the body and performing death care (Waugh 2013). Previously, around the time of the Great Depression in the 1930s, Canadian families commonly used their own vehicles to transport the deceased, and they cleaned and dressed the dead body, built coffins, used their homes as places where family and friends could view the body, performed burials, and arranged for deaths to be registered (Waugh 2013). Today, few families do these things; families have become much more reliant on other social institutions to manage death.

RELIGION

For centuries, religion has played a major role in dying and death. The concept of life after death is common in many religions; this is usually a comforting belief, particularly if reunification with loved ones is anticipated. Religion has also provided meaning for the dying process; for example, in some religions suffering is considered important for salvation and death is considered an avenue to eternal life. Religion has also established familiar patterns or rituals for human behaviour and thus provides direction during difficult times. Religious representatives are often still called to the deathbed to support the dying person and the grieving family. Last rites remain an important religious ritual for dying and grieving Catholics, for instance.

During the twentieth century, the influence of religion on dying and death declined considerably. In the past, religion was important to many people as health care could do little to prevent death, but scientific advances radically changed this. These advancements quickly led to the rising significance of hospitals and physicians in Canadian society. The increased success and prominence of health care tended to overshadow religious conventions regarding dying and death. A survey of Canadians in 2011 revealed that 24 per cent had no religious affiliation (Statistics Canada 2014a).

Science is not the only area that has reduced the role of religion in dying and death. The death care industry has also constricted the role of religion. Flynn (1993, 6–7) observed that "most religious groups have stepped back and allowed the funeral director to define the social customs of the burial rite. . . . Religious leaders have not recognized the need to set clear guidelines on funeral rites, and have not educated their clergy." Secularization has also led to professionals in the death care industry often taking over the roles that clergy once held (Emke 2002).

This is not to say that the institution of religion and religious roles or traditions in relation to dying and death are now irrelevant in Canadian society. Some dying individuals and grieving families still involve a spiritual leader in decisions over the use of life support or its discontinuation (Waugh 2013). Furthermore, priests, pastors, rabbis, imams, and other spiritual leaders still commonly preside over funerals and memorial services, which are frequently held in places of worship. Churches often have visitation teams to support dying individuals, and large hospitals commonly employ clergy to ensure dying individuals and their families receive assistance if needed or desired. Many religious-based groups offer bereavement support to families after a family member's death. In short, religion still has significance for individuals, but it is clearly more significant for some people than others.

Religion also influences dying and death at a societal level. Religious groups have provided leadership and advice on social and health policies related to dying and death. In the 1980s and 1990s, Canadian religious and health care organizations developed guidelines together for permitting the withholding and withdrawing of medical treatments that would only extend dying processes. At that time, life-supporting technologies were commonly used on all persons, regardless of their health or the possibility of benefit from these technologies (Canadian Nurses Association [CNA], Canadian Medical Association [CMA], and Canadian Hospital Association [CHA] 1984; Canadian Medical Association 1995). Furthermore, these guidelines indicated that withdrawing or withholding futile treatment should be done at all times in conjunction with "palliative care to alleviate the mental and physical discomfort of the [dying] patient" (CNA, CMA, and CHA 1984, 1357).

A more recent example is the actions of Catholic and other religious organizations in attempting to prevent the legalization of Medical Assistance in Dying (MAID) in Canada. Soon after the legalization of MAID in June 2016, a survey of medical students across Canada found that 89 per cent of those who indicated having no religious affiliation were willing to provide MAID as compared to 70 per cent of those who said they were Catholic or Jewish and 40 per cent of those who indicated they were non-Catholic Christians. Another revealing difference is that 89 per cent of those who never attended religious services indicated they were willing to provide MAID, as compared to 14 per cent of those who attended a weekly religious service and 40 per cent of those reporting monthly attendance (Falconer et al. 2019).

THE LEGAL SYSTEM

The law is highly influential with respect to dying and death in Canadian society. Civil and criminal law and other legal guidelines have developed in Canada in response to advances in health care and changes in society. Today, most large health care facilities, as well as government departments of health, retain lawyers to provide legal advice. Organizational policies that address life-or-death issues are likely to be formalized only after legal advice has been received. Legal advice is also frequently sought whenever there are questions about the adequacy of patient care, such as in the case of an unexpected patient death or when a medical error has jeopardized life. Governments also hold public inquiries over systemic issues, such as the 2000–2 *Commission on the Future of Health Care in Canada*, the "Romanow report" that investigated the sustainability of the public health care system (Commission on the Future of Health Care in Canada 2002).

The Criminal Code of Canada has had a substantial impact on dying and death. Until the Supreme Court of Canada's decision on 6 February 2015 to allow **assisted death**, both **euthanasia** ("mercy killing") and **assisted suicide** were criminally indictable offences. The Supreme Court of Canada's 2015 ruling specified the following:

> Section 241(b) and section 14 of the Criminal Code unjustifiably infringe section 7 of the Canadian Charter of Rights and Freedoms and are of no force or effect to the extent that they prohibit physician-assisted death for a competent adult person who (1) clearly consents to the termination of life and (2) has a grievous and irremediable medical condition (including an illness, disease or disability) that causes enduring suffering that is intolerable to the individual in the circumstances of his or her condition. (para. 147)

Although it would seem obvious that murder is a serious offence, mitigating circumstances influence how judges and juries view each crime and assign punishment. Every year, cases of "mercy killing" occur. For instance, after the MAID law came into effect in 2016, a Montreal man was charged with second-degree murder when he smothered his wife, long diagnosed with Alzheimer's disease, in a nursing home in 2017. Previously, a MAID request had been unsuccessful. At that time, a person had to be able to give consent to receive MAID and anyone with Alzheimer's dementia was deemed unable to do so. The husband was found guilty of manslaughter and sentenced to two years in a provincial jail along with three years of probation and 240 hours of community service upon his release (Montreal Gazette 2019). Crimes such as these, motivated by familial love, are often treated differently than other crimes.

It is not illegal to take your own life in Canada—3,811 people died by suicide in 2018 (Statistics Canada 2020c)—but it remains illegal to cause the death of another person or to assist in their suicide unless they have been approved for MAID (Government of Canada 2020a). An approved person can have one of two types of assistance in dying: (1) a nurse practitioner or physician directly administers a substance that causes death, typically by injecting a drug, or (2) a drug capable of ending life is prescribed and obtained from a pharmacist by the person who ingests the drug to end their life (Government of Canada 2020a). A 2020 amendment to the 2016 Act clarified how close to death people must be to qualify for MAID. People who can receive MAID are those who:

(1) are eligible for health services funded by the federal government or a province or territory in Canada (or have completed the applicable minimum period of residence or waiting period for eligibility);

(2) are at least 18 years old and mentally competent and able to make health care decisions;

(3) make a voluntary request for MAID that is not the result of outside pressure or influence;

(4) give informed consent to receive MAID at the time it is being delivered; and

(5) have a grievous and irremediable medical condition, which does not need to be fatal or terminal but where a natural death is reasonably foreseeable, where an advanced state of decline that cannot be reversed is evident, and unbearable physical or mental suffering is occurring (Government of Canada 2020a).

On 17 March 2021, additional MAID developments became law. These amendments removed the requirement that death be reasonably foreseeable. Further, the new legislation allowed persons approved for MAID to waive final consent if their death was reasonably foreseeable and they had qualified for MAID previously but may have subsequently lost the capacity to give final consent before receiving MAID. Finally, the new legislation means persons who are suffering solely from mental illness, who were not currently eligible for MAID, would become eligible in two years, on 17 March 2023 following the development of further guidelines and safeguards (Government of Canada 2021; Department of Justice Canada 2021a, 2021b).

By the end of 2019, almost 14,000 Canadians had received MAID since its inception in June of 2016 (Health Canada 2020). This number, which represents 2 per cent of all deaths in Canada in 2019, should be considered against the reality that almost all deaths in Canada occur after one or more treatments have either been withheld or withdrawn (Thurston, Wilson, and Hewitt 2012). Withholding and/or withdrawing treatment can allow death to occur.

Few physicians, health care administrators, or other health care workers in Canada have ever been charged for withdrawing or withholding care from dying persons. This is not to say that there are no issues over withdrawing or withholding treatment. In 2013, the Supreme Court of Canada was asked to address the question of who decides to withdraw life support in the contentious case of Mr. Rasouli, a 61-year-old man on life support since October 2010. Mr. Rasouli's wife, his substitute decision maker given that Mr. Rasouli could not speak for himself, fought to keep his physicians at Ontario's Sunnybrook Hospital from unilaterally deciding to stop life-supporting treatment. The family's cultural and religious background as Shia Muslims was said to influence Mrs. Rasouli's wish to have her husband's life support continued in the absence of any previously verbalized instructions from him or a written advance directive specifying his wishes. The Supreme Court of Canada (2013) ruled that life support termination required the consent of the family or a substitute decision maker and that disputes between doctors and family decision makers in Ontario must be referred to the Ontario Consent and Capacity Board.

Case law developments have also clarified rights and responsibilities on an individual level and set precedents for larger, societal-level rights and responsibilities, including the 2016 federal MAID legislation. Although American case law and other developments arising out of the sensational case of Karen Ann Quinlan and others since are of interest and have some effect on Canadian society, Canadian case law differs both in historical sequence and outcomes. One of the first precedent-setting cases in Canada was in 1992, when an Ontario physician was found guilty of assault and battery for insisting that blood be given to a woman of the Jehovah's Witness faith (*Malette v. Schulman* 1992). The physician knew the injured woman had signed a card indicating she did not want to receive blood. The ruling in favour of the plaintiff, whose life was preserved by the transfusion, identified personal autonomy in health care decision making as legally binding and morally compelling. In this and subsequent cases, the physician's judgement as to what is beneficial for the patient was not considered the key factor; instead, what the patient considered to be acceptable or appropriate treatment was deemed more important.

The *Malette* decision supported the withholding of life-sustaining treatment at the patient's request and was quickly followed by another major legal precedent, this time in regard to withdrawing treatment. **Withholding treatment** refers to not initiating treatment that is available, and **withdrawing treatment** refers to stopping treatment that has been initiated. In 1992, a judge was asked to grant a request by a young woman, Nancy B, who lived in a Montreal-area continuing care facility and wanted to have her life-supporting ventilator removed. After it had been determined that she was fully aware of the consequences of her decision to stop this life-supporting technology, her request was granted, and Nancy B died (Campion 1994; Sneiderman 1993). Since then, many competent adults and adults who have previously expressed their wishes verbally or through an advance directive that specifies treatment cessation in certain situations have had their life-supporting treatment stopped. Children as young as 11 years of age in Canada have had their wishes respected regarding treatment withdrawal (Mitchell, Guichon, and Wong 2015).

Thus, while criminal law in Canada prohibited assisted death before 2016, a dying person who is mentally competent has long had the right to refuse treatment, which may be withheld or withdrawn even though death results. Under these circumstances, withholding or withdrawing treatment is not defined as euthanasia or assisted suicide and, therefore, does not trigger prosecution under the law.

Withdrawal of and withholding treatment is an important consideration, as most terminally ill people can have their lives extended by health care therapies. People in comas, near-comas, or persistent vegetative states can be kept alive for years or even decades. For example, Karen Ann Quinlan was kept alive for 10 years by tube feeding after her American parents won the legal right to have her "life support," a ventilator, removed. Right-to-die groups, such as the Hemlock Society in the United States and Dying With Dignity Canada, have raised questions about the appropriate time to withdraw and withhold life-supporting treatments. Derek Humphry founded the Hemlock Society in the United States in 1980 and wrote a best-selling how-to book called *Final Exit: The Practicalities of Self-Deliverance and Assisted Suicide for the Dying* in 1991. On the other side of the debate, right-to-life or pro-life groups, including groups who represent disabled individuals and the unborn, raise the concern that life can be too easily ended.

Much of the debate over the use of life support to prolong life and the withholding or withdrawing of life support hinges on questions of human rights, most notably informed consent. In the past, physicians made many, if not all, health care decisions. Since the 1970s, greater awareness of the need for personal autonomy, punctuated by significant case law developments, has brought about a remarkable change in health care decision making. Today, competent individuals of almost any age can make their own health care decisions, even when these may not be considered by others to be the "right" decisions. This includes two 11-year-old children and their families who chose to stop chemotherapy. Both families were Indigenous, which brought additional cultural and racial considerations to the fore (Mitchell, Guichon, and Wong 2015).

Despite the emphasis on individual decision making, physicians, other health care professionals, and family or friends tend to influence many treatment decisions now. Physicians may even unilaterally make decisions, as some people want the physician to make the difficult "life and death" decisions. Alternatively, some people choose to refuse treatment or to demand treatment against physician advice. Nevertheless, health care professionals in Canada are not obliged to offer or provide futile care (Canadian Medical Association 1995; CNA, CMA, and CHA 1984) or non-beneficial and potentially harmful care (Kyriakopoulos, Fedyk, and Shamy 2017).

Advance directives allow competent individuals to indicate their preferences for care before care is actually needed and in anticipation of circumstances where the person might not be able to make or voice their own decisions. In other words, the advance care planning laws that have been enacted in every Canadian province enforce the right of individuals to direct their own health care even after they become mentally incompetent. Some confusion about terminology exists, as these may alternatively be called living wills, personal directives, representation agreements, health care directives, powers of attorney for personal care, or personal health care mandates, directives, or authorizations. Although advance care planning statutes vary across Canada, most allow one or more substitute decision makers to be named and allow instructions about health care to be left. These instructions must be followed or sanctions could be brought against those who do not abide by them, providing that the instructions are legal. These instructions are to take precedence over the preferences of family members and health care professionals.

The majority of adults in Canada do not have a written advance directive (Wilson, Houttekier, et al. 2013). These are advisable as they are intended to ensure that care preferences are carried out if individuals lose the ability to direct their own care. Unfortunately, many patients and their families are not certain today what should be done or not done in cases of serious illness and potential death (You et al. 2015). Whether or not to use **cardiopulmonary resuscitation (CPR)**, which has the potential to revive a person after death has technically occurred, is one of the most straightforward decisions. Other decisions, such as those that can hasten death (e.g., stopping kidney dialysis), are more difficult. Another major problem is that most, if not all, seriously ill and dying persons lose consciousness near death and thus lose the ability to direct their care at a time when decisions often need to be made (Wilson 1996; You et al. 2015). Other people are then in the position of having to make decisions, and these decisions may be difficult because written or verbalized instructions, if they exist, are often general in nature—such as the person saying that they do not want their life extended. Another major issue is that there can be differences of opinion among family members. Accordingly, some statutes permit the naming of individuals who should not become substitute decision makers.

Withdrawing or withholding care from the dying should not be confused with euthanasia or assisted suicide, which are two different ways of hastening death. The 2015 Supreme Court ruling in favour of assisted death follows the previous legalization of assisted suicide and/or euthanasia in the countries of Belgium, Switzerland, the Netherlands, and Luxembourg, as well as an increasing number of states in the United States starting with Oregon in 1997. The 2015 Canadian Supreme Court decision on hastened death reversed previous recommendations and rulings beginning in the early 1980s, when several law reform commissions recommended against legalizing euthanasia (Curran and Hyg 1984).

In 1993, the Supreme Court of Canada ruled against Sue Rodriguez's request for assistance in ending her life; Rodriguez's situation is discussed in more detail in chapter 5. Following this ruling, a Senate Committee was set up to study the issue of euthanasia and assisted suicide. The subsequent report of the Senate Committee on Euthanasia and Assisted Suicide (Senate of Canada 1995) contained several recommendations, one of which was that palliative care should become more accessible to dying Canadians. The committee assumed or felt that dying individuals would not request euthanasia or assisted suicide if their symptoms were managed and they were comfortable. It has not been established, however, that access to or experience with hospice/palliative care necessarily deters people from asking for assisted suicide or euthanasia.

In 1997, the Canadian Hospice Palliative Care Association published, for the first time, palliative care goals (these were later updated and enhanced in 2013, in "A Model to Guide Hospice Palliative Care: Based on National Principles and Norms of Practice Revised and Condensed Edition"). This was an important development as a second Senate Committee report in 2000, led by Senator Carstairs, continued to highlight concerns over the plight of dying individuals (Carstairs 2000). Carstairs's work led to the Compassionate Care Benefits Program being initiated in 2004 (Government of Canada 2017), and in 2018, the Government of Canada published a Framework for Palliative Care.

It is also important to point out that despite losing her case in 1993, Sue Rodriguez was helped to die at her home in British Columbia the following year. Her death is an example of **voluntary euthanasia** or assisted suicide, as it is not clear how she ended her life. No one was ever charged with this "crime." The circumstances surrounding her death can be contrasted with **nonvoluntary euthanasia**, as illustrated by another controversial Canadian court case. Robert Latimer, a Saskatchewan farmer, was found guilty of murder after he confessed to using carbon monoxide in 1993 to kill his severely disabled 12-year-old daughter, Tracy, who was mentally incapable of consenting. While some considered his actions to be a "mercy killing" to save Tracy from further surgery and from daily suffering, others felt he did not have the right to make this decision for his daughter. He served most of a 10-year jail sentence for second-degree murder.

It is not known how often unauthorized assisted suicide or euthanasia occurs now in Canada. Speculation also exists over unauthorized deaths in other countries, such as the Netherlands, where 4 per cent of deaths in 2016 were due to approved euthanasia or assisted suicide, with possibly an equal number of unauthorized cases occurring (European Institute of Bioethics 2020). In Belgium, the number of reported approved cases of assisted suicide has increased each year since 2003, although only 1.7 per cent of annual deaths

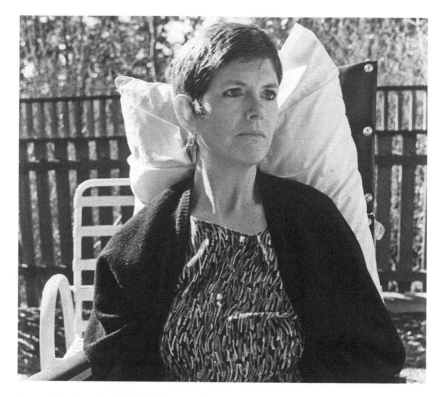

Image 3.2. Sue Rodriguez argued in 1993 for her right to assisted suicide, which was denied by the Supreme Court of Canada at the time (in a close five–four decision). In 1994, Rodriguez did end her life at home, although it is not clear how exactly she did so.
Source: Chuck Stoody/The Canadian Press. © The Canadian Press. All rights reserved.

between 2013 and 2016 were attributed to it (Dierickx et al. 2016). Over these same years, palliative care teams in Belgium were increasingly consulted and involved in the care of these individuals (Dierickx et al. 2016). In Oregon in the first year following the legalization of assisted suicide by prescription medications to end life in 1997, 15 people died after self-administering lethal prescriptions obtained from a licensed health care professional; in 2019, a total of 188 people died using medications obtained under the law, with 112 Oregon physicians writing 290 prescriptions. Similar numbers in Oregon are now occurring from year to year (Death with Dignity 2020). Moreover, most recipients of assisted suicide in Oregon are aged 65 or older, dying of cancer, receiving hospice/palliative care, and choose to die at home. The three most commonly expressed concerns contributing to their request for assisted suicide are loss of autonomy, decreased ability to participate in activities that made life enjoyable, and loss of dignity.

Clearly, considerable interest in assisted suicide and euthanasia is evident around the world (although Germany, the UK, and other countries experiencing referendums and tabled bills have so far not enabled either). This interest in death hastening may result from the increasing awareness of the futility of health care for preventing death and a related concern about enhanced or prolonged suffering during dying processes. Some time ago, Quill and Kimsma (2006, 10) emphasized this concern through this important question: "How much suffering is enough?" In another example, Dr. Donald Low had been the calm, reassuring voice on the evening news during the severe acute respiratory syndrome (SARS) outbreak in Toronto in 2003. Ten years later in 2013, at age 68, he was diagnosed with terminal brain cancer. In September 2013 he posted a YouTube video in which he made a passionate plea for "dying with dignity" and the legalization of assisted death. He died eight days later. Despite his plea, he stated that he thought it would be a long time before the law would be changed in Canada. He would have been pleased with the 2015 decision of the Supreme Court of Canada to allow Medical Assistance in Dying beginning in 2016.

In summary, a competent person of almost any age in Canada can request that life support be withheld or withdrawn, even if this hastens death. Similarly, a dying person who has become incompetent may have expressed their wishes in a written advance directive, which can result in the withholding or withdrawing of treatment. Moreover, Canadians who apply and meet the criteria for MAID can receive assistance to end their life earlier than if nature alone took its course. These are developments that have occurred over time, in a series of steps, within a society that was also clearly changing.

THE HEALTH CARE SYSTEM AND END-OF-LIFE CARE

Although all health care workers are expected to be prepared to deal effectively with dying and death, there is a long-standing concern that many do not feel adequately prepared to care for dying people or their grieving families (Brazil et al. 2006; Goodridge et al. 2005). Yet surveys of nursing and medical school curricula consistently show that all introductory programs contain content on death, dying, and supportive end-of-life care (Hall et al. 2006; Oneschuk et al. 2002; Wilson, Goodwin, and Hewitt 2011). Although thanatology (death) education is routinely provided in nursing and medical programs, this does not ensure that all health care professionals who provide end-of-life care feel confident in dealing with all aspects of dying and death.

In addition, many other types of health care providers besides nurses and physicians are involved in the care of dying individuals in homes, ambulances, emergency departments, hospitals, prisons, nursing homes, and all other places where dying and death can occur (Goodridge et al. 2005; Hall, Schroder, and Weaver 2002). These people may not have the thanatology education that nurses and physicians have (Brazil et al. 2006). Another challenging aspect of end-of-life care is that dying and death are not everyday events in many of the places where death occurs. Death is a rare occurrence in many health care specialties. Most health care workers are therefore unfamiliar with end-of-life care, and this unfamiliarity is increasing now that most deaths take place outside of hospitals (Wilson, Shen, and Birch 2017).

Of all health care providers, registered nurses and other nurses do the most direct, hands-on care for dying individuals. Through this work, nurses often come to know each patient's needs and preferences better than physicians and others who spend less time with the dying. Nurses often then become advocates for the patient. Moral distress is common among nurses (Gélinas et al. 2012) whenever futile or unnecessary care is provided because of a denial of the impending death by families or physicians (Palda et al. 2005; Zimmermann 2004).

Regardless, the culture of professionalism emphasizes a degree of emotional detachment to buffer the personal impact of caring for ill and dying patients. This detachment could help explain why Wilson (1997) found that most nurses and physicians working in a large Canadian hospital could not recall details about patients who had died recently under their care. In contrast, nurses and physicians working in a continuing care facility and two small rural hospitals were much more likely to recall details about the patient, the dying process, and the patient's family. This difference was related to the size and type of health care facility. In large hospitals, health care workers such as nurses, physician specialists, and physicians in training usually have very little contact with patients and their families. Contact is frequently limited to one hospital stay. In contrast, small hospitals are often situated in rural communities or less densely populated urban communities where there is a much greater chance of ongoing contact between health care workers and community residents, both in hospital over one or more admissions and outside the hospital. For residents in continuing care facilities, longer stays allow relationships to develop between health care providers and residents or their families when residents are unable to communicate. Dementia, other conditions such as stroke that impair speech or cognition, and serious health problems are common among continuing care residents (Cable-Williams and Wilson 2014).

Although individual health care providers vary in their preparation for and perspectives on dying and death, the context in which health care is provided has a powerful impact. Medical programs have long been criticized for training physicians to preserve life at any cost. For physicians, death may be perceived as a failure of medical care. Similarly, hospitals are primarily oriented to saving lives (Willison 2006). Indeed, the majority of health system funding is used for hospital, drug, and physician services that are largely oriented to the diagnosis and treatment of illnesses (Canadian Institute for Health Information 2014). The nature of the Canadian health care system, whereby access to hospitals and medical care is assured for all Canadians, has led to universal access to a wide variety of treatments that can support and extend life. One study found that active curative treatment normally continues until "nothing further can be done to preserve life" (Wilson 1997, 36). There is a long-standing concern that hospitals are oriented toward resisting death, not easing dying (Wilson, Anderson, et al. 1998).

There are many indications, however, that health care approaches to dying and death have changed and are continuing to change. The place of death has changed; only around 40 per cent of deaths take place in hospitals now (Wilson, Shen, and Birch 2017), with 35 per cent occurring in nursing homes (Statistics Canada 2014b), and most of the remainder taking place at home. Moreover, since the mid-1970s, hospitals and continuing care facilities in Canada have had policies that allow decisions about withholding life support to be made in advance of death (Choudhry et al. 1994; McPhail et al. 1981; Rasooly et al. 1994; Wilson 1996). By the mid-1990s, Wilson (1997) found that less than 3 per cent of adults who died in four Canadian hospitals and continuing care facilities had cardiopulmonary resuscitation (CPR) performed at the time of death. In 97 per cent of cases, a decision had been made to let death happen. It was clear that a curative orientation is both ineffective and inappropriate for patients who are terminally ill and dying.

Today, a **do-not-resuscitate (DNR) order** is often included in advanced care planning to clarify the preferred, if not legally mandated, care for when someone is terminally ill or actively dying. This care planning is routine now in nursing homes and hospices. Further, many patients now arrive in hospital with written advance directives that indicate their wishes about life support. A 2008 Canadian study found that nearly 20 per cent of people aged 70 or older visiting an emergency department had an advance directive (Gina et al. 2012). A 2010 study found that 44 per cent of adults in Alberta had an advance directive, and another 42 per cent were planning to write one (Wilson, Houttekier, et al. 2013).

Although increasingly planned for, deaths in hospitals and nursing homes are still largely hidden from conscious consideration. Many hospitals carry out a practice whereby deceased individuals are only removed from their rooms when the doors to other rooms are closed and in stretchers that conceal the body. Nursing homes can also downplay the occurrence of death onsite by transferring dying residents to a special room designed for family visitation that shields the dying person from the view of others. These actions reduce the effect of death on other people, as death is still an uncomfortable subject for many (Cable-Williams, Wilson, and Keating 2014). However, more nurses and physicians are specializing in hospice/palliative care, and the considerable dialogue about the 2016 implementation of MAID in Canada has helped to make dying and death a more open subject. Consequently, patients and families are less often asking for life supports to be used at or near the end of life (Canadian Institute for Health Information 2018).

The Canadian Hospice Palliative Care Association (n.d., para. 1) defines hospice/palliative care as "a specialized form of healthcare [that] aims to relieve suffering and improve the quality of life for those living with a life limiting illness, as well as their families. Hospice palliative care addresses the specific physical, psychological, social, spiritual, and practical issues, and their associated expectations, needs, hopes and fears on an individual basis." This aim is not oriented to preserving or lengthening life. Furthermore, hospice/palliative care is more holistic than curative care as it addresses the wide range of needs of the dying person as well as those of their family. Hospice/palliative care focuses on the prevention and management of symptoms to make the dying person as comfortable as possible. Hospice/palliative care is designed to improve patients' quality of life and prevent "bad" deaths from occurring (Wilson and Hewitt 2018). Hospice/palliative care is a highly interdisciplinary and team-based health care service that involves nurses, physicians, and other people who work together to achieve a good death in every setting (Canadian Hospice Palliative Care Association n.d.).

Unfortunately, hospice/palliative specialist services are still limited across Canada (Canadian Institute for Health Information 2018). The first palliative care units in Canada opened in 1975 in Montreal and Winnipeg hospitals. By 1985, approximately 300 hospital-based palliative care programs and 1,000 hospital beds were devoted to palliative care across Canada (Wilson and Woytowich 2014). Nevertheless, even now only a very small percentage of hospital beds are devoted to hospice/palliative care. Some large hospitals do not have palliative care units or their own palliative care specialist teams, a factor explaining differences in the care of dying patients across hospitals with or without this specialization (Cohen et al. 2012).

Growth in nonhospital hospice/palliative care has occurred instead across Canada, with around 100 hospices existing now and most home care agencies offering hospice/palliative care in their clients' homes (Canadian Institute for Health Information 2018). Home-based services are often critically important as most end-of-life care takes place at home (Wilson and Woytowich 2014). Respite care may be essential so family members can sleep, go to work, or leave the house for a few hours. Hospice/palliative day care, where the dying person goes to a care centre during the day, is another option (Wilson, Truman, et al. 2005). These options can help a wage-earning family caregiver keep working, which is an important consideration as there are many out-of-pocket costs associated with home-based end-of-life care (Chai et al. 2014). This issue was recognized by the federal government and led to the Compassionate Care Act being implemented across Canada in 2004 to support home-based care through partial wages and job security assurance for one family caregiver (Government of Canada 2020b). Moreover, in 2018, a federal Framework for Palliative Care in Canada was developed, along with a five-year action plan to advance policy and programs with the aim of increasing access to hospice/palliative care (Government of Canada 2019).

Although increasingly diversified in terms of care setting, the initiation of hospice/palliative care in hospitals created a competition for funding between curative and noncurative care. Issues of funding also plague publicly funded home care programs, as hospice/palliative clients typically receive more hours of care than other home care clients (Wilson, Kinch, et al. 2005; Wilson, Truman, et al. 2007). A growing number of freestanding hospices exist across Canada, built to provide inpatient and/or day care services for dying people and their families (Wilson and Woytowich 2014). Hospices were established in Canada in the late 1970s by community groups generally, and they are not yet considered a central component of the Canadian health care system. As a consequence, hospices must fundraise to support their daily operation, with this requirement limiting the number of services they can provide and the number of clients they can assist (Wilson and Woytowich 2014).

Regardless of this lag in the development of specialized hospice/palliative care services, the health care system, health care professionals, and families are increasingly recognizing and responding to terminal illnesses and active dying. As the number of people dying each year continues to increase, new developments in the organization and delivery of all types of specialist hospice/palliative and basic end-of-life care can be expected. An array of different programs is likely to develop as the needs for and possible options for programs within one community can be quite different from another. For example, small remote or rural communities and large urban communities are likely to develop different end-of-life programs. Moreover, the care needs of dying people often vary considerably (Wilson and Woytowich 2014). Hopefully, funding for these programs will not be as much of an issue as it has been. Canadian social values have traditionally emphasized rescuing people from death and thus preserving life, so diverting money from programs that save lives to hospice/palliative programs that facilitate dying is difficult. Additional health care funding specifically directed toward specialist hospice/palliative care programs and basic end-of-life care services may be needed instead.

Dying people can use a considerable amount of health care resources (Canadian Institute for Health Information 2020b). For instance, one study involving 2,074 Canadians who died of colorectal cancer found that 3.7 per cent received chemotherapy in the last two weeks of life, 12.5 per cent had multiple visits to an emergency department in the last 30 days of life, 9.5 per cent had multiple hospital admissions in the last 30 days of life, 2.2 per cent were admitted to an intensive care unit in the last 30 days of life, and 50.1 per cent died in hospital (Hu et al. 2014). Hospital care is approximately 10 times more expensive than care in a continuing care facility, which is itself usually double the cost of care in the home.

One further fiscal as well as ethical issue is the technological approach to care in hospitals. On admission, patients routinely have blood tests, X-rays, and other diagnostic tests done at considerable expense. Aggressive treatments are then common. Even when it becomes obvious that death is unavoidable, diagnostic tests and treatments may continue until death. In addition, dying people may be given oxygen to ease breathing, intravenous fluids to maintain hydration or deliver painkillers, antibiotics to reduce chest congestion, and other medications to strengthen the heart or other systems (Thurston, Wilson, and Hewitt 2012). As a result of these interventions, dying typically lasts longer. Although these procedures may cause pain or irritate the dying person, health care professionals and the public are often reluctant to adopt a noninterventionist approach during the dying process. Apparently, few trust nature to produce a good death. Interventionist care is occurring despite calls over the past 50 years for a more natural dying process, with pain medication alone used to ease suffering (Murray 1981; Pannuti and Tanneberger 1992; Turner et al. 1996). These issues and the fact that few deaths now are sudden and unexpected led to the June 2016 legalization of assisted dying for those who ask for it and meet the criteria for it. Although only about 2 per cent of deaths in Canada in 2019 resulted from Medical Assistance in Dying (Health Canada 2020), this development has opened the public discourse and made dying and death much more obvious.

Nevertheless, because death is so final and is viewed with such aversion in a youth-oriented and success-oriented society, the decision by the patient or the family or both to shift from curative care to hospice/palliative care is still often delayed (You et al. 2015). Some dying individuals and family members today are tremendously reluctant—given the possibility or hope of a medical breakthrough—to acknowledge that death is inevitable. Often this reluctance is expressed by a dying parent's adult child who has not seen their parent lately and so has not come to an understanding that their parent is irrevocably dying. A common situation involves an adult child who has moved far away from their parents and has had little direct contact over the years, returning only when a parent is facing death and thus finding themselves unprepared for the parent's dying. This child may be very much at odds with the other children in the family who have come to accept the certainty of impending death (Wilson et al. 2020).

Parents may also be reluctant to accept death for their children, although a study found parents of terminally ill children were more concerned about their child's pain and suffering than their death (Pritchard et al. 2010). Phillips (1992) was among the first to report a need to refocus our approach so that it does not appear that hospice/palliative care begins when treatment ends; instead, there should be a gradual and overlapping shift from curative care to hospice/palliative care.

Population aging has contributed a great deal to this shifting emphasis between curative care and palliative/hospice care. Cable-Williams and Wilson (2014) studied awareness of death for older residents (85+ years of age) in three long-term care facilities in Ontario. They noted that residents, staff, and family members all had a generalized awareness of the relative closeness to death for very old individuals. They knew that death might come tomorrow; however, they also knew that death might still be years away. Individuals who appeared to be dying occasionally rallied and lived on. Consequently, staff tended to predict death and adopt end-of-life care strategies such as palliative care only when residents were actively dying. Accordingly, the implementation of palliative care came very late in the dying process. Leung et al. (2012) noted this same delay in hospitals.

In summary, dying and death are largely, but inaccurately, associated with health care institutions, particularly hospitals and nursing homes; most end-of-life care in Canada today takes place at home. Nurses and doctors provide planning and care for the dying, with families continuing to have major roles in relation to end-of-life care. Although health care services are still too often oriented toward saving lives, withholding life support near death is common now. Furthermore, both hospital-based and community-based/home-based programs increasingly offer end-of-life care that facilitates dying. Finally, since 2016 in Canada, some dying persons have chosen death directly through MAID.

THE DEATH CARE INDUSTRY

The final stage of the dying process is an important time when most families want to be together with their dying family member. Following death, families typically also gather to demonstrate respect for the deceased person and to provide support to each other (Waugh 2013). Funeral and memorial services do much to assist those who are grieving by providing an opportunity to reflect upon the life of the person who has died and to publicly and collectively acknowledge that person's death. Following this, bereaved people have the option of accessing a wide range of bereavement services (Wilson and Playfair 2016), although only one in three do, with most of these individuals being female (Wilson, Cohen, et al. 2018). Bereavement grief may be severe and long-standing, such that the person is considered to have persistent or complicated grief, although most bereaved people recover over time.

One of the most profound changes in the death care industry is that over half of all deaths in Canada now involve cremation (Cremation Association of North America 2015). **Cremation** typically occurs when a very hot fire is used to reduce the body and its container to ash. Certain religious and cultural groups, such as Hindus, have long performed cremation. In contrast,

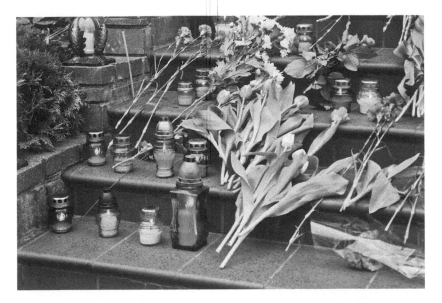

Image 3.3. Candles and flowers commemorate a death
Source: milka-kotka/Shutterstock.

other religious and cultural groups consider this inappropriate (Waugh 2013). Some people choose cremation because they are disturbed by the thought of the body decaying in the ground after burial (Cremation Association of North America 2015).

Cremations have become common in Canada for a variety of practical reasons. Cremations may be chosen over winter burials. Another significant reason is reduced cost. The average funeral in Canada costs between $5,000 and $25,000 (Cremation Association of North America 2015). There are charges for every service, including transporting the body, preparing the body for burial (which may or may not include embalming), providing the casket in which the body is buried and the cemetery burial plot or tomb in a **mausoleum**, and conducting the funeral service. Cremations typically cost less than half the cost of a burial (Cremation Association of North America 2015).

Cremation also allows for flexibility. Funerals usually take place soon after death—within one day for certain cultural groups, but most often within three or four days (Waugh 2013). Families typically are widely dispersed geographically, and gathering family members together quickly for a funeral can be difficult. Not only is the cost of travel on short notice high, but child care may have to be arranged, leaves of absence from work or study obtained,

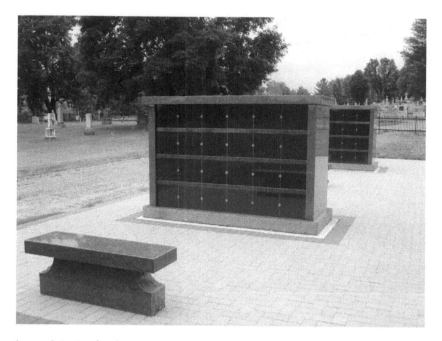

Image 3.4. A columbarium containing cinerary urns—urns holding the ashes of deceased individuals who have been cremated
Source: Robbie Gorr/iStock.com.

and many other personal circumstances attended to. Cremation provides the family with flexibility, as the urn containing the ashes of the deceased person can be easily transported to any location where a memorial service can take place at a time convenient to the family. There is less urgency, as well, in taking the ashes to their final resting place or in scattering the remains, in comparison to a body, which must be buried within a few days of death, kept "on ice" until a later burial, or embalmed.

Embalming is a semi-surgical process that replaces body fluids with liquid chemicals (formaldehyde and methyl or wood alcohol) to preserve the body (Waugh 2013). Embalming is not required unless the body is to be shipped across national or international borders or transported by public carrier. Bodies that have been embalmed and buried have been exhumed years later and found to be relatively unchanged.

The death care industry itself is an important social institution. This industry provides many people with employment and investment income (Industry Canada 2015). Caskets and urns have to be made; bodies need to be prepared for embalming, burial, or cremation; funeral parlours and crematoria have to be built and kept in good repair; and cemeteries and mausoleums have to be developed and maintained. In addition, other businesses benefit as notices of death and funeral services are usually published, flowers are sent, donations are made to charities, and travel is undertaken to attend the funeral or memorial service. This industry has long been considered recession proof (Flynn 1993), as most deaths involve a funeral or memorial service.

It should not be surprising that the death care industry in Canada is a large and profitable business. Doug Smith (2007) wrote about the "corporate deathcare" industry in his book titled *Big Death*, noting that corporations "dominate the Canadian funeral and cemetery business. . . . Together, they constitute Big Death" (55). In North America, approximately $9 to $10 billion a year was grossed in the early 1990s by businesses that provided death-related services (Flynn 1993). One of the most noteworthy facts about the death industry is that huge corporations largely replaced the local, family-owned funeral home during the 1980s and 1990s (Flynn 1993). Today, only a small number of large corporations supply most of the North American "death market." Service Corporation International (SCI), based in Houston, Texas, is the largest. SCI (n.d.) reports owning 1,900 funeral homes and cemeteries in 44 states, 8 Canadian provinces, Washington, DC, and Puerto Rico. SCI is listed on the New York Stock Exchange.

SCI and Arbor Memorial Inc. are the two largest death care providers in Canada (IbisWorld 2020). Funeral businesses come and go, however. Loewen Group Inc. based in Vancouver, British Columbia, once Canada's largest funeral company and the second-largest funeral business conglomerate worldwide, filed for bankruptcy protection in 1999. Too rapid expansion was blamed, but another factor was competition from firms selling "wholesale" caskets and "no-frills" funeral services, thereby reducing demand for expensive, full-service burials. For example, you can now buy your casket online or at Costco.

High prices, together with effective marketing to promote a wide range of end-of-life services, have made the death care industry very profitable. Other factors are also important, such as an increasing number of deaths accompanying population growth and the COVID-19 pandemic resulting in an increased demand for death care services (IbisWorld 2020).

According to Flynn (1993), "one-stop shopping," whereby families use one service provider to make all funeral arrangements, coupled with an increased range of services, has led to spiraling funeral costs. The amount of income available to the family impacts which ceremonies are held and which customs are followed. In a time of intense difficulty and pressure, families often must choose between a traditional, full-service funeral or an "alternate" funeral for which there is no standard format (Cremation Association of North America 2015). In addition, families typically must choose how elaborate the service and the casket or urn will be. The latter is a concern, as there is a substantial markup on these items (Flynn 1993). Some other common decisions that need to be made, if not made by the decedent before death, include whether to have a closed or open casket; whether to permit visitation or calling at the funeral home to see the body; whether to hold a funeral with the casket present or hold a memorial service at a later time; and whether the body will be buried, cremated, or entombed in a mausoleum. Given all these considerations, it is prudent to preplan a funeral to lower costs and ensure that important preferences, rituals and customs are upheld.

This advice is illustrated by the following story. The first author's mother died in November 2014. Her death was expected given her obvious health decline over several months, and her death was seen as imminent when she was placed in palliative care. What was not expected were the challenges of organizing her funeral. Following her death, a funeral home took her from the hospital. Family and friends were notified. Decisions had to be made, and family members were consulted extensively. She had prepaid her funeral in another city in another province. Nevertheless, the family had to first organize a service for people in her present location who wished to celebrate her life. A venue was booked, a casket chosen, flowers ordered, photos collected, a memorial card created for visiting guests, and an obituary published in a local newspaper. Her body was prepared and dressed for viewing. Several days later, she had to be transported across the Prairies to the city where she had spent most of her adult life and where she wished to be buried alongside her husband, who had predeceased her years before. Another funeral home took possession of her body, a funeral service was arranged in a local church, announcements were made, another obituary was published in the local newspaper, flowers were ordered, speakers and musical numbers were chosen for the funeral service, a program was printed, memorial cards and photos came from the previous service, a guest book was set out, food was ordered for the social gathering following the church service, volunteers were recruited to serve the food and set up tables and chairs, decorations for the tables were bought and configured, and the family and close friends were informed about the evening. It was another lovely time together celebrating her life and renewing relationships. It was also a huge relief when this final day of funeral activities was over.

All eight of her children and seven of the eight spouses made the journey to attend the final funeral service. Several grandchildren and great-grandchildren also attended. Her sons and sons-in-law carried her out of the church in her casket; grandsons carried her to her grave in the cemetery. A hotel at a convenient location had been booked to provide group rates. Costs to individual family members included airfares, hotel accommodation, food, car rentals, and gasoline. The local economy benefited substantially, and the funeral homes did very well. Despite a prepaid funeral, costs continued to rise. The two funeral homes submitted bills approaching $20,000 (including the prepayment of about $8,000 made years before). An extra charge for the funeral service and interment on a Saturday was included, along with extra costs for a winter burial in early December; apparently it is less expensive to be buried on a weekday in the summertime. Lingering around the grave past 4 p.m. on that cold December day would have resulted in another surcharge. A bitter prairie wind saved this extra cost, driving people back into cars and to the church for a much warmer social gathering and supper. The costs of the family members' travel added thousands of dollars beyond the costs of the funeral itself. Death is expensive. Her supportive care costs for the end of her life were yet another financial issue, with bills arriving after her death.

After the death, there was more work to be done. Her various sources of income had to be notified of her death, her bank accounts managed, her credit cards terminated, her outstanding bills paid, her financial investments withdrawn, her estate calculated, her taxes paid, her possessions disbursed, her estate distributed to her heirs, and so on. There was so much to do in the first two weeks following her death that there was little time for sorrow or grief. There was intense pressure to get things done, but little time for reflection. Her death was not a surprise, so perhaps this explains the limited feelings of grief at the time. Several weeks later, when things had settled down, family members finally had time to think about her death and miss her.

On occasion, when calling a business office to advise them of her death, a stranger would say "I'm sorry for your loss." Curiously, this conventional comment from a complete stranger would trigger emotion and make speaking difficult. Yet for the most part, grief was not present. This absence could be the result of advance notice, a sense that Mom's suffering had come to an end, and the pressures of organizing her funeral service and taking care of business. A request was made not to announce my mother's death at my work, as was customary, to avoid the heartfelt but superficial "I'm sorry for your loss." This resulted in a deprivation of my colleagues' support, since most of my colleagues did not know of my mother's death. Those who knew did not have licence to mention it to me. It would have been better to have the usual announcement and for colleagues to express the usual sentiment in the usual phrase. As trite and limited as these rituals are, they can leave one feeling supported. Funerary rituals, as the anthropologists would call them, perform many useful personal and social functions. In Canada today, these funerary rituals tend to incur considerable economic cost.

In summary, the death care industry is big business, offering a wide range of services to the family and friends of the deceased. Funeral plans can and should be made in advance. When this has not been done, the family of the deceased must make many decisions quickly at a time when decision making tends to be difficult. In such circumstances, the bereaved may pay more than they need to, may purchase more services than they can afford, or may end up with a service that does not meet their cultural needs and personal expectations. Cremation has become common in Canada, in part because it costs less than a traditional burial and because it allows for greater flexibility in planning.

SUMMARY

Dying and death typically take place in the context of the family and the health care system. The course of dying is shaped not only by terminal illness but also by decisions made by patients, family caregivers, and health care staff (physicians in particular). Although the hospital continues to have a major role in dying and death, the primary location of dying and death is shifting from the hospital to continuing care facilities, the home, and other locations such as hospices. Even in the hospital, the location of death is shifting from acute care wards to palliative care beds and units. Similarly, although health care workers may be primary caregivers for the dying in hospitals and nursing homes, the family is often heavily involved and are participants in end-of-life care decisions and actual caregiving.

The shift to a more normalized dying process outside the traditional cure-oriented hospital setting is occurring in large measure because of three major developments. The first is increased awareness of the limits of health care for curing illnesses and extending life. The second is the long-standing concern about inadequate and inappropriate end-of-life care in hospital, characterized by attempts to cure illness, prolong life, and deny death. Third is that hospice/palliative care has become increasingly established in Canada, with this and other end-of-life care strategies shifting the emphasis of care from extending life to providing a good death.

While dying and death typically take place in the context of the family and the health care system, the course of dying and death is also shaped by cultural, religious, legal, and funerary considerations. Cultural diversity and multiculturalism in Canada involve an increasing variety of expectations for dying and death. Furthermore, dying and death have changed as social institutions have evolved over time. For example, religion tends to play a lesser role in dying and death than in the past for many, but not all, people. Furthermore, legal developments have legitimized withholding and withdrawing care, the patient's right to refuse care, and the advance directive. Assisted death has been legalized in some countries, including Canada as of 2016. The funeral has moved from the home, church, and community to the profit-driven death care industry, where death processing has been professionalized and corporatized. These social changes have implications for the meaning and experience of dying and death for individuals, families, and society as a whole.

QUESTIONS FOR REVIEW

1. How has the family's role in dying and death changed? Why have these changes occurred, and what are the consequences of these changes? What issues in particular do LGBTQIA2S+ families face in the dying and death of their loved ones?
2. Discuss the role of religion in dying and death in past and present Canada. How does a family's religious beliefs and practices impact dying and death today? How do major religions influence the development and implementation of social policies associated with dying and death?
3. Examine the evolution of health care law in Canada. In particular, discuss issues involving advance directives, decision making rights, withholding

and withdrawing care, refusing care, futile care, palliative care, and assisted death.

4. The guidelines for Medical Assistance in Dying (MAID) have changed since MAID was introduced in 2016. What changes have been implemented? Has Canada gone too far or not far enough? Defend your position.

5. Discuss the rise of the death care industry. Consider the advantages and disadvantages of professional death care. Critically assess the increasing preference for cremation and for alternatives such as "green" burials.

6. Describe and evaluate the shift in end-of-life care from attempting to extend life to enabling a good death. That is, discuss the rise and role of hospice/palliative care in dying and death.

KEY TERMS

advance directive – A legal document that allows competent individuals to indicate their preferences for care before care is actually needed and in anticipation of circumstances where the person might not be able to make or voice decisions. Also referred to as a living will, personal directive, health care directive, representation agreement, or power of attorney for personal care. (p. 67)

assisted death – Usually involves providing a lethal substance, at the patient's request (or at the request of the patient's designated decision maker), that the patient consumes or that is administered to the patient with the intent of causing death. Includes both assisted suicide and euthanasia. (p. 63)

assisted suicide – Helping someone to die by suicide. (p. 63)

cardiopulmonary resuscitation (CPR) – Efforts made to restart a heart that has ceased functioning and to restore breathing. (p. 68)

cremation – The process by which a very hot fire is used to reduce the body and its container to ash. (p. 78)

do-not-resuscitate (DNR) order – A note on a patient's chart indicating that no attempt is to be made to restart the patient's heart if it stops. (p. 73)

embalming – A process that replaces body fluids with liquid chemicals (such as formaldehyde) to preserve the body after death. (p. 80)

euthanasia – Causing the death of another person. Sometimes referred to as "mercy killing" when done in the belief that the deceased was suffering and wanted to die. (p. 63)

good death – An optimal or ideal dying process and the end point of that process. (p. 59)

mausoleum – A building containing tombs for dead bodies. A columbarium contains niches for the cremains (ashes) of cremated bodies. (p. 79) nonvoluntary euthanasia – When a person who cannot express his or her wishes is euthanized on the assumption or assertion that he or she would prefer to die. (p. 69)

voluntary euthanasia – Euthanasia performed at the request of a person who asks for death and is competent to do so. (p. 69)

withdrawing treatment – Stopping treatment that has been initiated previously. (p. 66)

withholding treatment – Not initiating treatment that is available. (p. 66)

CHAPTER FOUR

Dying and Death in Canadian Culture

This chapter explores cultural constructions of the meaning of dying and death in Canada and the social responses associated with them. Cultural constructions are evident in many forms, notably literature, television, movies, the daily news, internet sites, social media, video games, everyday language, folklore, and the established processes of secularization, medicalization, professionalization, and bureaucratization of dying and death. Sociocultural responses to dying and death discussed here include making sense of death by means of shared **discourses**, distinguishing between different types of death, stigmatizing dying and death, and acknowledging ethnocultural diversity in end-of-life preferences.

It has been argued that Canadian culture, along with those of other higher-income societies, became death denying during the twentieth century (Ariès 1974, 1981; Becker 1973; Jalland 2006). Nevertheless, the reality of dying and death cannot be denied—dying and death do come to each person in turn. Regardless, in a death-denying culture, reactions to dying and death vacillate between denial and awareness, fear and fascination (Joseph 1994), and detachment and morbid obsession. Fascination with death is evident in cultural forms, including literature and television. This fascination has led several notable Canadian authors to explore the processes of dying and the mysteries of death.

SELECTED WORKS OF LITERATURE

Margaret Laurence, one of the most notable icons of Canadian literature, published *The Stone Angel* in 1964. This book begins with 90-year-old Hagar

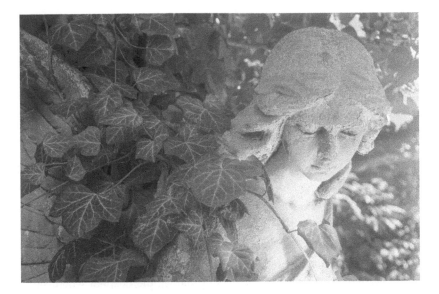

Image 4.1. Angel statue in a cemetery
Source: mojahata/Shutterstock.

Shipley's reminiscences of the stone angel standing over her mother's grave in a cemetery in the fictional town of Manawaka, Manitoba. This place is patterned after Neepawa, Manitoba, where Laurence herself was born. Through Hagar's memories, descriptions, and reflections, the reader is given a series of impressions about attitudes toward dying and death in Canada in the late nineteenth and early twentieth centuries.

Hagar remembers the stone angel and the inscriptions in the cemetery, and how strange and even amusing these things seemed to her as a young girl. As an old woman now, she recalls lives lived and largely forgotten and observes the tendency for weeds to overgrow the cemetery—a metaphor for how time obscures memories of the dead. Hagar also remembers sneaking into Simmons's Funeral Parlour with other children to look at Hannah Pearl's pale stillborn baby lying in a white satin box. Her brother Matt had told her that Mr. Simmons, the owner of the funeral parlour, drank embalming fluid. Hagar avoided the man, thinking of him as a ghoul. In these accounts, Laurence illustrates the paradoxical fascination and revulsion that people manifest with death and all that is associated with it.

Throughout the novel, Hagar remembers deceased ancestors and relatives including her dead mother and her teenage brother, four years her senior, who caught pneumonia and died in an upstairs bedroom asking for his long-dead mother. Hagar recalls the death from consumption (tuberculosis) of a school-mate's mother and the deaths of nonhumans as well: the pathetic death of a fighting cock and the gruesome euthanizing of some newborn chicks. As she reflects on her youthful emotions, she wonders why she could not then inter-vene to kill the chicks more humanely nor comfort her dying brother. In her youth, she recoiled and distanced herself from dying and death, both human and nonhuman.

The lily of the valley, both as a flower and as the name for the eau de co-logne she wears, reminds Hagar now of death. As she thinks back in her old age, her memories often focus on death, as if past deaths are a harbinger of her own. When her minister asks if she has many friends, she observes that most of them are dead. Her parents are long dead, as are her two brothers. Her husband and one of her two sons are dead as well. Hagar knows that her own death is near. She also knows that others—her remaining son and daugh-ter-in-law, and her doctor and the nursing staff in the hospital where she is spending her final days—are waiting, anticipating, and expecting her demise. Though no one speaks directly to Hagar of her impending death, she guesses the meaning of whispered conversations.

Throughout *The Stone Angel*, Laurence portrays death as both strange and familiar. While death is common and inevitable, it is also mysterious and repulsive. Laurence portrays death as something to be avoided and resisted as much as possible through cognitive, emotional, and behavioural distanc-ing and denial. Nevertheless, she also shows it to be intimately lived and highly personal. Finally, Laurence describes the common drama of mutual pretense. In this drama, everybody involved knows that death is imminent and yet nobody speaks openly or directly about it (Glaser and Strauss 1965). The dying person is discouraged from speaking of his or her own dying and imminent death.

Another Canadian literary great, W.O. Mitchell, described death in early twentieth-century prairie culture. His 1947 book *Who Has Seen the Wind* begins with a quote from Psalms: "As for man [*sic*], his days are as grass: as a flower of the field, so he flourisheth. For the wind passeth over it, and it is gone; and the place thereof shall know it no more." Mitchell then provides the reader with an explanation of the meaning of the story he is about to tell. The wind, he says, is a symbol of God, and the story to be told is about the mysteries of the cycle of life from birth to death for all people.

Mitchell tells the story of young Brian O'Connal, who grows up in a small town in Saskatchewan in the 1930s. Brian's family consists of his mother, father, grandmother, and a baby brother. The story begins when Brian is four years of age. His baby brother is very sick, and it is feared that he will die. Although the baby recovers, his near-death sets an ominous tone for the reader. Mitchell seems to be telling us that life begins and continues in the shadow of death; the possibility of death at any moment and its ultimate inevitability raise fundamental questions about the meaning of life.

A baby pigeon that Brian brings home is not as lucky as Brian's brother. When the pigeon dies, it is Brian's first experience with the demise of a being that had meant something to him. Several years later, when Brian is about eight years of age, his beloved dog is run over by a horse-drawn wagon. Brian sadly buries his dog under the prairie sod and grieves.

As the story unfolds, Brian approaches 10 years of age. His grandmother is now 80 years old and knows her death is near. At the same time, Brian's father gets sick and becomes jaundiced. Once again, the ominous tone moves from background to foreground, and the reader is left to wonder who will live and who will die. That summer, Brian's father dies. He is laid out in a coffin at home in the living room with blinds drawn against the light. Friends and neighbours come by with flowers, tears, and sympathy, and everyone observes that the deceased was a fine man. Brian's mother is quiet, stunned; his grandmother sits, looking frail.

The minister conducts the funeral in the living room. Afterwards Brian is sad, filled with longing, but he does not know what to do. He wants to cry because he feels it is the right thing, but even though he loved his dad, the tears are not there. Instead, he goes out to the prairie. As he thinks in his 10-year-old way of the endless cycle of the seasons, the endless cycle of birth and death, he realizes that his father is gone forever. He thinks of the irony that, although individuals are forever being born, at death the individual is forever gone. When he thinks of his mother grieving the loss of her husband he cries, but his tears are for the living as much as for the dead.

Following the funeral, Brian thinks often of his father and frequently dreams that he is still alive. As time passes, he feels guilty that he thinks of his father less often. The family visits the cemetery frequently, and during these visits Brian tries to think of his father. He grows closer to his mother, brother, and grandmother.

The story ends with the death of Brian's grandmother. Brian has reached the age of 12 and his grandmother has lived 82 years. Her death is not as traumatic as the death of Brian's father, who died prematurely in the prime of his life—an unexpected, shocking, tragic death. The grandmother's death is expected, legitimate, and bittersweet. Her long life and the frailty preceding her death justify her passing. In her own—that is, Mitchell's—words, her time had come. Nevertheless, losing her is not easy for the living, and Brian grieves her passing.

The story of Brian's childhood is thus punctuated with accounts of death and youthful attempts to make sense of life and death. Brian remembers the deaths of the baby pigeon, a gopher, his dog, a two-headed calf, his father, and his grandmother. He recalls the stench of a rotting cow. He reflects on his dead ancestors from whom his own life has come. Brian continues to live, hunger, and wonder about the sense of it all.

Who Has Seen the Wind explores the mysteries of life and death. The book suggests that death is omnipresent and yet ominous: mysterious, unwelcome, disturbing, distressing, and inevitable. All who live die. This observation is inescapable and yet hard to accept and even harder to understand. Mitchell suggests that if answers are to be found, they are ethereal, like the wind.

Mitchell also describes society's cultural and ritual ways of dealing with death, including churches, theology, philosophy, funerals and flowers, cemeteries and gravestone epitaphs, and sympathetic, if trite, sentiments expressed to the bereaved. In the end, though, the novelist suggests that individuals must come to terms with life and death on their own, in their own way, and in their own time.

Both novels—Laurence's *The Stone Angel* and Mitchell's *Who Has Seen the Wind*—are about the culture and experience of life and death in small towns and rural settings in Canada in the first half of the twentieth century. The urban experience of death both in the second half of the twentieth century and in the early twenty-first century involves a greater degree of distancing and denial (Ariès 1974, 1981; Becker 1973; Jalland 2006). Death is kept at a greater distance from the individual, family, and community.

LANGUAGE

The printed program for a funeral service for a colleague who died says "In Loving Memory Of" and then states his name. Under the heading "Born," his date and place of birth are listed. Under the heading "Passed Away," the date when and the city where he passed away are listed. The word "death" does not appear in the program. It is as if people are born, but do not die. People simply pass away. Nor was this colleague buried. According to the program, the funeral service was followed by an "interment," not a burial, yet a body was indeed buried.

Death cannot be completely denied, even in an allegedly death-denying culture, although convention can distance us from it. While one could speak directly, using terms such as "dying," "dead," "death," and "burial," the conventional language of death is often indirect and euphemistic. Speaking directly seems too harsh, too cold, even cruel. The direct language refers to a harsh reality, a reality that is known but that people prefer to soften rather than to acknowledge explicitly.

According to Webster's Dictionary, a **euphemism** is "the use of a word or phrase that is less expressive or direct but considered less distasteful, less offensive . . . than another." In Canadian culture, common practice indicates that it is less distasteful and less offensive to use euphemisms than to speak directly of death. Williamson, Evans, and Munley (1980, 434–5) present an extensive list of euphemisms for dying, death, and burial. The dead person is often referred to as the "departed" or the "deceased." The coffin is often called a "casket." When a person dies, it may be said that the deceased has "passed on," "passed over," "laid their burden down," "gone to a well-earned rest," "been called home," or "gone to heaven." Instead of saying the person has been buried, it might be said that they were "laid to rest." The corpse may be referred to as "the body" or "the remains"; an impersonal "the" is used instead of the personal pronoun "his" or "her." This depersonalization of the dead body disassociates the memory of the living from the evidence of death.

Rawlings et al. (2017) asked students in their 2016 massive open online course (MOOC) on dying and death to list euphemisms for dying, death, and dead. A total of 1,183 discrete euphemisms were listed by 471 students. The most common euphemisms were variations on "gone" (to heaven, to sleep, etc.), "pass/passed/passing" (e.g., passed away), and "loss/lost." A common colloquialism was "pushing up daisies" and a common dysphemism (the opposite of a euphemism and more likely to offend) was "kicked the bucket."

While the euphemisms for death tend to be tasteful and inoffensive to soften a harsh reality, there are dysphemisms that are at best humorous and at worst vulgar. Humour presents an alternative way of dealing with what makes us uncomfortable. Making light of something that terrifies us is one way of "whistling in the dark," of convincing ourselves that we can ignore or manage our fears. Humorous terms for death include "bit the dust," "kicked the bucket," "pushing up daisies," "your goose is cooked," "he croaked," and so on. Other slang sayings include "cold meat" for corpse, "bone box" for coffin, "bone orchard" or "marble city" for cemetery, and "planted" or "deep sixed" for buried (Williamson, Evans, and Munley 1980). In summary, by either distancing from death or making light of death, various euphemisms/ dysphemisms facilitate coping with the strong emotions that tend to accompany death.

FOLKLORE, POPULAR CULTURE, AND CONTEMPORARY MEDIA

Folklore embodies beliefs, customs, rituals, myths, legends, folk tales, stories, rumours, jokes, and sayings that are collectively shared and communicated verbally in both oral and written forms (Clifton 1991). Folklore tends to reflect popular culture. As such, some may judge the following stories and jokes to be in poor taste. Cultural constructions regarding death range from sensitive to insensitive, respectful to disrespectful, and tasteful to tasteless.

The following story illustrating this matter began circulating on the internet in the 1990s; its origins are unknown:

> A few years ago, in California, there was a raging brush fire. Once the fire was extinguished, the firefighters began the process of clean-up. In the middle of where the fire had been burning, they found a dead man wearing a scuba tank and wet suit. At first the firefighters were baffled as to why a man would be out in the middle of the countryside wearing full scuba gear. Upon further examination, it was determined that the man died from impact with the ground, not the fire. As best anyone can determine, this man was scuba diving and was accidentally picked up by one of the firefighting airplanes when it was refilling its water tanks.

Not only are the origins of this implausible story unknown, but there are also several versions of it, and if you search the internet today for this story you will find it along with disclaimers indicating that the story is not true. Stories that are not true but nevertheless circulate widely and are told as if they are true are called **urban legends** (Kendall, Murray, and Linden 2000, 648–9). Urban legends usually deal with topics that are particularly sensational from a culture's point of view, such as death or the threat of death. While the tale told above is ironic and perhaps amusing, folklore like this has the potential to define and instruct. If there is a message in this story, it is that death may come unbidden, unexpected, like a macabre prank played on an unsuspecting victim.

The above story illustrates a common belief that death will find you "when your number is up." There is a certain fatalism or notion of inescapable bad luck. Continuing with this theme, another story concerns a man whose car was blown off the road and into a river during a windstorm. As the car sank beneath the water, the man broke a window, climbed out, and swam to shore where a tree blew over and killed him. If there is a message in this story, it is that death cannot be avoided "when your time is up."

The following two urban legends were heard decades ago. Both stories concern medical students enrolled in the University of Manitoba's medical school, and the people who told these stories swore that they were true. According to the first story, some of the students from the medical school had taken an arm severed from a cadaver that they were dissecting in the course of their studies. They dressed the arm in a shirtsleeve, pasted a dollar bill to the hand, and boarded a bus. As the bus driver reached out to take the money, he pulled the whole arm off, had a heart attack, and died on the spot.

It is unlikely that this prank (or other versions of this story) ever actually took place. Yet it appears to be one of several similar stories that have circulated widely and been described as "cadaver stories" (Hafferty 1988). If there is a culturally mediated discomfort with the topic of death, there is a virtual taboo against contact with dead bodies. Students in the field of health care must not only break this taboo, but they must also learn to control their emotional revulsion about doing so. Cadaver stories are a vehicle by which medical students and others can acknowledge the problem of death and at the same time claim to have transcended their difficulties with death. In these stories, the students are usually portrayed as pranksters in control of their fears, while the victims of the pranks are portrayed as laypeople who are shocked. The underlying message is that death is horrifying, although some people can and must learn to overcome or at least manage their horror.

The second urban legend heard years ago contains a twist on the usual cadaver story. A medical student had been dissecting a corpse, starting at its feet, so the story goes. The body was covered with a sheet, and each part was uncovered in turn. Finally, the head was uncovered, and the student realized that he had been dissecting his own recently deceased father (or mother or other close relative—the details can vary as the story is told and retold).

In the first story, the medical students showed their emotional control by allegedly playing pranks on people who are easily shocked by death. In the second story, fate plays a trick on the medical student, reaffirming the horror of death. Although people can gain some control through strategies such as emotional distancing and depersonalization, the horror is still there and can suddenly overtake them. The message of this story is that death is horrible and there is no escaping that horror, especially when death takes a loved one.

Legends centred on death are widespread. Consider, for example, ghost stories and tales of haunted houses. Canada has its own deathly legends. The South Nahanni River in the southwest corner of the Northwest Territories is a place of such legend. The back cover of *Dangerous River*, R.M. Patterson's (1989, originally 1954) account of his time on the Nahanni, reads: "The Nahanni River follows its treacherous course between Yukon Territory and the mighty Mackenzie River. One section is dominated by Deadmen Valley, so-called because of the hair-raising legends about the fate of those brave enough to enter—and unfortunate enough never to return." In 1927, Patterson made his way by canoe from northern Alberta to the Nahanni. Many whom he met on his way told him about canyons with sheer walls thousands of feet high and treacherous currents. He was told that not many people came back alive to tell about it:

> There was gold in there somewhere . . . Deadmen Valley was tucked away in there some place . . . a valley between two canyons where the McLeods were murdered for their gold in 1906. No man ever knew what happened to them, but they were found—at least their skeletons were— tied to trees, with the heads missing. And enough men had disappeared in there since then that it was considered best by men of sense to leave the Nahanni country alone. (6)

Patterson was also told of the wild Mountain Men, who "lorded it over the wild uplands of the Yukon Mackenzie divide and made short work of any man . . . who ventured into their country" (7). Whether the alleged murderers were the mysterious Mountain Men or not, story after story told of the gruesome end that many came to in Nahanni country.

In 1946, stories about the "Headless Valley"—that is, Deadmen Valley— appeared in the *Toronto Star* and *Chicago Tribune*. According to Hartling (1993, 94), the stories were "a blockbuster. Nahanni became synonymous with unearthly phenomena. Stories sprang up in support of the reputation:

tales of hidden tropical forests, murder, head hunters, hot springs, canyons, waterfalls, and gold. Much of the reputation was based on fantasy, but an eager readership ate it up." A year later, Pierre Berton, then a young reporter for the *Vancouver Sun* and later a prolific author of books about Canadian history, led an expedition into the Nahanni. His reports fanned a national interest in the old legends. These stories resonate even today in the place names of the region: Deadmen Valley, Headless (mountain) Range, Funeral (mountain) Range, Sunblood Mountain, Broken Skull River, Hell's Gate, Hell Roaring Creek, and Headless Creek. In 1970, Prime Minister Pierre Elliott Trudeau visited the Nahanni, and in 1971 it became a national park (Hartling 1993, 99).

The stories of the Nahanni are part of Canadian folklore. They not only reflect the fear and fascination that people have with death, but they also foster that very same fear and fascination. While death for ourselves and our loved ones is usually unwelcome, bitter, and tragic, and while we often distance ourselves from the possibility or actuality of such death, death in general remains a topic of great interest. Finally, these stories serve as cautionary tales warning people to be careful lest tragedy befall them.

The invention of the internet provided a new medium for the circulation of folklore and popular culture. Since the early 1990s, stories about accidental deaths have been posted on internet websites and have circulated via email. Wendy Northcutt established her website Darwin Awards (www .DarwinAwards.com) in 1993. According to this website in 2021: "The Darwin Awards [named in honor of Charles Darwin, the father of evolution] salute the improvement of the human genome by honoring those who accidentally remove themselves from it in a spectacular manner!" These stories, circulated as humour, feature individuals portrayed as "idiots" who, in unfortunate and often stupendous lapses in judgement, bring about their own death. Readers smugly enjoy a laugh at the expense of the deceased but at the same time are reminded that they too are only a misstep away from a similar fate. Northcutt wrote a series of bestselling Darwin Awards books (2000 to 2010), and in 2006 a film called *The Darwin Awards* premiered at the Sundance Film Festival. Her website (2021) continues to post "award" stories.

The internet and social media have also played a role in the creation and circulation of rumours of celebrity deaths. Of course, such rumours circulated long before the internet. For example, the announcement in the news media in 1897 of Mark Twain's death occasioned the now-famous phrase ascribed to Twain: "The reports of my death have been greatly exaggerated." That phrase persists today and is used when a death is announced erroneously or as a metaphor to describe the alleged "death" of a project or idea (Winick 2018). In 1969, the news media announced that Paul McCartney had died three years earlier and been replaced by an imposter. Over the next half century, this celebrity death hoax and conspiracy theory gave rise to books, articles, websites, a Wikipedia page, and a 2018 comedy short film (Winick 2018). Celebrity death hoaxes persist today, revealing the public's adoration of celebrities and a fascination with the topic of death (Frank 2011, 180–8).

The contemporary news media not only reveal social constructions of dying and death but also play a role in creating, disseminating, maintaining, and changing those constructions. The news media report daily in great detail about death by crime, accident, disaster, and war. Visual images of death are frequent. At the time of writing in 2020, television reports repeatedly showed the gruesome, disturbing murder of George Floyd by a Minneapolis police officer, thereby highlighting violent deaths of Black men and women at the hands of police in the United States and elsewhere and triggering a widespread movement for change. The media's repeated reporting of phrases such as "Black lives matter," "Don't shoot," "I can't breathe," and with respect to the Indigenous population in Canada, "Missing and murdered women and girls," will hopefully help efforts to change racist practices and systemic abuses.

The role that the news media is thought to play in shaping collective definitions and motivating social responses to death is also illustrated by the following controversy. In late April 2006, the recently elected Conservative government led by Prime Minister Stephen Harper announced that media coverage of soldiers' bodies being returned to Canada following their deaths in Afghanistan (where Canadian soldiers had been deployed since 2002) would be banned. The rationale offered for the media ban was respect for the grieving relatives. Furthermore, the government announced that the flag on the Parliament Buildings in Ottawa would not be lowered to half-mast on the return of each individual soldier, but would be lowered once a year on Remembrance Day to commemorate all military personnel killed in wartime conflict. This practice, the government claimed, would be more consistent and equitable, treating all deceased military combatants—past, present, and future—with the same respect.

Considerable controversy erupted following this announcement. Opponents argued that media coverage was important to acknowledge and honour the newly deceased soldiers and their families. They also argued that the Harper government was attempting to muzzle the media and manage public opinion regarding the war by downplaying military deaths and eliminating disturbing and potentially opinion-shaping images from the evening news. It was alleged that the government feared that images of soldiers returning to Canada in coffins might lead to a decline in public support for Canada's military involvement in Afghanistan, a commitment that the Conservative government intended to maintain. A month later, after considerable and sustained public outcry, Harper lifted the ban and announced that media coverage would be left to the discretion of individual families and not placed under the control of government.

The deaths of individuals can have important social significance. The deaths of Canadian soldiers, for example, may be used by both proponents and opponents of a war as symbols mobilized to win support for their separate positions. Other deaths may also hold cultural significance. For example, Ramos and Gosine (2002) examined newspaper coverage of the death on 27 May 2000 of hockey legend Maurice "Rocket" Richard. English newspapers in Quebec and across Canada tended to emphasize Richard's greatness as a Canadian hockey legend, while Quebec francophone newspapers tended to emphasize his place as a Québécois cultural and political symbol. That is, the Quebec francophone newspapers focused on Richard's iconic status and its relevance to the development of a Québécois national identity. Thus, while death has personal significance for some, death as reported by the news media can have social, cultural, and political significance for a society. We were reminded of this again in 2014 by the news coverage of the death of Jean Béliveau, another hockey legend celebrated by both Quebec and the rest of Canada. Like Richard, Béliveau was portrayed as a Québécois icon in the francophone media. When Henri "Pocket Rocket" Richard, the Rocket's younger and smaller brother, died in 2020, another legendary hockey player (who won a record 11 Stanley Cups with the Montréal Canadiens) was remembered as an icon of francophone Québécois society and culture.

Clarke (2006) examined the portrayal of death in high-circulation English-language magazines available in Canada. She argued that portrayals of death reveal an underlying "frame" or discourse, namely, the optimistic notion that death is, can be, or should be under control (Clarke 2006, 157, 162). She concluded that the emphasis in magazine articles on the power, success, and potential of modern medicine presents an image of death as controllable and downplays the lack of control that most, especially the less privileged, have over death. Bayatrizi (2008) makes a similar argument, noting that modern discourses about death give "order" to it. These discourses define death as preventable and, when imminent, as manageable and orderly.

Clarke (2004) also examined the portrayal in English-language magazines in Canada of sex-specific cancers—breast cancer (which most often affects women after age 50), testicular cancer (which most often affects younger men), and prostate cancer (which most often affects men after age 50). She suggested that the mass media raise fears about these cancers, in part by portraying them as threats not only to life but also (and perhaps more importantly) as threats to one's femininity or masculinity, that is, to a person's gendered identity. Nevertheless, while media portrayals raise fears, at the same time they offer solutions such as early detection and treatment to alleviate these fears.

McWhirter, Hoffman-Goetz, and Clarke (2012) examined articles and accompanying images about breast cancer in Canadian women's magazines and fashion magazines. The images were typically positive in tone and featured younger, attractive, and healthy-looking Caucasian women. The accompanying articles were more balanced in tone than the accompanying images, discussing the various aspects of breast cancer experiences. Nevertheless, death was rarely mentioned or depicted. Articles and images rarely referred to people who had died from breast cancer.

In a similar fashion, Miele and Clarke (2014) examined articles about prostate cancer published in popular news magazines such as *Maclean's*, *Time*, and *Newsweek*. Miele and Clarke concluded that the articles reinforced traditional binaries such as male vs. female and masculine vs. feminine. They wrote: "The popular news articles reinforce dominant ideals and performances of hegemonic masculinity and male sexuality, traditional femininity, and heteronormativity" (15). Prostate cancer was represented as a "man's" disease and a threat to masculinity. While men were to take responsibility, get tested, get treated, and fight the "good fight," they were to do so with the help of their female partners, thus reinforcing both traditional male and female roles. These articles ignored persons with various other gender identities and sexual orientations, racialized minorities, and the economically disadvantaged.

Halpin, Phillips, and Oliffe (2009) examined newspaper articles about prostate cancer published in Canada's *Globe and Mail* and *National Post* newspapers. These authors found that the articles highlighted masculine ideals such as courage and stoicism but did not discuss negative topics such as fear, erectile dysfunction, urinary incontinence, or palliative end-of-life care. In addition, newspaper articles often mentioned that breast cancer fundraising and research spending greatly exceeded funding for prostate cancer, despite a similarity in the rates of occurrence of breast cancer and prostate cancer. The authors noted that some "worthy" cancers become the focus of popular attention and win public support while other cancers are associated with public discomfort and tend to be overlooked.

Henry et al. (2012) compared portrayals of cancer in Canadian newspapers in 2008 with portrayals 20 years earlier. These authors found that cancer had become a more common topic and discussions of cancer had become more positive. They also found that few newspaper articles examined end-of-life care for cancer patients or issues relating to dying, death, or bereavement. Most articles focused on prevention, effective treatment, advances in cancer research, and courageous patients who battled and overcame cancer. In summary, analyses of media portrayals of dying and death from cancer tended to emphasize the positive and minimize the negative, facilitating a degree of distancing from and denial of the realities of cancer as Canada's leading cause of death.

Popular culture such as television programming, movies, and novels (consider the success of horror-story writer Stephen King) regularly deal with death. It is ironic that, in an allegedly death-denying culture, contemporary movies and television programs are often preoccupied with dying and death. Indeed, popular prime-time dramatic series are commonly centred on health care professionals, including first responders, and their struggles to save the lives of the sick or injured, while others are concerned with law enforcement officers, crime scene investigators, and legal professionals who seek to bring justice for unjust deaths.

Perhaps dying and death make good dramatic fare because of the individual and collective fear they inspire. Dying and death get our attention and can provoke deep concern and great interest. While television often captivates viewers by capitalizing on fears of death, such programming tends to offer happy endings. In the hospital dramas, dying and death are usually managed successfully or at least humanely, and in the crime dramas the perpetrators of unjust deaths are typically brought to justice. In short, television programming raises fears of dying and death and then calms them. The message is that, despite the chaos of illness, accident, and crime, dying and death are manageable in a world that is, in the end, orderly, purposeful, and coherent.

DARK TOURISM

While people fear death, that very fear fosters a fascination with it. People often travel to places associated with death. Tourists go to battlefields

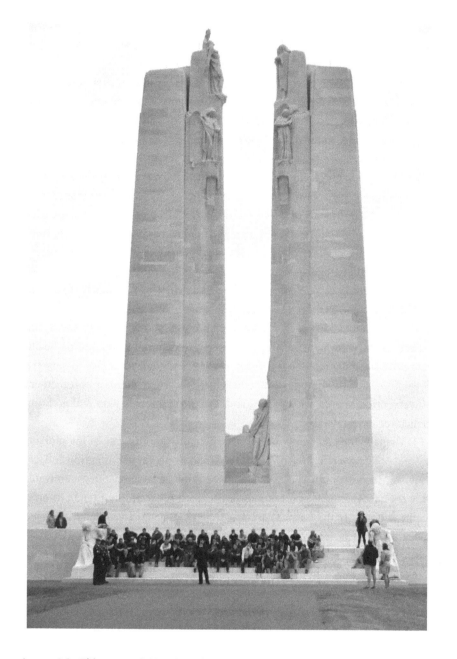

Image 4.2. This memorial in Givenchy-en-Gohelle, France, commemorates the battle of Vimy Ridge, which took place on 9–12 April 1917 during the First World War. Canadian casualties numbered 3,598 dead and 7,004 wounded. Memorials like this remind visitors of the human cost of war.
Source: Wikimedia Commons, Mike McBey – Vimy Ridge, CC BY 2.0.

such as Vimy Ridge in France, where almost 11,000 Canadians were killed or wounded in the First World War, or to Juno Beach, where Canadian troops landed in France on D-Day on 6 June 1944, or they visit concentration camps, such as Auschwitz in Poland, where millions were murdered by the Nazis during the Second World War. Tourists visit Eva Perón's mausoleum in La Recoleta Cemetery in Buenos Aires, Argentina. Perón (1919–1952) was First Lady of Argentina from 1946 to 1952 and subject of the 1978 musical *Evita*. Her legendary status continues today and draws tourists to the mausoleum that contains her remains. Tourists visit the Vietnam Veterans Memorial in Washington, DC, and the 9/11 Memorial in New York City. Some visit museums of terror, torture, and atrocity.

This phenomenon of people visiting places associated with death is known as "**dark tourism**" (Dermody 2017) and illustrates the fascination that death holds even in a death-denying culture. Note that the sites visited highlight the deaths of others, even though the tourists themselves may have difficulty accepting the inevitability of their own death.

Dark tourism has become a significant component of the tourism industry. Some refer to this as the "commodification of death" as part of the global tourist experience (Dermody 2017). The term "dark tourism" seems problematic, though, as does the alternative term, "morbid tourism." The labels sensationalize death, although perhaps that is the point: to sensationalize so as to commodify and create a tourist "attraction." We prefer the term "death tourism."

THE SECULARIZATION, PROFESSIONALIZATION, MEDICALIZATION, AND BUREAUCRATIZATION OF DYING AND DEATH

As discussed in chapter 3, religion has played an important role historically in making death meaningful and providing guidelines for dying persons, for their family and community, and for the management of the dead body. Increasingly, however, Canada is becoming a secularized society; that is, the importance of religion as a central social institution is declining. Church and state are separated, and weekly attendance at church has declined substantially since the mid-twentieth century. Death is also increasingly defined by secular rather than religious elements of society and culture. Doctors, nurses, philosophers, ethicists, psychologists, lawyers, and funeral home directors, for example, have tended to replace priests, pastors, rabbis, imams, and theologians as definers of the meaning of death. Similarly, the processing of the dead body is increasingly assigned to secular professionals rather than religious officials and family members. "Death care" has become a corporate industry (Smith 2007).

In addition to the church, the family and the community used to play major roles in assisting the dying, managing the dead body, and supporting the bereaved. During the twentieth century, however, dying, death, and even grieving came to be managed increasingly by professionals such as doctors and nurses, medical examiners and coroners, funeral directors, and grief workers like psychologists and social workers. Control of dying, death, and grieving shifted from people one knew to strangers, and from laypersons to professionals, particularly health care professionals. Furthermore, health care professionals have tended to define dying, death, and grieving as medical problems to be solved by therapeutic intervention. They have fought dying with increasingly sophisticated technology, defined death in medical terms, and recommended the management of grieving through counselling and prescription drugs. Dying and death were removed from the context of normal life and placed in the context of health care institutions to be managed by health care professionals.

Cultural rules and practices have developed to govern the process of dying, as well as the individual and collective responses to death. In bureaucratic settings, rules about dying and death are formally defined. As noted in chapter 2, in the twentieth century dying and death moved from the home to the hospital, an elaborate bureaucracy with diverse officials and formal roles and rules. The hospital bureaucracy assumed control over dying individuals, although the requirement for voluntary and informed consent leaves the dying person with some degree of control. Death is also bureaucratized. The dead body is certified and managed by various functionaries who work in the hospital or the medical examiner's office and the funeral home industry. These functionaries perform their services according to professional and governmental rules. **Bureaucratization** shifts control over dying and death away from the dying person, the family, and the community toward officials who are strangers and who operate according to bureaucratic culture rather than the individual's relevant subculture.

Kaufert and O'Neil (1991) were among the first to report on interactions between health care professionals and Indigenous peoples (Cree, Ojibway, and Inuit) in Winnipeg hospitals. In the hospital, health care professionals tend to take control of the dying patient. They impose predominantly Euro-Canadian, professional, and bureaucratic rules not only on the treatment of the dying person but also on the involvement of that person's family and friends, such as through enforced visiting hours. In addition, health care professionals apply bureaucratic rules regarding the processing of the body of the deceased. Indigenous communities find these rules inappropriate and inconsistent with their own cultural guidelines. Similarly, health care workers tend to find Indigenous cultural norms inappropriate. In short, neither group understands nor accepts the other (see Stephenson 1992 for a similar discussion involving Hutterites). The involvement of Indigenous interpreters who serve as language translators, cultural informants, mediators, and patient and community advocates in the hospital has helped to resolve this impasse.

Castleden et al. (2010) wrote about the difficulties of providing culturally sensitive end-of-life care to Indigenous persons in a rural area of British Columbia. The authors noted that Indigenous persons preferred to be close to nature, practise cultural ceremonies, eat traditional foods, and use traditional medicines. Hampton at al. (2010) asked Indigenous elders from southern Saskatchewan what non-Indigenous health care providers should know when providing end-of-life care for Indigenous individuals. The elders were Cree, Saulteaux, Anishinaabe, Métis, and Lakota/Dakota. The elders pointed out that the family and community gather around the dying person but that hospital policies tend to restrict the number of visitors and the hours or length of time for visitation. Further, hospitals tend to resist traditions such as burning sweet grass and smudging. Other Indigenous traditions include prayer and the singing of songs, which can be discouraged in hospitals. In addition, hospitals may control diet and resist family members' attempts to bring in traditional foods. The authors noted that Western medicine clashed with Indigenous culture, resulting in difficulties in communication and in discrimination. Further, the authors noted that institutional policies interfered with Indigenous families' sense of their traditional responsibilities to their dying family member.

Bablitz, Ahnadzadeh, and MacLeod (2018) reported the case of an Indigenous man, age 70, dying of cancer. He wanted to move from Edmonton to his reserve in northern Alberta in order to return home. In Edmonton, he had the support of his six children who provided interpretation—the dying man spoke Cree—and he had the support of a sympathetic palliative care team and an Indigenous cultural helper. In his reserve community, "the home-care services were only available during weekday business hours, no physician was present on a regular basis, and the closest pharmacy was more than 100 km away" (667). Nevertheless, he desired to return home. As a compromise, he moved from Edmonton to the rural hospital nearest his reserve, but "he was still isolated from his support network and he died lonely" (668). While the health care system had made many efforts to be culturally responsive, the limited availability of health care professionals, hospitals, and palliative care programs in rural and remote communities led to a disappointing outcome. This case study points out that **professionalization**, medicalization, and bureaucratization can be culturally responsive. The problem that this study highlights is the lack of availability of services in rural and remote communities. The solution is not less professionalization, less medicalization, and less bureaucratization, but rather more, as long as these are culturally responsive.

Building an effective and culturally responsible palliative care program in Indigenous communities requires "two-eyed seeing," where "one eye sees using Indigenous ways of knowing and the other sees using Western perspectives" (Kelley et al. 2018, S63). Doing this involves committees, policies, education and training, funding, health care professionals, community members, and traditional knowledge carriers (Caxaj, Schill, and Janke 2017; Fruch et al. 2016; Kelley et al. 2018). In other words, while processes of professionalization, medicalization, and bureaucratization have been widely criticized for being culturally insensitive if not inappropriate, these same processes can be used today to create a system of end-of-life care that is culturally responsive.

MAKING SENSE OF DEATH

Humans construct meaning to make sense of the world and to facilitate functioning in it. People everywhere have tried to make sense of death. While an individual's search for meaning is a highly personal endeavour, it is facilitated by systems of meaning that exist separate from the individual. These meaning systems are components of culture. Individuals often internalize cultural meaning systems without critical reflection through processes of socialization. For example, a person may be raised with a particular religious belief that provides this individual with answers to questions about the meaning of life and death. Systems of meaning are also found outside religion, in philosophy, psychology, schools of thought regarding therapeutic grief counselling, and so on.

Nevertheless, having a culturally based meaning system is no guarantee that death will be easily accepted. An individual may find that the circumstances of a particular death undermine their system of meaning; one such circumstance is when a young person is killed or dies suddenly without warning. In such circumstances, the living are forced to search for meaning and to make sense of the incomprehensible. If systems of meaning are socially constructed, they can also be deconstructed. Sometimes events in life do just that. Death, in particular, can be very destabilizing.

In Canadian culture, death is typically considered acceptable if—and only if—it comes at the end of a long life and ends a period of deterioration, illness, or suffering. Other deaths are not so easily accepted. Deaths by murder, suicide, and accident are typically seen as tragic and senseless, especially when these deaths are "premature." The death of a child, especially if that death is sudden and unexpected, can be particularly traumatic (Marchenski 2004). Commonly shared beliefs, values, assumptions, and rules that make the death of a child problematic include the following four tenets: (1) contemporary Western culture places a high intrinsic value on children; (2) children provide meaning and purpose for their parents' lives; (3) there is an expectation that life will be long and good and that death will come only in old age; and (4) there is a belief that if life is lived responsibly and correctly that things will turn out well and one will live into old age. In a cultural context such as this, parents lack a meaning structure through which they can make sense of the death of their child (Braun 1992; Chasteen and Madey 2003).

Furthermore, the death of a child may threaten other meaning structures that the parents have. Marriages end with the death of a child when the marriage is no longer meaningful or relevant to the grieving parents. The death of a child may also undermine faith in God. Parents who have believed all of their lives might find themselves asking, "If there is a God, and if God is good and all powerful, then why is our child dead?" While human beings crave and create systems of meaning, these constructions can be fragile. In the face of death, most people find themselves searching for meaning. Some find meaning in the cultural constructions of their upbringing while others find themselves separated from their cultural moorings.

DIFFERENT TYPES OF DEATH

Death is not simply a biological event. It is also a social and cultural phenomenon. Indeed, from social and cultural points of view, there are different types of death. The most obvious type is "biological death," which is death of the body. The death of the body is accompanied by "personal death"—that is, the death of the person. However, while the dead body decays, the dead person can seem to live on in the memories of survivors and may be believed to live on as a spirit or soul in a "life after death."

There are other types of death that may come to those who are not biologically dead. Sudnow (1967) wrote of people who were treated as if they were physically dead when they were still alive; he called this "social death." Years ago, following a disaster at a coalmine in Nova Scotia, 12 men were trapped underground for six and a half days, and another six men were trapped for eight and a half days. Lucas (1968, 2–3) records the following:

> On the fifth day a high-ranking official of the mining company pub-
> licly announced that there could be little hope that any man remained
> alive. The trapped miners although physiologically alive were socially
> dead. The wife of one of the trapped miners had ordered a coffin for her
> husband, had bought mourning clothes and prepared the house for his
> funeral. After rescue, the miner's comments on his social death were:
> "Well when I came home they talked about they had my casket ready,
> and then the wife she got sympathy cards, and when you think about all
> that it hurts you. [They] had you dead when you wasn't dead, you know."

Other examples of people who are likely to be treated as socially dead include those who are comatose, in a persistent vegetative state, institutionalized, senile, or socially derelict. The comatose can also be said to have experienced "psychological death" in that they lack consciousness (Doka 1995). Doka also writes of "psychosocial death," in which individuals are significantly changed so that they no longer seem to be the person they once were. Examples of psychosocial death include mental illness, trauma to the brain through head injury or stroke, organic brain diseases like Alzheimer's, drug or alcohol addiction, religious conversion, and even growing up. Parents may grieve when their offspring has suddenly, it seems, become a young adult and is no longer the little child who was loved so dearly. Finally, relationships are also said to die, as when a marriage ends in divorce or children are given up for adoption or taken into foster care.

In difficult or traumatic situations, some people appear to give up, lose the will to live, and die. This is called **psychogenic death** (Leach 2011). It has been observed in prisoners of war and in persons in disaster situations. It appears to involve a neurological and biological response to stress that results in death when death is not otherwise expected. Some survive such traumatic situations while others inexplicably die.

Legal death is yet another type of death. A person who is declared legally dead may or may not be biologically dead. In wartime, people missing in action may never be proven to be deceased but may be presumed to be so and declared legally dead. Such a declaration allows for the settlement of the missing person's property and terminates that person's legal relationships. For instance, a declaration of legal death ends a marriage relationship and makes remarriage possible for the surviving spouse.

Doka (1995, 272) said, "societies have sets of norms—in effect, grieving rules—that attempt to specify who, when, where, how, how long, and for whom people should grieve. Each society defines who has a legitimate right to grieve." Accordingly, cultural definitions and rules recognize some deaths as legitimate while others are "disenfranchised." The biological death of a close family member, such as a parent, grandparent, child, or sibling, is recognized as legitimate, and the bereaved are offered social support such as time off work, flowers and cards, and attendance at the funeral service. The bereaved are allowed to grieve because the death is perceived as a legitimate death. The biological deaths of more distant relatives, such as uncles, aunts, or cousins, tend to receive less legitimization and therefore less social support. No support at all may be offered for the biological deaths of ex-partners, extramarital lovers, roommates, friends, colleagues, clients, or pets—all of which tend to be disenfranchised. Similarly, other deaths that tend to be disenfranchised include spontaneous and induced abortions, and in some cases deaths by suicide and assisted deaths. Disenfranchised deaths are seldom acknowledged, publicly mourned, or socially supported (Thompson and Doka 2017).

Lawson (2014) observed that African Canadians in Toronto who have lost friends and family to gun-related violence tended to experience **disenfranchised grief** as a result of encounters with police and media reports about the deceased. Police investigations involving suspicions of guilt and media reports indicating that the deceased was "known to police" raised "questions about whose lives are worth grieving and whose are not" (2100). Police suspicions and media reports, even when unjustified and inaccurate, created the impression "that the deceased person is responsible for his demise and that the co-victims [e.g., family and friends] cannot legitimately grieve their loss" (2101).

Nonbiological deaths also tend to be disenfranchised. A person who reaches the later stages of Alzheimer's disease may illustrate social death, psychological death, psychosocial death, and the death of relationships. The partner of a person with advanced dementia may feel like a grieving widow or widower, but without a dead body, their grief is disenfranchised.

DYING AND DEATH AS SOCIAL STIGMA

A culture is a set of definitions and beliefs about reality, rules about how to behave, and evaluations about what is good and bad. These beliefs, normative rules, and values tend to be widely shared and persist over time. Some things are quite arbitrarily defined and evaluated as either good or bad. People who have characteristics defined as bad are socially stigmatized. Consider racism, where groups of people are defined as inferior on the basis of physiological characteristics like skin colour.

Death is generally defined as bad, repulsive, contaminating, and threatening. Accordingly, an ideology of beliefs has developed to justify these evaluations, and normative guidelines have developed to manage death. There may be good reason to evaluate death negatively. First, the smell of death—that is, the smell of rotting flesh—is highly disagreeable. Moreover, rotting flesh is associated with disease, pestilence, contamination, and contagion. Second, threats to life are generally feared and avoided; some dead bodies may be still infectious and risk the life of anyone in contact with them. Finally, the death of a loved one tends to be one of life's most emotionally painful experiences.

Nevertheless, the negative evaluations of death go well beyond the obvious. In many cultural groups, death, the dead, and places of death such as graves and cemeteries are negatively valued because of beliefs about the danger and malevolence of departed spirits or ghosts. Furthermore, death may be feared because of what might come after—religious constructions of everlasting torment in hell, for example. Even more curiously, people who are not dead but are merely associated with death may be negatively evaluated. Posner (1976) wrote that the widow, the orphan, the processors of the dead (such as the morgue attendant and undertaker), and the aged all tend to be negatively valued. Yet what offence have any of these people committed? None, except they have a relationship with the dead. The widow's husband is dead, the orphan's parents are dead, and the undertaker's clients are dead. What offences do the aged commit? None, except that age is a harbinger and reminder of death. The cultural logic seems to be that if death is bad, then anybody and anything that is associated with death is also bad. Such treatment is an example of what Goffman (1963) referred to as a **"courtesy stigma"**—a person is stigmatized because of a **stigma** attached to someone else with whom they are associated. Because death is stigmatized, almost anyone and anything associated with death is also stigmatized. The contamination is not literal, it is cultural (Posner 1976).

HIV/AIDS Pandemic

HIV/AIDS is an illustration of a stigmatized disease. The first cases of HIV/ AIDS occurred in Canada in the early 1980s at the time of a worldwide pandemic. An acquaintance of the first author was one of the first to die in Canada. He was handsome, charming, and accomplished; one of the nicest and most memorable individuals I have ever known. I did not know until after his death that he was gay. At that time, HIV/AIDS was new, mysterious, and deadly. Today, thankfully, HIV/AIDS is not the death sentence it once was (Orsini, Hindmarch, and Gagnon 2018).

HIV/AIDS is typically sexually transmitted or a result of unsafe injection drug use. It is largely associated with marginalized groups including homosexuals, sex workers, injection drug users, and the poor (Orsini, Hindmarch, and Gagnon 2018). It is contagious, although only through contact with infected bodily fluids. It used to be deadly, following a trajectory of illness and decline that was particularly devastating. An illness such as HIV/AIDS has social and psychological consequences that go far beyond the illness itself and reflect the socially stigmatized nature of this particular disease. While HIV/AIDS is better understood today, less stigmatized, and antiretroviral drugs are now available to manage HIV infection and prevent it from progressing to AIDS and death, Hindmarch, Orsini, and Gagnon (2018, 346) argue that "we must continue . . . to recognize the social and structural inequities that underpin and facilitate the spread of HIV, and the persistently inadequate policy response to these inequities."

Stigmatization is a social process, and what society stigmatizes, society can also destigmatize, that is, normalize. HIV/AIDS, cancer, mental illness, and non-heterosexual orientation are examples of previously stigmatized but increasingly destigmatized subjects.

Issues in Dying for Same-Sex Couples

Laws recognizing same-sex couples are relatively recent, beginning in Sweden in 1987 and in Canada in 1992 (Augcr 2003). Because heterosexual couples have been recognized for a much longer time, heterosexual and same-sex couples may have different experiences at the end of life (Auger and Krug 2013). Where same-sex relationships are not recognized or if same-sex couples choose to maintain their privacy and not acknowledge their relationship to family and co-workers (i.e., remain "in the closet") or if a couple rejects institutionalized forms of being a couple, then end-of-life matters may involve difficult issues for the same-sex couple. This point applies more generally to the lesbian, gay, bisexual, transgender, queer, intersex, two-spirited (LGBTQI2+) community.

Aging LGBTQI2+ persons have particular concerns about long-term care and end-of-life care (Wilson, Kortes-Miller, and Stinchcombe 2018). They may feel that the staff and residents of long-term care facilities will not understand or accept them. They may fear discrimination, stigmatization, harassment, and rejection. They may have concerns about who will be allowed to help them make end-of-life decisions. In short, they worry that they might be "forced back into the closet," forced to hide their sexual orientation and gender identity in order to obtain quality end-of-life care.

When a heterosexual couple experiences dying and death, there is no question about who has the right to visit the dying person in the hospital, to participate in end-of-life decisions about care, or who has claim to the body of the deceased. There is no question about who has the right to grieve and mourn or to organize and attend a memorial service. Inheritance, taxation, claims on the property of the deceased, and survivor benefits from insurance and public and private pensions are unambiguous. The survivor's relationship with the couple's children is not questioned. All of these issues become problematic where a same-sex relationship is unrecognized or unacknowledged. While all couples should anticipate and plan for these end-of-life issues, it is particularly important for same-sex couples to do so. In the absence of a recognized relationship, there is a tendency for the blood relatives of the deceased to take over and exclude the same-sex partner.

When a partner in a heterosexual relationship dies, family, co-workers, employers, and community members recognize and accommodate the loss and grief of the surviving partner. When a partner in an unrecognized or unacknowledged same-sex relationship dies, the surviving partner may experience disenfranchised grief. That is, the grief of the surviving partner may not be recognized, and the survivor may not be accorded the right to mourn openly (Auger and Krug 2013).

It follows that same-sex couples should be vigilant about implementing the necessary legal safeguards to protect the interests of the dying partner and the surviving partner (Auger and Krug 2013). These safeguards include having a financial will; designating beneficiaries for pensions, investments, insurance, and property; having an advance directive specifying who has the right to participate in end-of-life decisions; and providing guidelines about what can and should be done before death. The details of a memorial or funeral service can also be specified, including who will speak, what music will be chosen, and so on. In the absence of these formal arrangements, the relatives of the deceased may intervene and assume they have the right to make these decisions. In the worst-case scenario, the same-sex partner is excluded, ignored, trivialized, or denigrated.

THE SOCIAL CONSTRUCTION OF DYING AND DEATH

In his social history of dying, Kellehear (2007, 3) divided human history into four ages and argued that dying and death were different in each age, reflecting "the economic and cultural character of the time." According to Kellehear, the first age was the hunting and gathering economy of the stone age, when lives were short and death came quickly. The cultural response focused on helping the spirits of the deceased to journey successfully from this world to the next world, the otherworld of spirits.

The second age, according to Kellehear, was the pastoral age, a time of farms, domesticated animals, and villages. People tended to live longer lives and experience slower deaths, allowing people to anticipate death. The sociocultural emphasis shifted to preparing for death and the afterlife. People aspired to a good death in which worldly affairs were settled. Kellehear states, "The Good Death is a moral dying, a dying that can be done well or badly as a social performance" (86), and according to social norms, beliefs, and values of that time.

A third age followed—the age of the city. The good death became the well-managed death aided by professionals, including the physician, lawyer, and priest. Wild, out-of-control, unmanaged death was feared, and efforts were made to manage and tame death.

Kellehear labelled the fourth age—our present time in history—as the cosmopolitan age. He describes this age as a global mix of "wealth and poverty, long and short life expectancies" (7). He suggests that deaths in the cosmopolitan age "are neither good nor well-managed" (8). Death in our present era, he argues, is shameful. He suggests that death is often either too early or too late. Poverty, famine, war, genocide, and pandemics such as HIV/AIDS and COVID-19 bring premature death. Deaths in very old age in nursing homes can come too late, although the COVID-19 pandemic highlighted the dismal organization of nursing homes that contributed to the premature death of thousands of frail seniors. Kellehear noted that old age, frailty, and dementia are stigmatized and experienced as undignified, humiliating, and embarrassing. He pointed to nursing homes where older people are abandoned, isolated, lonely, depressed, ignored, and infantilized. Their deaths are viewed by all, outsiders and the dying themselves, as shameful.

Kellehear argued that as the cosmopolitan age unfolds in the twenty-first century, the major challenge for dying is the problem of identifying the "right time to die" (233), and to accept dying when it is evident or near. Kellehear concludes, "Across our entire human history we have provided . . . support to our dying through the social offerings of recognition, presence, giving and receiving, and ritual. Sadly, those deep-seated responses toward our dying now increasingly seem endangered" (256).

Philippe Ariès (1974, 1981) surveyed portrayals of death in Western European culture over time. He suggested that until the early Middle Ages (through the twelfth century), death was "tame" or omnipresent, familiar, and accepted as the natural order of things. Later, death became "wild" and was increasingly feared and resisted. By the twentieth century death had become dirty, ugly, shameful, hidden, and denied.

Alternatively, Stroebe et al. (1995) characterized nineteenth-century Western culture as romantic. Romanticism emphasized the soul, love, and enduring commitment to intimate human relationships, even after the death of a loved one. Accordingly, "to grieve was to signal the significance of the relationship, and the depth of one's own spirit. Dissolving bonds with the deceased would not only define the relationship as superficial, but would deny as well one's own sense of profundity and self-worth" (237). From the romantic perspective, grief could legitimately last a lifetime and indeed was expected to do so.

Stroebe et al. (1995) described twentieth-century Western culture as modernist, in contrast to the romanticism of the nineteenth century. Modernism emphasizes efficiency, progress, and rationality rather than emotionality. Bayatrizi (2008) makes a similar point about the early twenty-first century, arguing that death has become increasingly orderly and ordered. Stroebe et al. (1995, 234) state that from the modernist point of view, "bereaved persons need to break their ties with the deceased, . . . form a new identity of which the departed person has no part, and reinvest in other relationships." From the modernist perspective, grief is to end.

Postmodernism takes the view that romantic and modernist conceptualizations of death are products of cultural and historical processes; that is, they are socially constructed (Stroebe et al. 1995; see also Marshall 1986). Nevertheless, it is not clear that one perspective is more correct than any other or that one perspective has better therapeutic outcomes than another. Each perspective defines death differently, and each prescribes different courses of action for the bereaved. What is defined as appropriate in one culture may be inappropriate in another. What "works" for the individual, then, often depends on that person's cultural frame of reference. It follows that the meaning of death for the individual and the individual's reaction to death must be understood in a cultural context. It also follows that, when support or therapy is offered to an individual, the support must be tailored to the individual and must fit with that person's cultural point of view. In an increasingly diverse society like Canada, death has different meanings for different subcultures, and reactions to death will vary depending on the subcultural frame of reference.

SHAMEFUL DEATH

Kellehear (2007) argued that the ideals of the good death and even of the well-managed death are seldom achieved. Indeed, he characterizes the typical death in our time in history as "shameful," falling far short of the ideal. But is death ever ideal? The reality of death is complicated, not a simple acting out of a few idealized steps. People generally prefer life rather than death, and even when they embrace death it is often in the sense of accepting the least worst alternative. Nevertheless, to illustrate Kellehear's point, four case studies are worth considering.

Story 1: Grandpa X

Grandpa X had a rare wasting disease that "progressed" (which hardly seems like the right word, but that word is commonly used to indicate the worsening of an illness) over a couple of years and was ultimately fatal. In the course of the disease, his kidney function was destroyed and he relied on kidney dialysis to keep him alive. He made three trips each week to the hospital for dialysis. He endured dialysis; he did not enjoy it. As his disease progressed, he was occasionally hospitalized. He alternated between home and hospital. He would be admitted to the hospital, be released home, have a crisis, and return to the hospital. In the final months of his life, he spent more and more time in hospital. He complained that a succession of doctors asked him the same questions over and over, each with their own theory about how best to care for his rare disease. He was irritated by these conversations, feeling that he was not getting effective care. He wanted to go home. He felt he would be better cared for there, attended by his wife and adult children. He even intimated that he believed he might recover his health if cared for at home. But his children had busy lives and his wife could not cope with his care at home. So, he spent much of his final months in hospital. He spoke of the shortness of time remaining but never indicated that he was ready to die. The last time I saw him, he was in a cavernous and windowless room receiving dialysis. He was propped up in bed, but slumped to one side, asleep. He was alone. He died the next day.

Grandpa X did not want to die this way. He raged against his disease and time slipping away. He wanted to go home. He wanted to be surrounded by family, at home. He was critical of the hospital experience. He railed against the dying process that he did not choose but was forced to endure. This is an example of Kellehear's criticism of dying and death in our present day.

Story 2: A Beloved Mother

As the first author's mother's independence became increasingly compromised in her old age, she moved into an assisted living facility. Over the next year or so, she experienced a series of small strokes and each time was moved to the hospital. Finally, her team of health care workers (including her physician, nurse, occupational therapist, physical therapist, speech therapist, and social worker) and several family members decided that she could not go back to assisted living but would have to go to a nursing home. However, there was a long waiting list, so she stayed in hospital. A government official had recently and pejoratively characterized patients like my mother, waiting in hospitals for placement in nursing homes, as "bed blockers." A recent stroke had robbed my mother of her ability to form sentences, but she could manage one-word responses. She did not want to be in hospital. When told that efforts were being made to release her, she could only say "Hurry." Then she had another stroke. The doctor and one of her sons consulted. They selected palliative care. They stopped feeding her. They stopped hydrating her. Late on the third day, she took her last breath.

She did not want to die this way, or at this time. She had planned to live to be 100, so she was not ready to die at 92. While she had agreed to a do-not-resuscitate order in the event her heart stopped, she never endorsed any strategies to hasten death. She did not want to be in hospital. She wanted to be in her own apartment surrounded by her familiar possessions. And she did not want to die—she never spoke of a desire for death or a readiness to die.

Is this a shameful death? Like Grandpa X in the previous story, she did not get the death she wanted. Nor apparently did she get the death that public officials preferred. "Bed blockers" are not supposed to languish in expensive hospitals. She lost control to professional caregivers, bureaucratic rules, and family members. She died the way they dictated, not the way she chose. Kellehear (2007) labels deaths such as this as "shameful," implying that there is a better way to die. But perhaps dying is never ideal, never exactly what one wants. Perhaps the best we can expect is a "good enough" death or a "least worst" death. Her death was bittersweet. One wishes it could have been different, better, and according to her wishes, but reality constrains and compromises ideals.

Story 3: The RCMP Officer

The third story is about an RCMP officer in Alberta, David Wynn, who was shot in 2015 by a person with a long history of criminal behaviour. The news media immediately reported that the officer was not expected to recover. His wife made a tearful and heroic statement to the public about his imminent death. A day later it was announced that he had died. One can assume that he laid in hospital on life support while his family, friends, and colleagues said goodbye. An RCMP official publicly complained about the failures of the criminal justice system in keeping dangerous individuals off the street. Kellehear (2007) would call this death shameful as well; certainly, in an ideal world, nobody would die this way, leaving a wife and young children behind. And yet in the wife's public statement, there was nobility in her open acceptance of death. Although death comes unbidden, this story suggests that the challenge is to rise to the occasion, deal with it as well as one can, make the best of a bad situation, and thus turn a bad, senseless, "shameful" death into a good, heroic death.

Story 4: The Death Seeker

One of the most recent social phenomena to impact dying and death is Medical Assistance in Dying (MAID). Many different social contexts and components are illustrated in the stories of those who have sought and gained a hastened death. One such story was provided by a nurse practitioner known to the second author. This nurse practitioner had never envisioned participating in death hastening of any kind, let alone being the agent to deliver a fatal drug cocktail. This action required her to ensure the person did indeed want it done, and that all bureaucratic forms and formalities to have it done were correctly carried out. She also needed to check and certify death. Her story is one of personal and professional values and expectations in flux, and of compassion for those who are suffering.

Further, the middle-aged person who died by MAID had fought bravely, as expected, against a cancer that could not in the end be cured or managed. When she and others important to her became aware that all treatments had failed and death would occur in the near but unknown future, she raised the possibility of assisted death. Those she spoke with provided no support for this option, and as she was in a Catholic hospital at the time for pain control, she needed to be forceful and assert that she be moved to a location where she could be assessed for MAID and perhaps also receive it. She was able to choose her home as her last living place. A select few were invited and gathered with her in her final hours. These were people who ranged in age, gender, and culture. They varied in support for her wish for death, including those who abhorred her choice but respected her right to have MAID performed, and those who were fully supportive of what they considered was a carefully chosen, orchestrated, and sanctioned death event. She said her goodbyes to each, and in this and other ways could be thought of as having a "good" death, as MAID ended a dying process that had already begun and that was neither pleasant nor controllable. All were comforted by the end of her suffering, but all were left with much to ponder as cultural rituals and normative actions did not exist to help them. Only afterward, through familiar funeral and burial rituals, were the watchers or witnesses (as they described themselves) released from what they commonly characterized as their "numbness."

This story raises questions concerning dying and death in Canada. Is MAID a practice that will become common and will it then make death less shameful? Will MAID embody the ideals of the good, or at least better, death and the well-managed death? Will MAID provide for the well-timed death, chosen by the dying person, neither too early nor too late? Will rituals emerge that will guide the implementation and experience of MAID? No doubt, many masters theses, doctoral dissertations, academic analyses, and journalistic reports will examine these questions over the following decades.

SOCIAL RITUALS ACCOMPANYING DYING AND DEATH

Major changes in an individual's life and social status tend to be publicly acknowledged and celebrated in rituals known as rites of passage. Examples of rites of passage include the christening of a newborn baby, the bar mitzvah for a Jewish boy who has reached the age of 13 or bat mitzvah for a Jewish girl who has reached the age of 12 or 13 (depending on the particular Jewish sect), the quinceañera for a Latina girl turning 15 years of age, high school graduation, post-secondary school graduation, marriage, retirement, and death. Regarding death, Posner (1976, 46) wrote:

> In a culture such as ours which abhors death, it is not surprising to find that we attempt to deny it or at least repress the emotional responses which accompany such occasions. It is appropriate to conclude that funeral rituals represent a rather clever attempt to deal with a paradoxical situation. On the one hand, death must be denied, covered or played down at all costs. On the other hand, the occurrence of death must be tactfully disclosed so that members do not inadvertently touch upon contaminating topics.

Funeral rituals acknowledge the death of a member of the community, acknowledge the grief of those who have lost a loved one, and provide guidelines for the public display of emotion. These guidelines describe what emotions should be shown, and where and when and how they should be shown. Furthermore, funeral rituals provide guidelines as to how to proceed with the disposal of the dead body and how members of the community are to provide support to the bereaved. As Posner notes, funeral rituals have a dual and paradoxical function: they simultaneously allow for the display of emotion but also control emotional displays. In addition, funeral rituals simultaneously acknowledge disruption of the normal social order but also provide a mechanism for re-establishing social normality. (For a discussion of the funeral industry in Canada, see chapter 3.)

Post-death rituals in Canada typically acknowledge both the deceased and the mourners. In many funeral services, a **eulogy**—a selective and idealized reconstruction of the life of the deceased—is given. Furthermore, the grief of the mourners is discussed openly. Support is offered in the form of attendance at the funeral or memorial service, flowers, sympathy cards, donations to charities or research organizations, and verbal expressions of sympathy.

In addition to the eulogy, a formal speech is often given at the funeral service, generally by a religious official, that constitutes a message for the living about the meaning of life and death. Burial or cremation typically follows the funeral service. Alternatively, instead of a funeral service, a memorial service may follow a burial or cremation. At the conclusion of these formal rituals, community members return to their normal lives, with little to no residual grief, and the bereaved, despite having major ongoing grief, are expected to return to public normality shortly thereafter.

Memorial services, rather than religious funeral services, are increasingly common in Canada. Jesse's story is illustrative. Jesse (name has been changed) and his family had long been active members of a church community. A typical funeral service at church would have included Jesse, who would have been present in his casket, a eulogy presented by a family member or friend, a sermon presented by the church official who was head of the local congregation, and some musical numbers. This ritual would have been followed by Jesse's burial in a nearby cemetery, and a meal shared back at the church.

Instead of the traditional church service, however, Jesse's family opted to have a memorial celebration. It started with a buffet lunch in the church hall. Jesse was not present. His body had already been "disposed of." After everyone present had filled their plates with food and sat down at the many tables, family members stood up one by one and told stories about Jesse. The stories were moving and often very funny. The audience teared up and more often laughed out loud. A slide show followed featuring photos from the family's albums collected over the years.

While this memorial service was held in the church, the tone was very different from the usual church funeral. And most notably, the claim that the church has had on funeral rituals over the centuries was ignored. No church official preached the usual religious sermon that attends funerals and focuses on the theological meaning of life and death and life after death. The family was clearly in charge and they did things their way. The church and church officials relinquished control. This story illustrates the **secularization** and personalization of the contemporary memorial celebration of life.

Memorialization of the dead is connected in part to the physical remains of the dead and the location of those remains. Memories of the dead are often linked to landscape (Baptist 2010). These landscapes include cemeteries, roadside memorials, battlegrounds, and places where the cremated remains of the dead are placed or scattered. Visiting and tending to these sites, or simply reflecting on them, give the living a tangible connection with the dead. Baptist notes that "ritual activities within deathscapes" create a "relationship between the living, the dead, and the landscape" (304). Landscape provides a place for memory, an embodiment of memory, and an embodiment of grief. The unmarked graves of hundreds of Indigenous children discovered in 2021 on the grounds of former residential schools they were forced to attend and where they died away from their families and communities violates this expectation that landscapes memorialize the dead.

CULTURAL CONSTRUCTIONS OF DYING AND DEATH

Canada is a diverse society (Statistics Canada 2017b). Canadians report over 200 different ethnic origins. Immigrant languages in Canada represent 23 major language families. Canadians report a wide variety of religions including Christian, Muslim, Hindu, Sikh, Buddhist, and Jewish, as well as many reporting no religious affiliation. And there is diversity within each of these major groupings. Christians may be Catholic or Protestant, and Protestants may be Anglican or other, such as United Church members. Muslims may be Sunni, Shia, or Ismaili. Jews may be Orthodox, Conservative, or Reform. And individuals may be more or less "observant" of the traditions, practices, and beliefs of the groups with which they identify. Finally, many Canadians are racialized "visible minorities."

Indigenous groups in Canada include First Nations, Métis, and Inuit peoples (Statistics Canada 2017b). There are over 60 Indigenous languages in Canada representing 12 distinct language families. The most common Indigenous languages are Cree languages, Inuktitut, and Ojibway. Indigenous cultures are not uniform but encompass a wide variety of beliefs, traditions, and practices.

Culture influences personal beliefs, subjective perceptions, and the meanings that individuals assign to dying and death. Cultural rituals dictate how the family and community help the dying person to die and, depending on cultural beliefs, to journey from this world to the otherworld where spirits are believed to reside. Cultural rules direct the processing of the dead body and provide guidelines for public mourning. These dying, death, and post-death rituals vary from one culture to another. Furthermore, individuals identified with a particular ethnocultural group may follow tradition, modify tradition to fit the contemporary Canadian context, or reject tradition altogether.

It is important to be culturally sensitive, culturally responsive, and "culturally competent." Because it is impossible for any one individual to become an expert on the many different cultures in Canada, it is necessary to be humble and to be open to conversation with diverse others about what they believe, expect, and prefer. Further, it is necessary to focus on the individual and avoid cultural stereotypes (Nayfeh, Marcoux, and Jutai 2019; Thompson 2017a).

It is important to ascertain which rituals and practices the individual, family, and community follow. Furthermore, there are differences in the ways that individuals engage in their cultures. The following accounts illustrate Canada's cultural complexity and the challenges this presents for dealing with dying and death.

A Coast Salish Case Study

This case study illustrates the ethnocultural diversity that can exist *within* an ethnocultural group. The Coast Salish are an Indigenous people living on the West Coast of Canada. Joseph (1994) studied their cultural values and rituals regarding dying and death. Salish people combine traditional beliefs with Catholic and other Euro-Canadian beliefs. Furthermore, beliefs vary from one individual to another among the Salish people, as they do in any other community. Joseph noted that in traditional Salish culture there is a belief in the continuity of life from this world to the spirit world and in the connection between these two realms. The deceased lives on in the spirit world and is taken care of there. It is believed that the living and the deceased can communicate through rituals and in dreams, and that the spirits visit the living from time to time. These beliefs do not lessen the pain of grief, but they do facilitate healing.

In her study of the Salish, Joseph records the recollections of two sisters concerning the death of their father following a series of strokes. The two sisters were members of the Squamish Nation living on a reserve in North Vancouver. Joseph notes that, while one sister relied on a Christian church and prayer to deal with her grief, the other sister relied on traditional Salish cultural rituals, going to the Longhouse to engage in socially supported ritualized emotional expression for the purpose of healing. Other social rituals included the use of water, cedar, and devil's club (a shrub) for purification, as well as the grieving circle, smudging, a pipe ceremony, and burning (to send selected items to the deceased). The sister who relied on Salish traditions also received ministrations from a medicine man.

The dying of this elder was described as a time for family gathering. As is customary, on the third day after the elder's death a wake was held where the body of the deceased was viewed. On the fourth day, a funeral at the church was followed by a graveside service. The church service combined elements of both Catholic and Salish tradition. Not long afterward, the family had a burning to send their loved one's clothes and other items that they thought he would need in the spirit world.

The sisters thus selected different cultural elements to shape and assist their grieving and mourning. Both exercised their faith, although faith in different cultural elements. It is an oversimplification to assume that culture is necessarily a monolithic homogenizing force. Instead, there is a diversity of cultural elements from which individuals select. Molzahn et al. (2004) make the same point with respect to the diversity of Coast Salish values and beliefs about organ donation following death. In short, culture tends to shape but also permit a diversity of individual responses.

The Inuit of Nunavut

Laugrand (2019) discusses Inuit views of the afterlife. The traditional Inuit understood the person to be comprised of the physical body, the double-soul (tarniq), and the name-soul (atiq). At death, these separate. The body decays while the double-soul goes to the land of the dead and the name-soul lives on in newborn infants who are given the name of the deceased. Traditional views have merged to varying degrees with Christian and Western views including notions of the soul, heaven, and hell. Laugrand nevertheless suggests that traditional views have a continuing influence, in particular, the notion that the afterlife can be preferable to this life when faced with difficulties such as severe illness. In the past, this belief justified suicide and euthanasia. In the present, Laugrand notes that it is important, especially for young people, to resist "seductive calls to participate in the mysterious beauty of the afterlife" (366).

A Study of Conflict between Western and Islamic Cultures

Hebert (1998) examined Western and Islamic cultural definitions and prescriptions regarding perinatal death, that is, the death of a baby before or shortly after birth. In Western societies, fetal death (miscarriage) is often unacknowledged, and grief following such a loss tends to be disenfranchised (Doka 1995). However, Hebert (1998, para. 12) wrote:

Consistent with the Muslim attitude toward life and death, the death of a fetus or neonate is not minimized as it tends to be in the West, nor does it carry with it the same onus evident in Western societies—that of being an illogical, unnatural, and incomprehensible event to be quickly forgotten as soon as possible. Rather, the loss is regarded as being just as significant and meaningful as the loss of someone later on in life and the fetus is treated with the utmost dignity and respect by all.

Prayers in the case of Muslim infant deaths are said at the site of death, which may be the hospital. The baby is given a name. Autopsy, cremation, and embalming are prohibited by the Muslim faith. The family prefers to take the baby quickly for preparation for burial. This preparation may include ritual washing and shrouding. The burial takes place soon after death, usually within 24 hours. Uncontrolled emotional outbursts are discouraged, as grieving parents are encouraged to accept the will of Allah. The official mourning period is 3 days, but unofficial mourning may go on for 40 days, with visits to the grave on Fridays, the Muslim holy day.

Hebert described a case involving a Muslim family and a perinatal death that occurred in a Montreal hospital. The mother had a miscarriage and lost her baby of 22 weeks gestational age. A bereavement support team, including a social worker, was called in. The following are excerpts from the case report:

A conflict . . . was brewing. The nurses had offered the patient [the mother] an epidural, which her husband had refused outright, and [the nurses] were becoming increasingly frustrated with the men, their loud chatter in the hallway, and their seemingly controlling and unsympathetic attitude toward their patient. . . . The first successful intervention centred on the need to find a female physician. Once found, [the father] seemed to calm down. The mother was asked if she would like to hold the [dead] baby. [The father] refused for her, saying that it would be too painful. He, however, would hold the baby, which he did lovingly and tearfully. . . . He was horrified when offered a snippet of the baby's hair. . . . One family member declared that there should be no autopsy, that the body should be kept, unwashed, with the placenta, and that formalin [a preservative] should not be used. . . . The men's loud praying, once again, became disturbing to the staff . . . and the social worker had to find an empty room in which they could continue their prayers. The nurses felt that [the father], because of the time he spent with the men, was unsupportive of his wife. To make matters worse, within an hour after the delivery, [the father] was asking to take the baby home. The nursing team became extremely upset. . . . On clarification, it was discovered that [the father wanted to take the baby] to the Islamic Centre for preparation for burial. . . . Finally, after much negotiating and compromising, the baby was ready for transport. (Hebert 1998, para. 27–9)

These excerpts from the case report reveal the frustration felt by the hospital nurses. These "Western" nurses were reluctant to set aside practices to which they were committed as modern women, and also as directed professionally and bureaucratically. Furthermore, while the nurses were sympathetic to the mother, they were extremely critical of the father and the other Muslim men. From the Western point of view, the father and other visiting men were authoritarian and overbearing, and the nurses felt that the mother was oppressed and abused.

While this case report does not portray Muslim men sympathetically, the reader can extrapolate that the Muslim men also felt a great deal of frustration. They had to fight every step of the way to follow their cultural and religious practices. This case study reveals how difficult interactions can be when cultures collide.

East Meets West: Chinese in Canada

Bowman and Singer (2001) interviewed elders in Toronto who had immigrated to Canada from China. These older individuals were asked about their attitudes toward end-of-life decisions including, in particular, their views regarding advance directives. The seniors rejected the notion of the advance directive and gave the following reasons, which reflected their cultural values:

• It is important to maintain hope and a positive attitude and not focus on the negative.
• Advance health care planning focuses on the negative and can have undesirable consequences.
• Decision making should be done collectively and should involve a consensus of family members.

The authors suggested that the views of these Chinese individuals can be understood through the lens of Confucian, Taoist, and Buddhist traditions rather than from Western points of view.

Molzahn et al. (2005) interviewed Chinese Canadians in the greater Vancouver area about their values and beliefs regarding organ donation. These authors found considerable diversity in beliefs, reflecting a mix of Confucian, Buddhist, Christian, and Taoist teachings. They noted that a blend of cultural, philosophical, and religious perspectives, more than formal religious dogma, influenced beliefs about organ donation. Because the Chinese have a tradition of not discussing matters relating to dying and death, organ donation was usually not discussed and therefore was unlikely to occur. Nevertheless, Nielsen et al. (2013), who studied Chinese immigrants dying at home in Toronto, cautioned readers that the issues of receiving palliative care at home were not necessarily ethnoculturally specific, so health care providers need to avoid making stereotypical cultural assumptions and focus instead on the individual circumstances of the dying individual and their family.

East Meets West: Ethnic Viet and Lao Hmong in Canada

While the following study is dated, it illustrates the complexity of colliding cultures. Schriever (1990) compared medical and religious belief systems related to dying for ethnic Viet and Lao Hmong refugees in Canada. Ethnic Viet refugees (not to be confused with ethnic Chinese refugees from Vietnam) arrived in Canada from Vietnam in the late 1970s. About the same time, Hmong refugees arrived from Laos. Schriever discusses the intricacies of the traditional Viet and Hmong beliefs and practices regarding dying, death, and mourning. She observed that it was not clear to what extent these refugee groups in Canada maintained their traditional beliefs and practices and to what extent they had incorporated Western beliefs and practices. In a multicultural society, there is a tendency for one culture to borrow from another. This fusion of differing belief systems is known as "syncretism." It follows that individual Viet and Hmong immigrants may be traditional, syncretic, or Westernized. Schriever encouraged Western professionals to ascertain the belief system of their clients rather than proceeding on the basis of stereotypes or limited understanding.

Schriever (1990) offered several suggestions for workers providing palliative care to dying Viet or Hmong patients. She recommended using bilingual and bicultural interpreters, including the extended family in care and decision making, and not isolating the patient from the family. Schriever observed that health care workers should expect that the patient and family will use dual medical systems (traditional and Western) and should not assume that traditional remedies are inconsequential. The workers should not dismiss accounts of dreams or encounters with spirits as having no meaning or relevance and should be aware that emotional distress may be reported in physiological terms. It is important to note that the individual's surname is often placed first instead of last, and that several gestures may be inappropriate. For example, it is rude to touch an adult's head, to show the bottoms of one's feet, to snap one's fingers, or to beckon with an upturned finger (fingers should be pointed down instead). Referring to the deceased by name may also be inappropriate.

Health Care Providers and Cross-Cultural Care

Nayfeh, Marcoux, and Jutai (2019) interviewed doctors and nurses about the challenges they faced in providing end-of-life care in an increasingly diverse ethnocultural Canada. The authors noted the following:

> Research has shown that some ethnocultural groups view the idea of patient autonomy as disempowering and isolating, informed decision-making as violating the protective role of family decision-making, truth-telling as inducing the nocebo [detrimental] effect and with it the risk of a premature death, and taking control of the dying process as an offense to a plan that is dictated by God. (307)

The challenge, then, is for health care providers to develop "effective cross-cultural communication and culturally competent skills" (307). The health care providers noted that it was important to ask the dying patients and their family members about their values and goals for care and for a meaningful death. Further, it was important not to generalize or stereotype but instead recognize that there is variation within ethnocultural groups. The health care providers spoke about the importance of establishing "common ground," that is, creating mutual trust between health care provider and the patient and their family. The health care providers acknowledged that it was counterproductive to try to convince others to accept the provider's point of view. It was generally better to try to understand each other and respect the other's point of view, even though this could be frustrating at times, and could even lead to "moral distress" wherein the health care provider felt that they were compromising their ethical obligations to the dying patient. In short, ethnocultural diversity requires sensitivity, openness, and **cultural competence** from health care providers dealing with the dying person and their family members. This can be a challenging and sometimes frustrating experience for all involved in matters of dying and death in the context of Canada's increasing ethnocultural diversity.

SUMMARY

This chapter explored cultural constructions of the meaning of dying and death in Canada and the resulting social responses. Canadian culture became a death-denying culture in the twentieth century, and reactions to dying and death vacillate between denial and awareness, fear and fascination, detachment and morbid obsession. While death cannot be completely denied, convention can distance us from it. Indeed, the conventional language of death is often indirect and euphemistic. For example, few die today; most simply "pass on." Alternatively, humour presents a way of dealing with what normally makes us uncomfortable. By either distancing us from or making light of death, various euphemisms, sayings, and stories facilitate coping with the strong emotions that death evokes. While death is usually unwelcome, and while we often distance ourselves from its possibility or actuality, death in general remains a topic of great social, individual, and cultural interest. The contemporary media, including television, online news, and social media not only reveal social constructions of dying and death but also play a role in creating, disseminating, and maintaining those constructions. While media portrayals raise fears, at the same time they offer solutions to alleviate those fears. The message is that, despite the chaos of illness, accident, and crime, dying and death are manageable in a world that is, in the end, patterned, orderly, purposeful, and coherent. Nevertheless, having a culturally based meaning system is no guarantee that death will be easily accepted. Individuals may find that the circumstances of a particular death undermine their own system of meaning and their ability to cope. In such circumstances, they are suddenly forced to search for meaning and make sense of the incomprehensible.

Death is increasingly defined by secular rather than religious elements of society and culture. Further, while the family and community used to play major roles in assisting the dying, managing the dead body, and supporting the bereaved, during the twentieth century dying and death were removed from the context of normal life and placed instead in the context of health care institutions to be managed by professionals. There are indications, how-ever, of a growing tendency in the twenty-first century for individuals and their families to reclaim dying and death and return them to the home and community.

It follows that death is not simply a biological event—it is also a social and cultural phenomenon. From such points of view, there are different types of death, and each society defines who has a legitimate right to grieve. Death is generally defined as bad, repulsive, contaminating, and threatening; the cultural logic seems to be that if death is bad, then anybody and anything that is associated with death is also bad. In terms of social responses to death, fu-neral rituals acknowledge the death of a member of the community, acknowl-edge the grief of those who have lost a loved one, and provide guidelines for the public display of emotion. Funeral rituals have a dual and paradoxical function: they simultaneously allow for the display of emotion and control emotional displays. In addition, funeral rituals simultaneously acknowledge disruption of the normal social order and provide a mechanism for re-estab-lishing social normality. In an increasingly culturally diverse Canada in the twenty-first century, these definitions and guidelines vary among different ethnic and religious groups.

QUESTIONS FOR REVIEW

1. In what ways is Canada a death-denying society? In your answer, discuss the paradoxical orientation to death of "fear" and "fascination."
2. What are euphemisms and dysphemisms? What role do they play in Canada's cultural orientation toward death? Discuss the role of news media, television programming, urban legends, folklore, and popular culture in constructing Canada's contemporary cultural orientation toward death.
3. What is "dark tourism"? Is dark tourism consistent or inconsistent with the argument that contemporary societies deny death?
4. Discuss the various kinds of death that exist including biological, social, legal, psychogenic, and disenfranchised death. What are the social con-sequences of these different kinds of death?
5. Discuss past and current ethnocultural diversity in regard to dying and death in Canada. What is meant by "common ground" and "cultural competence" and how do they affect end-of-life care?

KEY TERMS

bureaucratization – The establishment of extensive formal rules to govern procedures and division of labour in a complex organization such as a hospital. (p. 104)

courtesy stigma – When a person is stigmatized because of a stigma attached to
   someone else with whom he or she is associated. (p. 110)

cultural competence – Being aware of and responsive to cultural differences in ways
   that are sensitive, caring, and supportive. (p. 127)

dark tourism – The phenomenon of people travelling to places associated with death
   such as battlefields, cemeteries, memorials, and Second World War concentration
   camps. Also known as morbid tourism and death tourism. (p. 103)

discourse – A widely shared set of beliefs, assumptions, values, and so on. (p. 88)

disenfranchised grief – Grief that is not recognized as socially legitimate. The bereaved person is not accorded the right to mourn openly. (p. 109)

eulogy – A selective and idealized reconstruction of the life of the deceased. Presented at a funeral or memorial service. (p. 119)

euphemism – A word or phrase that is used when a more direct statement would
   make people uncomfortable. (p. 93)

folklore – The beliefs, customs, myths, legends, folk tales, stories, rumours, jokes,
   and sayings that are anonymously produced, collectively shared, and communicated in both oral and written forms (Clifton 1991). (p. 94)

memorialization – Various ways of remembering the dead. (p. 120)

professionalization – Defining an occupation as professional involves extensive specialized training, licensure or certification, and adoption of the values and practices of the professional group. (p. 106)

psychogenic death – Giving up and dying in difficult or traumatic situations. Losing
   the will to live. (p. 108)

secularization – A decline in the importance of religion as a central social institution.
   (p. 120)

stigma – An attribute that disqualifies a person from full social acceptance (Goffman
   1963). Stigmatization involves being socially excluded as a result of that stigma.
   (p. 111)

urban legends – Stories that are not true but nevertheless circulate widely and are
   told as if they are true. (p. 94)

PART THREE

The Individual Response to Dying and Death

CHAPTER FIVE

Individual Perspectives on Dying and Death

Death presents an existential problem for the living: as an individual becomes more and more aware of the inevitability of their death, questions often arise about the meaning and purpose of one's existence. How should one live, given that life ends in death? What is the meaning of life? What is the meaning of death? Furthermore, for dying individuals and their family members, questions arise about how a person should die and how dying itself can be made meaningful.

EXPECTATIONS OF DYING AND DEATH

The possibility of dying can be assessed in both statistical and psychological terms. Statistically, babies born in Canada 100 years ago had a much higher likelihood of dying in infancy or early childhood than do babies born now. Today, death typically comes in old age, and the death of a child is unlikely.

In psychological terms, very young children have a limited awareness of the possibility of dying. At birth, a newborn child cries when it experiences cold, hunger, thirst, pain, and fear. Crying expresses the baby's discomfort and distress and typically elicits caregiving responses from people in the baby's social environment. In other words, the baby has an innate capacity for dealing with threats not only to its comfort and well-being but also to its very existence. Nevertheless, it may be some years before the young child can conceptualize dying and death (Aiken 2001, 229–35).

Hadad (2009) provides an overview of the development of the psychology, understanding, and experience of dying and death across the course of one's life. She noted that infants from birth to about three years of age react emotionally to separation from people to whom they are attached. They experience pain, anger, and sadness as a result. It is interesting that while adults are able to assess death in cognitive terms, their emotional reactions reflect the infant's anger, sadness, and pain.

Hadad (2009) also observed that in early childhood, from three to five years of age, children have a limited and often inaccurate conception of death. For example, they typically do not see death as final or universal. They tend to exhibit what has been called "magical thinking" (Didion 2007; Hadad 2009). They puzzle over death, ask probing questions, and expect the dead person to come back to life. While this puzzlement and magical thinking in children is said to reflect their stage of limited cognitive development, it also reflects the tendency of adults not to provide direct explanations to children and to deflect children's questions about death. Telling a child that grandpa is in heaven may reflect sincere beliefs, but it also allows the child to believe that grandpa is alive and capable of dropping by for a visit, leading to some confusion when he does not. The first author's four-year-old grandson announced regularly and with considerable gravity that his maternal grandfather had died, echoing the grief that his mother and family experienced earlier that year. My grandson then followed his announcement with questions about where grandpa was, when we would see him next, and so on. Clearly, he was trying to figure things out and having some difficulty processing the information he received and the emotions he had felt and witnessed in others.

Hadad (2009) also discussed middle childhood, from 5 to 10 years of age. She noted that during this life stage, children begin to comprehend that death will come to all, and that death is final and this means that the deceased is no longer living and breathing; they also begin to understand causes of death. During this stage of development, the death of a pet may be instructive. Indeed, children today often have a closer attachment to a pet than to a distant grandparent, for example, and may grieve the death of a pet more than the death of their relative (DeSpelder and Strickland 2011). It follows that the death of a pet can be a significant event in a child's life, introducing the child to the nature of death, including its finality and irreversibility.

Hadad (2009) observed that adolescents 10 to 16 years of age have a more sophisticated, complex, and abstract understanding of death. At age 12, the first author's grandson teased me regularly about my closeness to death. He would ask me how much money I would be leaving him and if it would be enough to buy the car he fancied. We all laughed. But he understood death. And when his younger brother asked probing questions, my then 12-year-old grandson and his 10-year-old sister gave me a knowing look and a complicit silence as his parents "answered" the four-year-old's probing questions: Grandpa is in heaven and it will be a long time before we see him again. My 10-year-old and 12-year-old grandchildren knew that this is one way of representing death. They had additional knowledge and insight into the duality of these discourses about death. They knew that grandpa may be in heaven; they also knew that he is buried in the cemetery. This insight of the older children is reminiscent of their awareness and complicity in cultural myths, including the tooth fairy, the Easter Bunny, Santa Claus, and sexuality and birth (consider the European mythology of storks delivering babies to welcoming homes). Older children have figured out the differences between the mythic world and the nonmythic world; they have been admitted into the adult's conceptual universe and, with a knowing wink, participate in the perpetuation of mythic and magical thinking that is used to deflect but ultimately "inform" younger children. Gorman (2019) pointed out that understanding children's knowledge of death and their reactions to death requires paying attention to the child's social context, as well as to the child's stage of development. As Gorman puts it, "context matters," including social, cultural, familial, and religious contexts that inform the child. The experience of a death depends not only on the child's age and stage of development but also on who dies and how close the child was to the deceased. The death of a grandparent will therefore be experienced differently than the death of a mother or father or sibling, or even the family pet.

Children and young adults give little thought to the possibility of their own death (Ens and Bond 2007). Nevertheless, fear of death may underlie this distancing from death. Thus, while young people may rarely think of death, they may fear dying when they do think about it. Because young people often perceive death to be removed from them, they can simultaneously fear death and put it out of their minds. In contrast, middle-aged and older people, who because of their age are closer to death, are more likely to think about dying and death. Yet older adults are less likely to fear death than middle-aged or young adults (Major et al. 2016). Indeed, older people may welcome death. It appears that proximity to death in old age may motivate one to think of death, and not necessarily fear it.

Claxton-Oldfield et al. (2005) asked young adults enrolled in introductory psychology courses in New Brunswick about their willingness to volunteer in a classroom, nursing home, food bank, or palliative care setting. Most expressed a willingness to volunteer in a classroom, food bank, and nursing home; they were much less likely to express a willingness to volunteer to work with dying people in a palliative care setting. Male undergraduate students were less likely than female undergraduate students to indicate that they would be willing to become a palliative care volunteer. Both young men and young women feared that volunteering with the dying would be too demanding emotionally and too stressful, and that they would not know what to do as they lacked the skills and the inclination for this kind of volunteer work. This study suggests that many, although not all, younger university students tend to distance themselves from dying and death.

However, Buckle (2013) asked the university students she taught in a psychology of death and dying course in Newfoundland about their reasons for taking the course. The students stated that they took the course because they had a desire to learn more about death as they had limited knowledge and experience of it; they hoped to achieve personal growth, awareness, and insight. They also hoped that the course would be relevant to their future careers and their desire to help others. At the end of the course, students commented on feeling more comfortable thinking and talking about dying and death.

Chow (2017) surveyed university students in Saskatchewan about death anxiety and its correlates. He found that students generally reported a moderate level of anxiety over death. In terms of correlates, Chow found that females, non-Caucasian students, and students with a higher socioeconomic status reported more death anxiety, while students who had a clear sense of purpose in life, a strong self-image, and psychological well-being reported less anxiety. Students who had religious beliefs and participated in a religious community also reported less death anxiety.

A colleague of one of the authors died at the age of 45 and another at age 57. At these ages, death seems inappropriate because it is premature. When a child dies, it is even more incomprehensible and unacceptable (Martin 1998). Some years ago, death at earlier ages was more expected. Consider a man and a woman born on the Prairies in 1912 and 1922, respectively, who married in 1946 and who in the early 1950s bought three grave plots—two for themselves and one for a child they expected to lose to an early death. Eight children and over 70 years later, the extra grave is still unused. It seemed prudent years ago to expect death at any time. Now, Canadians generally do not expect death except in advanced old age.

DYING TRAJECTORIES

In one sense, we all begin to die from the moment we are born. However, children, adolescents, and young adults do not think of themselves as being on a trajectory ending in death. Similarly, while awareness of one's mortality does tend to become more acute in middle age, and particularly after any deaths of family members or friends, the healthy middle-aged do not think of themselves as dying (Marshall 1986, 137–8). The everyday phrase "over the hill" is significant, then, as it reflects the perception that one has reached the zenith of one's life and has begun the inevitable decline into old age and ultimately death. Nevertheless, the concept of the "dying trajectory" is reserved for those who are perceived to have a disease with an explicit terminal prognosis; that is, death is clearly anticipated given the circumstances of that person's current health.

The dying trajectory refers to the course that a person follows over time as they move through the dying process to death. Glaser and Strauss (1968) noted that there are various dying trajectories. In unexpected deaths, such as sudden infant death syndrome (SIDS), accidental death, homicide, suicide, or fatal heart attack, the dying trajectory is precipitous and brief: death comes quickly. Alternatively, the dying trajectory may be long, as with Alzheimer's disease, for example, or may be complicated by remissions and relapses, as can be the case with cancer.

People who are undergoing a long dying trajectory may express concerns about being or becoming a burden on others. McPherson, Wilson, and Murray (2007) interviewed Ottawa residents who were receiving palliative care for advanced cancer. All but one were cared for at home, and in most cases the primary caregiver was their spouse. All of these palliative care recipients expressed concerns about the physical, social, financial, and emotional burdens they felt they had created or might create in the future for their caregivers. This perception of being a burden resulted in feelings of guilt, regret, sadness, frustration, anger, loss, failure, dependency, uselessness, and lowered self-esteem. As a result, the dying often tried to find ways to contribute to their own care, concealed their own needs, focused on the needs of their caregiver, and engaged in planning for their death. Some eventually achieved a resigned acceptance while others focused on the positive aspects of the caregiver–care receiver relationship or expressed a sense of previously earned entitlement in an effort to reduce their feelings of being a burden. This study shows that a long dying trajectory can change previous roles and relationships in such a manner that the dying experience distress if they perceive they are becoming a burden for their familial caregivers. Similarly, McGregor et al. (2017) surveyed frail older people receiving home-based care in Vancouver, British Columbia. These individuals often commented on their fears of becoming a burden and gave expressions of gratitude to their family caregivers who they felt they had burdened.

Because dying trajectories typically unfold over weeks, months, and even years, family caregiver burden is a commonly reported outcome of providing care to dying family members. Studies of the benefits for both the family caregiver and care recipient are less common, but they are growing in number. These benefits include a feeling of satisfaction resulting from opportunities to discharge duties and responsibilities that are gratefully accepted. Enhanced relationships through meaningful last conversations are also likely. Awareness and acceptance of inevitable death is another noted outcome for both the caregiver and care recipient.

PREFERENCES FOR DYING AND DEATH

Despite the benefits of having time to prepare for death, a shorter dying trajectory that results in quick death is preferred over a long and lingering or dwindling dying trajectory. Indeed, the ideal death is often described as sudden and painless, occurring in one's sleep, and following a healthy and happy long life. It can be illustrated by a story told by a barber. One day, a gentleman in his nineties came in for a haircut. After the man had been in the chair for a while, the barber noticed that he seemed to have drifted off to sleep. In fact, he had quietly died. He had peacefully passed from life to death. Stories like this are told to illustrate the preferred way to die and contrast accounts of ways of dying that are less preferred.

Another example of preferences for death is seen in a story discussed in chapter 4. You will recall that Lucas (1968) interviewed men who had been trapped underground for days in a coalmine disaster in Nova Scotia. The miners had run out of food, water, and batteries to power their lights. They were surrounded by their dead and dying co-workers. The men began to speculate that death would come to them either from starvation, thirst, or suffocation from deadly gas or lack of oxygen. They had little fear of death itself but were concerned about how they might die. They hoped to die painlessly, to just "go to sleep." They seemed to expect that poisonous gas would come eventually, with gas the preferred mode of death. The miners knew that if the gas came, they would drift off to sleep, and death would follow quickly and painlessly.

As mentioned in chapter 3, the dying and death of Sue Rodriguez received a great deal of public attention in the 1990s (Bartlett 1994; Ogden 1994; Wood 1994). In 1991, Rodriguez, an athletic woman who was just past 40 years of age and who was the mother of a young son, began to experience symptoms that would eventually be diagnosed as amyotrophic lateral sclerosis (ALS). This disease leads to a progressive loss of muscle control, ending in paralysis, with death often coming from suffocation. Told by doctors that she had from two to five years to live, Rodriguez said that at first she felt panic, then numbness and shock. She began to notice older people, envying them because she would not get to experience old age (Bartlett 1994). Although she was briefly defiant, thinking that she would beat the disease or at least live longer than predicted, its relentless progression soon put an end to those thoughts. Instead, she decided she would end her own life at some future time when the quality of her life was sufficiently compromised. As she became increasingly dependent, however, she realized that she would need help to die and so began a much-publicized and, at that time, ultimately unsuccessful campaign to legalize assisted suicide in Canada.

The CBC program *Witness* (Bartlett 1994) followed Rodriguez through her final 18 months of life. The program intimately revealed to viewers both Rodriguez herself as a person as well as the devastating effects of her disease. Rodriguez assessed her situation in a straightforward manner. She did not want to die, and had she not gotten ALS she would not be seeking to end her life. However, she had observed that ALS is an awful disease to live with and from her point of view was a gruesome and unfair way to die. She wanted some control over her destiny and wanted a better death than the one that the disease promised. Early in 1994, completely dependent and barely able to speak, Rodriguez achieved her "better," though still illegal, death through the assistance of an anonymous person. She was 43 years old at the time of her death, having lived not quite three years from the time she first experienced symptoms.

Like Sue Rodriguez in Canada, Professor Morrie Schwartz, an American, died of ALS. Also like Rodriguez, Schwartz faced his disease with great courage and dignity and with a desire to make his death meaningful. He spoke of the lessons learned in dying, lessons shared with and recorded by a former student. Indeed, the professor and his student collaborated on a book about the professor's experience with dying, his "last thesis" (Albom 1997). As was the case with Sue Rodriguez, Schwartz's dying became public. In 1995 he came to the attention of the host of the American television program *Nightline*, and interviews were aired on three different occasions as his disease progressed and death approached. The book about his dying and death, *Tuesdays with Morrie*, became a bestseller and in 1999 was made into a movie of the same name starring Academy Award–winner Jack Lemmon.

Unlike Sue Rodriguez, however, Morris Schwartz did not campaign for assisted suicide. While both sought to gain control over their dying, they did so in different ways. Rodriguez wanted to control her dying and avoid a bad death through assisted suicide. Schwartz first acknowledged and then set aside negative emotions such as self-pity and concentrated on positive emotions such as love. Schwartz accepted a natural death and made no effort to control its time or cause. In contrast to Rodriguez, who died at home from an assisted death, Schwartz died at home from the suffocating end of ALS, an end that Rodriguez had described as gruesome and unfair.

Although most people would say that ALS is not a good way to die, both Rodriguez and Schwartz could be cited as having "good" deaths. Their manner of dealing with their terminal illness can be applauded and portrayed as exemplary. As discussed earlier, however, dying peacefully in one's sleep in old age also tends to be considered a good death. In this scenario, there is only death—no lengthy dying, no pain, no suffering, no need for coping, and no test of character. It is an ideal death because it is an easy one. Note that the aim of hospice/palliative care is to ease suffering and promote a good death—one in which pain and other problems are prevented or successfully addressed.

Dying from ALS and many other chronic illnesses is not easy: it is a dying that tests, shapes, and reveals one's character. Cultural ideals value dignity, fortitude, courage, endurance, self-control, and making the best of the worst situations. Public accounts of people such as Rodriguez and Schwartz are designed to move others emotionally and provide moral inspiration. Dying is not simply a biological process; it is also a process with psychological, social, moral, spiritual, and occasionally, as in the case of Sue Rodriguez, political dimensions. Public accounts of people who die exemplary deaths remind us of these various dimensions and serve to describe and define the various pathways to a "good" death.

Professor Diana Austin at the University of New Brunswick, in an article originally published in the *Globe and Mail* (16 July 1997), described the dying and death of her mother. She "began her journey to death" when she experienced sudden liver failure at the age of 70. Her unexpected recovery from that initial event "led to a three-year celebration of life in the shadow of death." Austin also wrote that her mother "continued to laugh and shop" and that "she chose to gauge the quality of her existence by the joy she found every day in her interaction with others." She resisted death, and even near the end said resolutely, "I am not going." Noting that dying does not necessarily mean a quick and quiet death, Austin concluded, "Mom died slowly, but she died well" (quoted in McPherson 2004, 439–40).

Austin's account shows that the dying process, despite its many drawbacks, can be a rewarding and meaningful time for the dying person, their family, and for others such as professional caregivers whose lives are touched by the dying person. It also illustrates a particular style of coping with dying. In this case, coping involved living life to its fullest extent, given the circumstances, and resisting death by fighting the good fight and never giving in. In this regard, Austin's mother illustrates a cultural ideal: the person who exercises her will to live, to extract as much meaning as possible from life, while holding death at bay for as long as possible. The notion that willpower can extend life is part of our cultural mythology and reflects the social expectation that a person should make every effort to resist death. Although we cannot know the extent to which Austin's mother was influenced by cultural prescriptions, the telling of the story tends to reinforce these prescriptions. Increasingly, these prescriptions are seen in eulogies indicating that the deceased had battled disease or old age to live longer and also to live better while dying.

While Sue Rodriguez's campaign to legalize assisted suicide in the early 1990s resulted in the 1993 Supreme Court of Canada decision against legalization, in 2011 Gloria Taylor became the public face of a renewed attempt to legalize assisted suicide, initiated by the British Columbia Civil Liberties Association. Like Rodriguez, Taylor was diagnosed with ALS. Like Rodriguez, Taylor campaigned publicly to win the right to have the option of choosing an assisted death. While Taylor died naturally in 2012, her campaign culminated in the 2015 Supreme Court of Canada decision to legalize MAID, or Medical Assistance in Dying (see chapter 3 for more details). Gloria Taylor's heroic campaign was the subject of a CBC *The Fifth Estate* documentary in 2012. This documentary portrayed Taylor as an average Canadian who found meaning, purpose, and a quiet heroism in her dying trajectory.

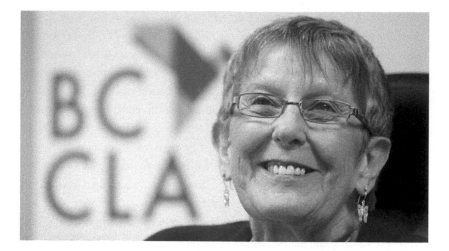

Image 5.1. Gloria Taylor, who suffered from ALS (amyotrophic lateral sclerosis), smiles during a news conference at the British Columbia Civil Liberties Association in Vancouver on 18 June 2012. The Supreme Court of British Columbia had granted Taylor the right to a physician-assisted suicide. This decision led to the implementation of MAID (Medical Assistance in Dying) in Canada in 2016.
Source: The Canadian Press/Darryl Dyck.

Further, Professor Kathleen Venema at the University of Winnipeg, in an article published in the *Globe and Mail* (9 May 2019; see also Venema 2018), described her mother's experience with Alzheimer's disease from a diagnosis in 2005 to her death in 2017. By 2008, Venema's mother spoke often about ending her life; however, she needed help to end her life and that was not legal in Canada until MAID was legalized by the Government of Canada in 2016. And even so, the initial 2016 legislation did not allow MAID for persons with dementia because they are unable to give consent to the act of death hastening. Venema observed in 2019 that people with dementia "still cannot choose—as my mother could not choose—the conclusions to their own stories" and argued that "this needs to change." The 17 March 2021 MAID legislative changes addressed that concern by instituting a "waiver of final consent," often referred to as "Audrey's Amendment." Audrey Parker, a 57-year-old woman who lived in Halifax and who was dying of cancer, chose to receive MAID early in 2018 because she feared losing her final decision-making capacity.

The importance of dying well, as evident in the stories of Rodriguez, Schwartz, Austin, Taylor, and Venema is not solely a manifestation of

Euro-Canadian values. The Cree living in Quebec near James Bay also value self-control and composure in the face of death (Preston and Preston 1991). A story is told of a Cree man, Jimmy Moar, who was old and blind, and who one evening announced his impending death by saying to his daughter, "I'm almost falling off from my chair. That's all I can [do to] sit here. I am very tired." He then told his daughter how much he loved her and his granddaughter, put on his best clothes, went to bed, and died (Preston and Preston 1991, 142). This story is told as an example of a good death and a preferred death. Goodbyes were said, relationships were affirmed, and death was met with dignity and quiet acceptance.

FEAR OF DYING

The preference for a quick death suggests that dying is perceived as distressing, even more than death itself (Frank 1991, 43; Lévy, Dupras, and Samson 1985, 31; Lucas 1968). Although most people prefer living to dying, some people on a dying trajectory may find living on that dying trajectory so unpleasant that they wish to die and ask for death. Indeed, following their demise it is commonly said of such people that death was a "blessing" because it brought their suffering to an end.

Fear of dying is driven by concerns about loss and suffering (Frank 1991, 43; Lucas 1968), and the possibility of a long or lingering and unpleasant dying trajectory. A person entering such a dying trajectory faces loss of health, loss of control and independence, loss of mental competence, loss of status and social roles, loss of future plans and goals, and impending loss of life. Furthermore, fear of dying is motivated by concerns about prolonged suffering and, in particular, about pain (Frank 1991, 43; Lucas 1968).

Another concern associated with fear of dying is loss of dignity. Chochinov et al. (2002) studied palliative care recipients in Winnipeg, the majority of whom reported that they were able to maintain their sense of dignity. Only a small number (8 per cent) reported frequent feelings of shame, degradation, or embarrassment. Those with a lessened sense of dignity tended to be younger rather than older, and they were cared for in hospital rather than at home. The authors noted that a person's sense of dignity appears to be "a particularly resilient construct and, in most instances, is able to withstand the various physical and psychological challenges that face patients who are terminally ill" (2002, 2028). Nevertheless, it was noted that alterations in physical appearance coupled with feelings of being a burden, needing assistance with activities such as bathing, being in pain, and being hospitalized can undermine the dying person's sense of dignity, competence, autonomy, self-esteem, and sense of self-worth (Chochinov et al. 2002, 2029).

AWARENESS OF DYING

People who are dying may be unaware that they are dying because they have not been informed of a terminal prognosis, or because they are in denial. According to Glaser and Strauss (1965), two of the first researchers to examine dying and death in this modern era, people who are aware that they are dying have two options. On the one hand, a drama of mutual pretense may be enacted in which dying persons and the people around them do not speak of the dying process or of impending death, although everyone is aware that death is near. On the other hand, people may prefer to discuss the terminal prognosis openly. Today, dying individuals are more likely to prefer to talk openly of dying and death (Corr, Corr, and Doka 2019), although some ethnocultural groups have social norms that discourage open communication (Nayfeh, Marcoux, and Jutai 2019).

For instance, some cultures hold that if a person is told they are dying, that person will give up hope, and this loss of hope will hasten death. A student reflected on this recently. The student wrote that her mother, who had immigrated to Canada from China, had been open with her mother (the student's grandmother) about the grandmother's dying (per Canadian culture). The student's mother now lived with guilt and regret, as she felt she had deprived her mother of hope and caused her death (reflecting Chinese culture).

Not speaking of dying and death, it is argued, maintains denial, hope, normalcy, and dignity, while avoiding unpleasant topics. On the other hand, openly acknowledging dying facilitates the obtaining of information, allows for the expression and sharing of feelings, helps with decision making, and allows one to settle one's affairs and make final arrangements. This dilemma impacts health care providers in Canada, as they must obtain informed consent to provide care. Any cultural requirement that a dying person not be informed they are dying will create a moral and at times practical dilemma for health care personnel.

The internet provides many opportunities now for people to increase awareness and communication about dying and death. People can use the internet to find information about any symptom or diagnosis, and to connect with others who share their experiences or concerns about illnesses. Radin (2006) studied online cyberspace communication about potentially fatal breast cancer. Radin argued that this form of communication breaks down established professional information monopolies and old ways of communicating. She observed that it provides a safe and supportive environment that allows people with breast cancer and their supporters and also survivors to communicate with each other about the various aspects of the disease and their experiences with it. This peer-to-peer communication can provide emotional support and encouragement, facilitate the exchange of information and insight, empower laypeople, provide a forum for advocates of change, and may facilitate social activism.

THE DYING PROCESS

Dying is a process that takes place over variable lengths of time. Elisabeth Kübler-Ross (1969), the physician who helped bring conversations about dying into the open, interviewed dying individuals and, from these interviews, theorized that people typically experience "stages" in the course of their dying. This theoretical model is a generalization and does not necessarily apply to every individual. Furthermore, the model has been misused as a prescription about how one *should* feel in the course of dying and about how one *should* proceed through that process.

Kübler-Ross's model indicates a typical initial reaction to a terminal diagnosis is denial. As reality overcomes denial, anger is the typical second reaction. A third stage involves "bargaining" for more time. In the fourth stage, depression sets in as the person reacts to their many losses and prepares for further losses. Finally, cognitive and emotional resistance gives way to resigned acceptance. In other words, the stages might be characterized in the dying person's voice as: "Not me!" "Why me?" "Not yet," "Poor me," and finally "I give in."

David Kuhl (2006, 2), a palliative care physician in Vancouver, suggested that "what dying people want is the same as what living people want." Both, Kuhl argued, want to feel good about themselves, experience closeness to significant others, and feel that their lives are meaningful. Accomplishing this for the dying depends in part on controlling physical symptoms and facilitating open communication and fostering new and old relationships.

In 2003, a documentary titled *Dying at Grace* provided an intimate view of the dying and death of five patients in the palliative care unit at Grace Hospital in Toronto. Each had a terminal cancer (ovarian, bladder, breast, lung, and brain). Nichols (2005, 143) reviewed this documentary and observed that it "is a poignant, in-depth exploration of the process of dying." Nichols further observed that "dying is seen as a gradual loss of control" and that "death is seen as an anticlimax—the end of struggling for breath, the end of pain or suffering, a time of quiet after much activity, and the notable absence of struggle often after a prolonged period of suffering."

PERSONAL ACCOUNTS OF "BRUSHES WITH DEATH"

Occasionally people have an experience where they think that they might be facing dying and death, but they do not die. A middle-aged man told the following story:

> In my early thirties, I began to experience frequent, extreme, and unexplainable fatigue often accompanied by anxiety, depression, and difficulty coping with everyday tasks. Visits to the doctor produced no explanation. Indeed, visits to the doctor were so unproductive and frustrating that at one point I swore I would never go back to a doctor again. I assumed that I was under stress from my employment and needed to develop better stress management strategies. However, nothing seemed to help.
>
> Things got worse over several years. I thought I might be losing my mind. In time, I became convinced that I was dying. The thought that I was dying came as a clear and certain realization. I remember being surprised that I felt no emotion attached to this realization. I was neither afraid nor angry. I was dying, most likely, and that was that. Indeed, I felt so miserable that death seemed to be the solution and dying seemed to be the explanation. I still wondered exactly what was wrong with me, but nevertheless, whatever was wrong, I felt that it was killing me.
>
> I was pretty desperate when my wife made a doctor's appointment for me with a new doctor and told me that I was going to see him or else. I went. The doctor told me that I was probably losing my mind but agreed to do some blood tests. A week later he diagnosed Hashimoto's thyroiditis and shortly afterwards a specialist diagnosed pernicious anemia as well. I had a double whammy.

It seems melodramatic now to say that I was dying. These diseases are perfectly treatable today. But I was dying. A hundred years ago, I would have gone mad and then died. It would have been an unpleasant death for myself and for those around me, in particular for my wife and young children. While these two diseases will not kill me today, I find myself wondering what will. Someday, sooner or later, I will get another diagnosis, and next time I may not be so lucky.

For this storyteller, personal self-diagnosis was more a cognitive exercise than an emotional one. While there was much emotional turmoil in his life, he exhibited an emotional detachment as he assessed his health status, concluded that he was dying, and attempted to deal with that realization. This story also reminds us that death has a certain capriciousness about it: many who are now reading this would already be dead if born at an earlier time in history or in some place where modern health care is not available. Many of the diseases that killed our ancestors are now either preventable or treatable. Similarly, those diseases that today are most likely to kill us may yet be rendered impotent. When we die and how we die is in part a function of our time and place in history. Yet the storyteller himself did not dwell on such academic observations. His concerns were more pragmatic: his perception was that he was dying, and his concern was what to do about it.

People who confront dying are often said to show anger, revealed in part in the form of questions such as "Why me?" or "Why now?" (Kübler-Ross 1969). Such questions imply resistance and an unwillingness to accept fate. The storyteller above seems to be more fatalistic. It is as if his reaction is a bemused acknowledgment that these things happen haphazardly, and so "Why not me?" and "Why not now?"

Another brush-with-death story is told by a woman in her thirties, who was an emergency nurse and who found some lumps behind her ear:

I was thinking the worst. What if these [lumps] were cancerous tumours? . . . I phoned my family doctor. I told the receptionist that I needed to see my doctor that day. They got me in to see him later that afternoon.

My doctor was not able to explain the lumps. His facial expression said it all, and then he started asking me a lot of questions. Questions I had heard over the years from my nursing experience. Questions that centred on signs and symptoms of cancer. I asked him bluntly. Is it cancer? He said he wasn't sure what they were, but he didn't like what he saw. In his attempt to be reassuring, he said, "If it is Hodgkin's disease, you are lucky. It is one of the best types of cancer to get. You could have up to a 10-year survival rate." Why was it that I wasn't feeling too lucky? Ten years did not seem like such a long time when I had one daughter in Grade 2 and the other in Grade 3.

[The next day] I had an appointment with a surgeon. I was due to work the night shift but I called in sick. The charge nurse . . . called me back at home and asked me what was wrong. . . . She was very understanding.

The next day was as fearsome and tense as the day prior. Waiting. Always waiting and wondering. I saw the surgeon. Again, the visit was not very encouraging. He thought the lumps looked suspicious. The only way to get a diagnosis would be to have a biopsy.

You may be wondering what was going through my mind these long days and nights. Well, I guess the first thing was fear. Not fear for myself, but fear for my daughters. If the news ends up being bad, what will happen to my girls? My husband works out of town, which means that they would have no mother and would see their father infrequently. Essentially, they would be raised by a stranger, perhaps by a nanny. This is not something I wanted for my daughters. . . .

Another concern was how to tell my children if the lumps turned out to be malignant. How do you tell your school-age daughters that their mom has cancer and may die? . . . I decided to tell them the truth. "Mommy is having minor surgery to see if these lumps on my neck are cancer." They took the news very well. . . . Now I realize that they were trying to be strong for me.

The waiting game wasn't over. My surgery was two weeks away. Two more weeks of thinking and trying to prepare myself for the worst-case scenario. I couldn't cope with working so I called the nurse manager. . . . Once again, I had a lot of understanding from my immediate supervisors. But the support given to me by my husband was different.

I don't want to say that my husband wasn't supportive, I guess he thought I was getting myself all worked up for nothing. "Wait until we see what the results are. It may be nothing." My husband didn't go with me to either of my doctor appointments. I guess he thought that he wouldn't be much use to me. After all, I was the health care professional, not him. He wouldn't know what the doctor was saying anyway, so why miss a day's work. He also did not go with me to the hospital for my surgery. Again, he felt that we wouldn't find out the results that day and he wouldn't be able to go in the treatment room so he chose once again to go to work. My mother knew that this would be a difficult day for me and drove me to the hospital, waited in the waiting room (picked my girls up from school while I was having my biopsy done), and drove me home. . . . I know my mom was as worried about the outcome as myself. I don't think my mom knows how much that meant to me having her there, and I also don't think my husband knows how hurt I was not having him there. . . .

What was frustrating during that week [waiting for the results of the biopsy] was the attitude of the surgeon. I knew he had no idea what I was going through emotionally and mentally. What was equally infuriating was that when my results did reach the surgeon's desk, he shuffled them aside when he saw that the diagnosis was benign. He did not call me with the results. He waited until I called him. When I asked him if he had the results he said yes, but couldn't remember what the report said. As he shuffled through the reports on his desk, he finally found mine. Oh yeah. The news is good. Nothing to report.

. . . I wasn't going to die from Hodgkin's disease. . . . [But] the scar behind my ear is a constant reminder of those very stressful few weeks in my life and of my mortality.

A casual reading of this story suggests that the storyteller was afraid that she might have cancer and that she would die. She highlights the anxiety and fear that she felt while waiting for a diagnosis. But what is she really afraid of? She indicates that she did not give any thought to death in purely personal terms. Instead, she focused on her children. Her greatest fear was that her young daughters would be left motherless, would be raised by a stranger, and might suffer because of the loss of their mother.

The storyteller discusses her relationships during the time she waited for a diagnosis. She describes the women in her life as being very supportive: her daughters, her supervisor at work, and her mother are all sympathetic, understanding, and helpful. Her male family doctor sees her almost immediately and tries to be reassuring. The other men in the story are not perceived as being supportive. Her male surgeon does not acknowledge her concern or her need to know her diagnosis. Her husband minimizes the situation, refusing to get upset over something that "may be nothing." Not only does he distance himself emotionally from the situation, but he also distances himself physically by going to work.

The differences between the males and the females in this story can be explained in part by sex role socialization. Social norms for females legitimize emotional expression and nurturing responses. In contrast, social norms for males define emotional displays as deviant and unacceptable. Although these roles are changing, males are still less likely to show their emotions and less likely to acknowledge the emotions of others (Symbaluk and Bereska 2019).

The storyteller finishes her account by pointing out that, in the end, the experience served as an ongoing reminder of her mortality. This event brought death into focus in a very close, personal, and threatening manner, when previously it had been only a distant eventuality. Death had become threatening because the storyteller wishes to raise her young daughters herself. She has an agenda—unfinished business—and death would disrupt her plans for the future. Death for this storyteller means suffering, not for herself, but for the daughters she would leave behind. For this reason, death is feared.

Another story about people who thought they were likely to die returns us to the Nova Scotia coalminers referred to earlier in this chapter. Trapped underground, for the first three days the men tried to dig their way to safety. When their battery-powered lights gave out, they waited in total darkness. They would either be saved or they would die. Before becoming trapped, the miners had not discussed death with each other and seldom thought of it individually, although they knew that coalmining was dangerous work. Even when trapped in the mine, the coalminers maintained a psychological distance from dying and death by directing their lights away from the dying and dead and by speaking of the dying as if they were already dead, thereby using social death as a substitute for physical death. Furthermore, the miners knew that they were expected "to die 'like [men]' with little expressive outcry, but with stoic determination" (Lucas 1968, 16). Haas (1977) observed the same behaviour among the "high steel ironworkers," who erect superstructures for high-rise buildings. While the ironworkers would cognitively assess the danger of a given situation, they never discussed or showed emotions such as fear.

The coalminers did express certain regrets about dying. They spoke of things they had planned to do but would have to leave undone. They mentioned their roles as husbands, fathers, and providers and expressed concern about not being able to fulfill these roles and the consequences for the survivors. In this regard, the miners were like the mother in the earlier story who worried more about the daughters she would leave behind in the event of her death than about herself. Finally, the miners engaged in a review of their lives in an attempt to affirm "that their achievements were creditable" (Lucas 1968, 13). In summary, the miners who faced death did not express fear about their own impending deaths. They did, however, express concern about how they might die, hoping for a quick and painless death, and about the consequences that their death would have for those left behind.

Arthur Frank (1991), a professor at the University of Calgary, published a personal account of his own experiences with two very different "brushes with death." When he was 39 years old he had a heart attack, and at 40 he was diagnosed with cancer. He survived both life-threatening illnesses and wrote to tell his story. Frank noted that serious illnesses take a person to the edge of life. He referred to life-threatening illnesses as a "dangerous opportunity" to clarify what is important about life. The danger, of course, is that one might die; however, there is opportunity as well. Standing at the edge of life, at the boundary between life and death, changes one's perception of both life and death. When death becomes personal, an immediate and real possibility, questions are raised about how one has lived one's life and how one should live one's life in the future should the illness not prove fatal.

Recovery from his heart attack meant that Frank returned to his previous life "as if nothing had happened." Of course, something had happened, but his inclination was to put the whole experience behind him. The diagnosis of cancer was different. The sense of being in remission rather than fully cured, coupled with the lengthy and demanding experience of cancer treatment, was transformative. Neither Frank, nor his life, nor his wife, nor their life together were the same again.

In analyzing his relations with his doctor, Frank observed that their communication involved a detached language of medical objectivity rather than the language of personal experience and subjective perceptions. In other words, health care communication was "cool" rather than emotional, impersonal rather than personal. Furthermore, interactions focused on the management of the disease rather than on the experience of it. In short, both doctor and patient conformed to cultural rules that emphasize professionalism, and technical and personal competence. In our society, emotionality is associated with incompetence. As a result, people facing death tend to be denied legitimate expression of their fears, frustrations, and experiences.

Frank also wrote about the coherence and incoherence associated with serious illness. Incoherence is the loss of order in one's life and the loss of connection with others whose lives are ordered. Illness, pain, and dying separate a person from the normal biological and social order of life. Because perceptions of order help a person make sense of life, incoherence involves the loss of a sense of understanding and meaning. Coherence involves gaining or regaining a sense of order, connection, and meaning. Frank observed that communication with others can facilitate the construction and maintenance of coherence. However, he distinguishes between communication in the form of detached medical talk, which promotes a sense of incoherence, and the communication of personal experience to sympathetic others, which promotes a sense of coherence.

Antonovsky (1987) argued that a sense of coherence is important to health and well-being. Coherence, he suggests, has three components: comprehensibility, manageability, and meaningfulness. Comprehensibility refers to the ability to make sense of things, to understand, to explain, and to predict. Although things may be either good or bad, it is helpful if they are at least understandable. Manageability is the perception that one has adequate resources and supports to deal with problems. Meaningfulness is the ability to find meaning, purpose, and motivation. Life-threatening events, terminal illnesses, and the death of others can undermine a person's sense of coherence. From the perspectives of both Antonovsky and Frank, the challenge for the person facing death is to hang on to or re-create their own sense of coherence.

Frank describes the experience of a potentially terminal illness as alienating: one is separated from future plans and goals, from past health, from roles and relationships, and from "innocence"—that naive sense of security that persists as long as death remains distant and abstract. Frank notes that all of these losses must be mourned. Yet society tends to dictate the terms of mourning, and these are not always consistent with the needs of individuals who grieve for their losses in their own way and in their own time. Similarly, Frank complains that the health care system tends to take control of one's body, disease, identity, and even experience. One's identity becomes the disease; one's personal experience, expressed in subjective terms, is treated as largely irrelevant. The challenge for individuals facing death is to hang on to their personal identity and acknowledge their personal experience in their own terms.

Robert Hughes (1999) described his brush with death in a severe automobile accident. He remembered the hours he was trapped in the wreckage. Gasoline was leaking, and he begged a friend to shoot him if the car caught fire. Nevertheless, he desperately wanted to live. Hughes's story gives voice to the common assumption that individuals have a strong will to live. Indeed, it has been argued that, in a nonreligious age, the terror of death and the fear of nonbeing have led to the widespread denial of death (Becker 1973). Nevertheless, Hughes's story also points out that some types of death are preferred to other types, especially to avoid unacceptable suffering.

The story of the car accident contrasts in many ways with the other stories reported above. Hughes's brush with death was sudden. In the other stories, the storytellers have more time to contemplate death's approach. Hughes's concerns are immediate and personal, and he has little time to come to terms with death. The other storytellers, perhaps because they have more time to contemplate death, come to terms with their own death. If they resent dying, they do so more for the disruption that it will cause the loved ones they will leave behind.

FEAR OF DEATH AND DENIAL OF DEATH

In Kübler-Ross's (1969) model of the dying process, denial is the initial reaction to learning that one is dying. This suggests that, initially, death is unwelcome and unthinkable. In the last stage of her model, however, the dying person accepts death. There is a paradox here. People who are closer to death apparently fear it less than those more removed from it. Furthermore, dying may be feared more than death itself.

According to Becker (1973), another early theorist, fear of death is fundamentally motivating and at the same time denied. Becker rewrote Freud's thesis by arguing that awareness of one's mortality, rather than one's sexuality, is the fundamental human motivation. Furthermore, because awareness of one's mortality gives rise to terror, it is also the fundamental repression. Becker thus argued that people repress their awareness of their mortality so that they can avoid the anxiety this awareness provokes.

Becker further argued that an awareness of one's mortality provokes terror not only because it ends the individual life but also because it potentially invalidates the life lived. The individual prefers to believe that their life is significant and has meaning and purpose. In Becker's terms, people have a need to see themselves as "heroes." The eventuality of death creates a problem for heroism, in that it calls into question the value of the individual's life. In other words, awareness of one's ultimate demise creates an existential crisis centred on questions about the meaning of life. To deal with these unsettling questions and emotions, Becker argued that individuals either search for answers of their own creation or, more often, find answers in the form of socially constructed solutions such as religion, notions of romantic love, or cultural prescriptions about how one can live a good and respected life. These ready-made answers provide direction and rationale that help the individual gain a sense of heroism, a sense that their life is meaningful.

Becker's thesis has some merit. People distance themselves from death. Young people act and feel immortal, even if they are cognitively aware of their mortality. Death raises existential questions and anxieties, and dying individuals typically attempt to make sense of their impending death and their life in the face of death. Terror management theory (TMT) is an extension of Becker's thesis. Major et al. (2016, 262–3) noted that, according to TMT, "the primary way humans manage the fear of death is through cultural worldviews and self-esteem. Cultural worldviews are humanly constructed, shared-symbolic conceptions of reality that infuse human existence with a sense of meaning, order, and permanence. Self-esteem is the general sense that one is valued within the context of the cultural worldview." It follows that when people are reminded of their mortality, they tend to affirm their faith in a cultural worldview. This provides them with the assurance that their lives are significant and that they can transcend death either in the belief of a life after death and/or a belief that their contributions to significant others and to society will live on as a legacy after their death.

Major et al. (2016) noted that strategies used to find meaning and purpose in the face of death develop and change across the life course. Furthermore, the effectiveness of these strategies changes as people age. The authors observed that older people appear to be more effective than younger people at managing death anxiety. They noted that older adults are less afraid of death than younger persons even though they think about their own death more. One way they do this is by emphasizing "generativity." Generativity includes "passing knowledge and skills to others, making contributions to community, engaging in activities that create a lasting legacy, being creative and productive, and caring and taking care of others" (269).

Major et al. found that thinking about death increases the importance of generativity for older people. This finding implies that older people use generativity—by emphasizing the well-being of their grandchildren, for example—as a way of enhancing self-esteem, fostering meaningful relationships, and maintaining their beliefs and worldviews, all of which provide a sense of immortality, legacy, meaning, and purpose.

Major et al. suggested that Erikson's theory of psychosocial development explains the different strategies that younger and older people use to manage death anxiety. Erikson (1959) argued that the challenges of adult development involve achieving intimacy in the form of meaningful and satisfying relationships with others, generativity by making meaningful contributions to others and to society, and finally ego integrity.

Ego integrity during the last stage of life involves transcending the self and finding meaning and purpose in supporting others—in particular, future generations—and in advancing abstract principles such as cultural ideals and values. Erikson, Erikson, and Kivnick (1986) referred to this as grand-generativity, and Tornstam (2005) wrote about the related concept of gerotranscendence. **Generativity**, in the sense of contributing to future generations, is a means of pursuing immortality strivings, attaining symbolic immortality, and transcending death.

ACCEPTANCE OF DEATH

Zimmermann (2012) noted that acceptance of death rather than denial of death has become part of the contemporary discourse about what constitutes a good death and the correct way to die. She suggested that acceptance of dying and death has become a goal and expectation imposed by health care personnel on dying patients and their families. The emerging discourse regarding the acceptance of death imposes a moral imperative on the dying, a new commandment: thou shalt accept thy death. Acceptance counters the often-quoted refrain from poet Dylan Thomas (1971): "Do not go gentle into that good night. Rage, rage against the dying of the light." Thomas's poem articulated the twentieth-century discourse regarding denial of death and the prescribed stance toward death: nonacceptance, resistance, anger, and struggle. Dying individuals then were encouraged to go to battle with death and to fight valiantly, and health care providers were to encourage and facilitate that struggle. Today, instead of encouraging the good fight and its struggle and resistance, the prescriptive discourse now suggests that the dying embrace death, welcome it, make peace with it, and accept it. Sirois (2012) noted, however, that not all dying people are able to accept their impending death. Some rage, resist, complain, and deny. However, these individuals may be described as "difficult" and as falling short of the culturally prescribed ideal of the good patient.

Acceptance of death may come easily for many. Clarke, Korotchenko, and Bundon (2012) interviewed frail elderly individuals who had multiple chronic conditions. Assuming that these people, who were near death, would not want to talk about dying and death, these researchers were surprised when these elders brought up the topic in interview after interview. Furthermore, these men and women were comfortable discussing dying and death. They spoke of how many of their relatives and friends had died; the inevitability of death; their hopes for a good, swift, and painless death; their fears of a prolonged dying process with pain and suffering; and the plans they were making for death. They complained that family members and health care personnel often were unwilling to engage in discussions about dying and death. While they emphasized living life well and enjoying the time they had left, they also spoke of death as an inevitable and welcome end to suffering, dependency, and becoming a burden on family and society. The authors concluded, "We have become strongly aware of the importance of providing a space for older adults to speak about their thoughts, feelings and concerns regarding death and dying rather than assuming that these are undesirable and unmentionable topics" (1415).

Molzahn et al. (2012) reported similar findings in their interviews with people with chronic kidney disease. These individuals were very aware of the possibility of dying from their illness and were comfortable discussing dying and death. They spoke of the importance of living life but also of making plans for death, including, for example, advance directives and funeral plans. In contrast, the authors observed that dialysis facilities in hospitals tend to have a death-denying culture and the patients they interviewed indicated that their health care providers were often uncomfortable discussing dying and death. Once again, we see the paradox that those who are far removed from death avoid acknowledging it more than those who are in close proximity to it. Those who are closer to death tend to be more accepting of it and more comfortable discussing it.

THE RELIGIOUS SOLUTION

Becker (1973) identified the "religious solution" to the problem of death as the most pervasive and enduring sociocultural mechanism for defining death in terms that reduce anxiety. However, this solution may be irrelevant for those who do not have faith. Furthermore, the religious solution to the problem of death has been undermined by secular trends. Interestingly, people who have strong religious beliefs and people with no religious beliefs tend to report less fear of death than people with weak religious beliefs (Mirowsky and Ross 1989). It appears, then, that religion can make death palatable for those who firmly believe, and that those with no religious faith whatsoever also seem to be able to come to terms with death.

THE SPIRITUAL SOLUTION

In a secular era, religion has little force in the lives of many individuals, yet many continue to emphasize spirituality. While spirituality may reflect religious discourses, in the twenty-first century spirituality is often linked with nonreligious constructions that are designed to assign special meaning and significance to selected experiences, such as dying and death.

Thompson (2017b, 337) defined spirituality as a "sense of meaning, purpose and direction." He observed that while religion is a source of spirituality, it is not the only source. Thompson suggested that both religious and secular spirituality connect people to something significant and greater than the individual. Durkheim ([1915] 1965) observed that things and experiences can be defined as ordinary or special or, in Durkheim's terms, as profane or sacred. Thus, to construct a definition of something as having special significance and meaning is to define it as sacred. Once something is defined as sacred, it tends to elicit reverence, respect, and deep consideration. Today, there is a tendency to define life as sacred and to give the end of life special consideration. The search for meaning and for significance in dying may be inherently a spiritual quest.

NEAR-DEATH EXPERIENCES

Many people who die briefly and are brought back to life, and people who come very close to death without actually dying report a variety of sensations that have been labelled **near-death experiences (NDEs)**. Some of these NDEs include "out-of-body" experiences. Some believe that these experiences are evidence of the soul and life after death. Others assume these experiences are biological and psychological phenomena that have no metaphysical or theological significance. Rodabough and Cole (2003) reviewed the literature on near-death experiences and indicated that reports of NDEs tend to include various combinations of the following: hearing someone pronounce them dead, feelings of peace, having some sort of auditory sensation, travelling through a dark space or tunnel, seeing themselves and others from a place outside of their own bodies, meeting people who have died previously, inter-acting with a being of light, seeing a review of their life, experiencing a line of demarcation (a border or boundary), and coming back into their body and back to life. The authors concluded, "Those who believe in a life after death and those who do not will find nothing in NDE studies to contradict either belief" (146). In other words, the evidence is inconclusive, and belief in the afterlife continues to be a matter of faith.

One of the experiences associated with a NDE is seeing "spirits"—people who have died previously and are usually known to the dying per-son. Betty (2014) discussed these deathbed or near-death visions and noted that, whether real or hallucination, the experience is usually reassuring and comforting for the person who is near death. The terror of death is ab-sent, death is approached with a sense of peace, other people—whether real or imagined—greet and accompany the dying person, and the dying person gains a sense of an afterlife and afterworld. Sociologists often note that whatever is believed to be real, whether it is real or not, is real in its consequences. Near-death experiences are an interesting and consequential phenomenon; however, from an academic point of view their exact nature remains an open question.

RISKING DEATH

Gerald Kent (1996) described himself as "yuppifying rapidly: 33 years old and somewhat paunchy; four young children; a ten-year marriage; a passion for golf and curling; and a busy law practice in Cranbrook, British Colum-bia." He wrote: "I needed a weekend away! The stress and strain of home and practice was calcifying my soul" (81). His solution involved climbing Little Robson, a rock outcropping partway up Mount Robson, the highest peak in the Canadian Rockies. This was his first experience rock climbing.

"After the descent," Kent wrote, "the relief and happiness of being alive flooded my soul and I initially vowed never to return. I would stick to golf and curling and succumb to domestication at home with a thankful heart. Life was too precious to risk" (81). However, a year later he attempted a dangerous solo ascent of Mount Robson. He worried about leaving his children without a father and wondered how to deal with those who would ridicule him for risking his life. So why did he make the climb? He explains that he thought it "a great way to protest our society's obsession with physical health and security and its willingness to wink its eye at everything that is destructive to spirit and soul" (82).

Paradoxically, and metaphorically speaking, the moral of the story is that one can lose one's life while living it and find one's life by risking the loss of it. Kent was engaging in **"edgework"** (Lyng 1990, 2005a). Note that Kent characterizes his quest in spiritual terms, as an activity to free the spirit and to decalcify the soul. The experience is transcendent: the edgeworker transcends his or her own limitations and the petty circumstances of everyday life. Becker (1973) suggested that an awareness of our mortality undermines our sense of heroism, that is, our definition of ourselves

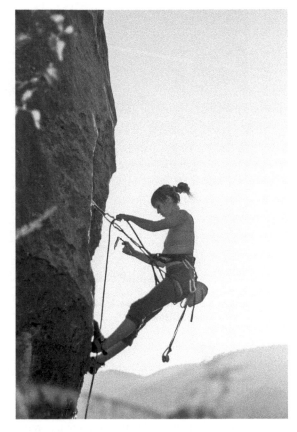

Image 5.2. Doing edgework: Climbing
Source: mmpile/iStock.com.

and our lives as significant. Ironically, in edgework, coming face to face with mortality by purposely risking one's life is a means of achieving heroism and finding significance for one's life.

Edgework is evident in the current trend toward extreme sports, including skydiving, hang gliding, BASE jumping, auto racing, dirt biking, mountain climbing, mountain biking, whitewater kayaking and rafting, cave and deep-water scuba diving, downhill skiing, heli-skiing, ice climbing, and bungee jumping. Edgeworkers acknowledge the risk of dying. Part of that acknowledgment typically involves making the sport as safe as possible— there is no death wish operating here. Edgeworkers want to live—they want to *really* live! They risk death because it makes them feel alive.

Edgework theorists have identified a paradox (Lyng 2005b). On the one hand, edgework is viewed as a way of escaping from and resisting the

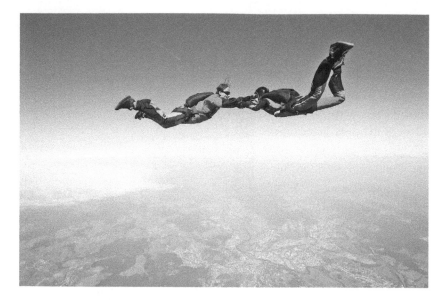

Image 5.3. Doing edgework: Skydiving
Source: vuk8691/iStock.com.

strictures of contemporary society. It is argued that many of these strictures have been designed to promote safety and order, but end up producing alienation, boredom, depression, and malaise. Edgework, then, is an attempt to find excitement and authenticity in an otherwise soul-crushing social context. Edgework is valued because it revitalizes the human spirit that has been deadened by an overly protective and controlling society. On the other hand, it is argued that contemporary society increasingly values risk taking—note the contemporary emphasis on innovative risk taking in business, industry, research, firefighting, and warfare; the emphasis on wealth generation through speculative investment in stocks, bonds, and real estate; the downloading from employers to employees of the risks of funding future retirement; the devolution of the social welfare state; and so on. From this point of view, extreme risk taking reflects the central values of a society that increasingly values and individualizes risk. That is, edgework is emerging from and reinforcing the increasing valuation of individual risk taking as a core social value. In this sense, edgework may also be called "centre work."

BASE jumping (BASE stands for building, antenna, span, earth, which represent four categories of surfaces one can jump from) is a relatively new form of voluntary risk taking (Forsey 2012). While skydiving involves parachuting from an airplane high above the ground, BASE jumping involves parachuting, sometimes illegally, from tall buildings, antennas, bridges, or cliffs. From these limited heights so close to the ground, there is little time or room for error.

Forsey (2012) examined BASE jumping as a social and gendered activity. She noted that BASE jumping involves a mix of efforts to ensure safety while at the same time undertaking extreme risk. She pointed out that this is consistent with core values in contemporary society, values that are particularly expected of men. That is, males are socialized to engage in a variety of risk-taking activities—from firefighting to stock brokering, from soldiering to finding new sources of wealth—and are expected to manage the associated risks. While women are increasingly assuming these risks, Forsey noted that BASE jumping at present is a predominantly male activity.

She commented that "BASE jumpers actively seek risk in order to give meaning to their lives" (99) and in so doing reflect both social and gendered values. Forsey (2012, 100) also noted the irony that while risk taking and risk management are central social values, BASE jumpers develop and practise both on the social periphery. As Lyng (2005b) pointed out, edgework and centre work are not mutually exclusive but instead are compatible and mutually reinforcing. What appear to be highly individual activities and values derive from and reinforce widely shared social activities and values. Forsey (2012, 100) concluded, "Participation in high risk activities such as BASE jumping might therefore be more appropriately understood as an opportunity to learn, practice and perfect the skills necessary for overcoming the insecurities in [contemporary] society." People risk death to both stand out and fit in, and to find self-esteem, identity, meaning, and purpose in life.

Forsey (2012, 101) also pointed out the complexities and contradictions of masculinist prescriptions and proscriptions regarding risk taking and risk management in BASE jumping: "On the one hand, cautious men are celebrated because they avoid injury; however, in some contexts they are feminized and rendered subordinate for expressing fear. Similarly, badass men are revered for the willingness to crowd the edge, but when they go over they are deemed idiots by fellow jumpers." These contradictions echo the larger social world of risk taking and risk management.

CHOOSING DEATH

The affirmation of life through edgework highlights the value of life both for the individual and for others in general. Nevertheless, while some people risk death to affirm their life, some choose death voluntarily and purposely. The choosing of death may suggest that life has no value. Because others tend to think of life as inherently worthwhile, it can be particularly difficult for those who have lost a loved one who has died by suicide to understand and accept the decision of the person who chooses death. Note that death resulting from refusing health care treatment, choosing hospice/palliative care or MAID, or engaging in altruistic behaviour or risk-taking behaviour that results in death are not considered death by suicide (MacNeil 2008).

Why would a person choose death over life? As noted above, dying generally tends to be feared more than death. In death, there is no life, no living, and therefore no pain, suffering, humiliation, and so on. Dying is feared when it involves a life with pain and suffering. In such a situation, the dying may prefer to "get it over with," and death may be viewed as a relief or a blessing.

While dying may involve suffering, living may also involve suffering to the point where life does not seem worth living. Suicidal ideation—that is, thinking about suicide—is common. People who are not otherwise facing death may prefer to actively seek death for a variety of reasons: depression, mental illness, grief, loneliness, unhappiness, chronic illness, pain, guilt, shame, bullying, low self-esteem, or feelings of failure (Kastenbaum 2007, 195–231). Alternatively, death may be chosen to escape social sanctions, such as imprisonment or public humiliation.

It might be expected that the worst circumstances of old age, including sickness, suffering, pain, isolation, loneliness, indignity, loss of control, death of loved ones, societal ageism, a sense of futility, a lack of meaning, and so on, would lead to depression, despair, and suicide (Monette 2012). This may be the case for some very old men but few older women. Figure 5.1 shows that both women and men in Canada in 2014–18 had relatively high rates of death by suicide in the age groups from 45 to 59. However, compared to women in these age groups, men were about three times more likely to die by suicide. In addition, figure 5.1 shows that females from age 70 onward, compared to all other age groups, had relatively low rates of death by suicide. In contrast, males 75 years of age and older had relatively high rates of death by suicide. In summary, these data indicate that middle age is associated with the likelihood of death by suicide for both males and females and, in addition, old age is associated with the likelihood of death by suicide for males. Youths, by comparison, have low suicide rates.

Préville et al. (2005) examined a group of people 60 years of age and older in Quebec who died by suicide and found that, in comparison to a matching control group of elderly people who had died from natural causes, elderly

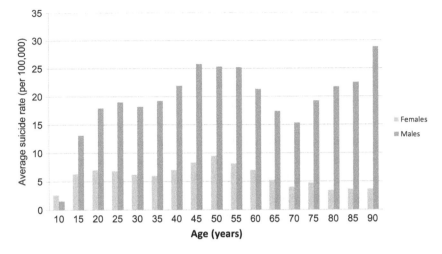

Figure 5.1. Suicide rates in Canada, by sex and age, 2014–2018
Source: Statistics Canada. 2019. Deaths and age-specific mortality rates, by selected grouped causes. Table 13-10-0392-01. Average rates calculated by author (HN).

people who died by suicide were much more likely to have been suffering from psychiatric disorders, particularly depression. It is notable, however, that the people who ended their own lives, compared to those in the control group who did not, did not differ in the number of their chronic physical health problems.

Achille and Ogloff (2003–4) surveyed people in Canada, the United States, and Britain who were dying from ALS about their attitudes toward assisted suicide. The majority (70 per cent) indicated that they felt assisted suicide was morally acceptable, and 60 per cent favoured legalization. Respondents who endorsed assisted suicide emphasized self-determination, dignity, avoiding dependency, and not becoming a burden to others. Respondents who opposed assisted suicide tended to hold a religious perspective. This study also suggested that there is an association between depressive symptoms and the desire for assisted suicide.

Nissim, Gagliese, and Rodin (2009) interviewed people dying of advanced cancer about their desire for a hastened death. Almost all contemplated the option of hastening death hypothetically "as a future exit plan when all other means of controlling the illness had failed, and when they would be in a state of 'lingering' or 'wasting away.' This hypothetical exit plan was generated as a reaction to the multiple fears participants [anticipated] regarding the final active dying phase, including that it would be an undignified and painful process, which would inflict suffering on both patient and family" (168). In addition, these dying cancer patients also reported desiring death during times of severe pain, despair, and demoralization. At these times, desire for a hastened death was temporary; it came and went with the waxing and waning of pain and a sense of despair. Finally, for those who had reached the last weeks or days of their lives and were actively dying, a desire to hasten death acknowledged an acceptance of the inevitability and imminence of death and a letting go in the sense of "capitulation to death and disengagement from life" (169). This is consistent with Kübler-Ross's (1969) last stage of dying that she described as resigned acceptance.

Farand et al. (2004) determined that adolescents involved with the child welfare and juvenile justice systems in Quebec were much more likely than adolescents in general to end their own lives. Factors thought to contribute to an increased risk of adolescent suicide included family disorganization, family violence, physical and sexual abuse, substance abuse, behavioural problems, psychiatric disorders, and intervention by the juvenile justice system or child welfare services (e.g., removal of the adolescent from the family home and placement in a foster home).

A content analysis of Canadian newspaper articles about youth suicide noted that the Canadian media did not report individuals who died by suicide but rather discussed the issue of youth suicide in general terms (Easson et al. 2014). The authors observed that media did not glamorize, sensationalize, or normalize youth suicide but rather emphasized that there is hope and help available for youth contemplating death by suicide. This stance was in contrast to media discussions of suicide for elderly individuals and media reports about the movement to legalize assisted suicide, where the emphasis was often on the importance of the right to choose the circumstances of one's death. Similarly, the terminally ill cancer patients studied by Nissim, Gagliese, and Rodin (2009) wished that assisted suicide would be legalized and made available as an option should their dying become unbearable.

Not all people who attempt to die by suicide or who do die by suicide want to die. For some, suicidal behaviour is a desperate attempt to obtain help. Death by suicide can even be "accidental" (Kastenbaum 2007). Some who did not intend to die may have engaged in behaviour such as the "choking game" (Linkletter, Gordon, and Dooley 2010) or in autoerotic asphyxiation that resulted in death. Others may intend to survive an attempt to die by suicide but miscalculate the lethality of the means employed or may expect to be rescued but are not found in time. Death by suicide may also result from a momentary impulse when, for the most part, the person would prefer living. In summary, while some who end their life suffer chronically and reject a life without quality, others may be more ambivalent about the relative merits of life over death.

Molzahn et al. (2012) reported that people in their study of chronic kidney disease often contemplated ending their own lives. They tended to equate stopping dialysis treatment, which leads to death within a few days, with death by suicide. These researchers pointed out that there are important distinctions between refusing life-sustaining treatment and death by suicide. Semantic distinctions matter when death by suicide is stigmatized.

In the past in many societies, death by suicide has been stigmatized and even criminalized. Some major religions including Christianity, Islam, and Orthodox Judaism have considered suicide to be a sin. Some religions continue to oppose the legalization of assisted suicide. Suicide has been decriminalized in Canada since 1972 and assisted suicide (known more euphemistically as Medical Assistance in Dying, or MAID) has been legal in Canada since 2016. Furthermore, there are ongoing attempts to destigmatize death by suicide, along with attempts to destigmatize mental illness, and psychological and psychosocial distress more generally. Nevertheless, death by suicide has been defined as a public health issue to be prevented and efforts are made to support individuals in distress.

The following story illustrates the movement to destigmatize death by suicide and redefine it as a mental health issue. A middle-aged woman had ended her life. Her funeral service was held in a Christian church. A high-ranking church official spoke. Knowing that some in the congregation would view her death by suicide as an offence to God, he emphasized some of the details of her life that led to her death. He made a passing reference to her experience of childhood abuse. He spoke of her ongoing, unresolved struggle with chronic, clinical depression. And then he very explicitly argued that no one should judge her or blame her and that all should sympathize with her suffering. He noted that her death by suicide should be understood in mental health terms.

Many Indigenous cultures around the world have long accepted death by suicide, assisted suicide, and euthanasia for people in difficult situations such as illness or frailty or in times of famine (de Beauvoir 1973). In Canada, Christian missionaries and the police suppressed these practices as immoral and criminal, especially among the Inuit in Canada's North. It is ironic that MAID, legalized in Canada in 2016, now allows a person to ask for self-administered lethal medications or clinician-administered lethal medications. What was normal for the Inuit years ago was deemed immoral and criminal, and now what was defined as immoral and criminal has been normalized once again. These definitions are contingent, varying from time to time, and from one sociocultural context to another.

There has been concern that media reports of death by suicide, either in the news media or on social media, will lead to imitative ("copycat") suicides and to suicide clusters, even though suicide clusters are relatively uncommon (Haw et al. 2013). When they do occur, suicide clusters typically involve young people under 25 years of age and may be specific to a local community (point clusters) or to a specific geographical location such as a bridge or railway station. There is also some evidence that clusters may appear in elevated rates in a population (mass clusters) following media reports of the death by suicide of a high-profile person (Cox et al. 2012; Haw et al. 2013). For example, the highly publicized accounts on television and in newsprint of the 1999 death by suicide of a popular journalist in Quebec is thought to have had a dramatic effect on suicide rates in that province in the weeks that followed and over the course of the following year (Tousignant et al. 2005).

Accordingly, guidelines have been developed for news media reporting of death by suicide. These guidelines typically include instructions to avoid sensationalizing, glamorizing, or romanticizing death by suicide, to avoid giving the story undue prominence, to avoid providing specific details about the death, and to use the story to educate and provide information about supports for the vulnerable (Pirkis et al. 2006; John et al. 2014). Note that controlling the presentation and discussion of death by suicide on the internet and on social media platforms is much more challenging than controlling reports in news media (Gunn and Lester 2012).

News media occasionally report the occurrence of suicide clusters involving youth in Indigenous communities in Canada. Niezen (2009) lived in the Indigenous reserve community of Cross Lake, Manitoba, in 1998–2000. This community had a population of about 4,500. During that time, there was a cluster of nine deaths by suicide over a six-month period. In addition, there were numerous suicide threats, suicide attempts, and incidents of self-harm. There had been a previous suicide cluster over a six-month period in 1986–87. At that time, there were seven deaths by suicide and many attempted suicides. Suicide of course affects family and friends and the entire community. Consequently, these suicide clusters were devastating for this small community.

Niezen (2009) suggested that explanations for suicide clusters among Indigenous youth include belonging to a group with a shared identity, ideas, values, and outlook on life coupled with a view of life as hopeless and without meaning or purpose; disengagement from community and negation of life and self; a normalization and positive valuation of self-harm and self-destruction as a central value of social life; and ending one's life as a public expression and way to achieve recognition, acceptance, sympathy, notoriety, and love. This youthful malaise, angst, anomie, alienation, and nihilism occurred against the backdrop of, and arose from, colonialism, residential schools, collective trauma, racism, family dysfunction, alcoholism, drug addiction, and abuse. It is important to note that not all Indigenous communities exhibit patterns of suicide clusters. Niezen (2009) reported that there is considerable variation in the occurrence of death by suicide in Indigenous communities.

PREFERRED LOCATION OF DYING AND DEATH

A "good death" has several possible characteristics. As discussed above, most individuals prefer a quick and peaceful death. Dying individuals may also want to be conscious, informed, and free to openly express themselves and to exercise some control by participating in all decision-making processes. Finally, a good death may be seen as one that takes place at home, where one's surroundings are familiar, comfortable, and meaningful and where family and friends can freely congregate (Leming and Dickinson 2016). Such deathbed ideals were firmly enshrined in pre-twentieth-century literature and art (Ariès 1974, 1981). However, as discussed in chapter 2, during the course of the twentieth century the rise and successes of modern health care resulted in dying and death being moved from the home to the hospital (Ariès 1974, 1981). In the later twentieth century, the hospital was perceived as a good place to be saved from death but not as a good place to die. The health care community itself has also increasingly questioned the appropriateness of the acute care hospital for the dying. Furthermore, those witnessing dying in the hospital have tended to characterize a hospital death in negative terms, using adjectives such as cold, technological, antiseptic, and impersonal.

By the late twentieth century and now into the early twenty-first century, the preferences of the dying and their caregivers are resulting in dying being returned to the home, perhaps with palliative home care, and to more home-like institutional environments such as freestanding hospices (Kastenbaum

2007). Hospice/palliative care, which administers to the family and to the dying person's physical, emotional, psychological, spiritual, and social needs (Novak, Northcott, and Kobayashi 2021), is increasingly preferred over futile attempts to maintain life. Dying persons are typically more interested in comfort, dignity, and social support than they are in prolonging their life when prolongation means additional suffering, indignity, and impersonal care.

The National Film Board of Canada (NFB) documented the work of one of the first palliative care units (PCUs) in Canada, established in 1975 at the Royal Victoria Hospital in Montreal. This unit was opened specifically to treat the terminally ill, a new care concept at that time. Another PCU was opened around the same time at the St. Boniface Hospital in Winnipeg, Manitoba, and additional ones, as well as free-standing hospices, have been established since that time across Canada. PCUs and hospices serve not only the dying person but assist the grieving and bereaved family as well.

The NFB documentary was titled *The Last Days of Living* (Gilson 1980) and featured several PCU clients who were dying from cancer, including elderly and middle-aged men and women as well as a man in his early twenties. The filmmakers showed the needs of the dying and caregiver responses to those needs. The clients' responses to their terminal illnesses ranged from angry questioning and discouragement to philosophical acceptance. A middle-aged woman who had a mastectomy could not fully accept what had happened to her: "It is just not right," she says. One elderly man declined an invitation to go out on the patio on a sunny day. He said that it held no interest for him and that it would not do him any good. Another elderly man said that he felt lousy and complained that he could not even change his position in bed half an inch: "You ask for death," he says. A young man decided to forego further treatment in hospital and go home to die. He talked matter-of-factly about his impending death, observing that he finds it easier now that he knows he will die in comparison to the "roller coaster" phase when he and his family lived with uncertainty and vacillated between hope and despair: "We are all going to die," he says, and it is only the how and the when that differ. As he expressed it, "there is no right age to die; any age is the right age." His parents observed that his dying had scared his friends away—they had stopped visiting. The documentary showed the young man and his parents sharing meaningful times together until his death at home.

The Last Days of Living had two central messages. The first is that death comes to us all and comes in its own time—it can come early in life, in middle age, or in later life. The prominence in the documentary of the young man who died at home emphasizes the capriciousness of the timing of death and highlights the vulnerability of people of any age. Furthermore, this young man's story suggested that dying at home can be a positive experience for all involved. This is the second central message of this documentary—it was an attempt to describe the good death or at least a better death. Dying with the assistance of hospice/palliative care, whether in a hospital PCU, hospice, or at home, was implicitly contrasted with dying in the hospital's intensive care unit while enduring heroic attempts to prolong life. Although this contrast was not made explicit, it was shown that hospice/palliative care can make dying less painful and less lonely, thus helping the dying achieve a better death.

Wilson, Birch, et al. (2013) found in a survey of Albertans that 71 per cent of respondents preferred to die at home and another 15 per cent preferred to die in a hospice/palliative care facility. Only 7 per cent indicated a preference for dying in hospital, 2 per cent in a nursing home, while 6 per cent did not have a preference. However, dying at home requires adequate support from family members who are able and willing to serve as caregivers. Stajduhar et al. (2008) asked seriously ill patients in five hospitals across Canada together with their family caregivers about their preferences for location of death. Just over half of the patients (54 per cent) and half of their family caregivers (50 per cent) preferred death at home. Yet only half of the patients and their family caregivers agreed on the preferred location of death, whether in home or in hospital.

A study of people dying of severe chronic obstructive pulmonary disease in Montreal noted that they preferred to die in hospital, where they felt they would receive the care they required to prevent excessive suffering and where they would not be a burden on their family (Hall, Legault, and Côté 2010). Campbell (2013) pointed out that the preferred place to die depends on the circumstances, including the kind of caregiving required, the availability of caregivers, the intensity of required care, the length of time that care is required, and the costs involved. In a hypothetical and ideal world, people prefer to die at home cared for by loving and competent family members; in the real world, people assess their circumstances and decide where death will be most appropriate. And in the real world, family caregivers and dying family members will not always agree on the best place to die. Dying people also may have no family members, or they may not have family caregivers who are available and willing to provide care.

Topf, Robinson, and Bottorff (2013) interviewed family caregivers in Western Canada who had promised to care for a dying family member at home but were unable to keep their promise. While the family caregivers were committed to keeping their promise in principle, the caregivers found themselves unprepared, overwhelmed, and unable to access sufficient additional support and the necessary resources. As a result, dying persons were moved to a hospital or hospice. While death in the hospital or hospice was described as peaceful, the family caregivers reported feeling regret, guilt, and a sense of failure for being unable to keep their promise that death would occur at home.

In contrast, Robinson et al. (2017) interviewed family caregivers in British Columbia who were able to facilitate a family member's death from cancer at home. Several factors enabled their commitment to providing dying family members with the death they desired at home. Despite the challenges of providing ongoing care, their determination to provide a home death was enabled by their willingness to ask for help, considerable assistance from formal hospice/palliative care professionals, assistance and respite provided by other family members and friends, and a fierce determination to make the health care system work for the dying person at home. Virtually all said that they would do it again (with just one exception out of 29 family caregivers).

LIVING WITH DYING

Two documentaries from the National Film Board of Canada show that living with dying can be a long process with both positive and negative aspects. In the documentary *Living with Dying* (Dolgoy 1991), the audience is introduced to Albert and Margaret Kerestes. Albert Kerestes was in his early sixties when told by a cancer specialist that he was terminally ill and had only weeks or perhaps months to live. Kerestes said that it was difficult to learn that he had only a couple of months of life left. He noted that, initially, he was emotionally upset, but he "got over it." Despite his acceptance, this was a difficult time for him and his wife. Their calendar was full of appointments at the cancer clinic, at the hospital, and with doctors. These appointments and treatment regimens took control of their lives. They were glad when this phase came to an end and they were able to stay home and regain some control over their own lives. Their home care nurse emphasized the importance of people having a sense of personal control in such situations.

Albert Kerestes's dying trajectory did not go as expected: his cancer went into remission. Although he still suffered many limitations and his prognosis was still terminal, he was now living longer with dying, and the time of his dying was no longer predictable. The home care nurse began to describe him as a chronic palliative care client. Her initial focus had been on managing pain and symptoms and providing needed physical aids like a wheelchair. During his long remission, she shifted her focus from active care to surveillance.

Albert Kerestes benefited from the care he received. At home he benefited, in particular, from the care of his wife and from the visits of the home care nurse. The local pharmacist helped with Blue Cross to facilitate payments for medications. Other supports came from the Kerestes's extended family (grown children, grandchildren, siblings), friends and neighbours, church officials and fellow parishioners, and a move to a government-subsidized senior citizen apartment that charged a fixed percentage of the Kerestes's income for rent and was at ground level with no stairs to negotiate. Family and social gatherings and activities were frequent and enjoyable. The Kerestes indicated that they never felt alone.

In short, Albert Kerestes had expected to die, and the remission of his cancer was unanticipated. He subsequently lived for years following his original diagnosis. His home care nurse said in the documentary that he wanted to live, and that his wife and family wanted him to live. She noted that he defied the experts and stayed alive because he was a fighter.

This reference to the will to live is common in discussions about dying, reflecting a widespread belief that people have some control over the course of their dying and can will themselves to live or alternatively to die. There is some risk in making this assertion. For example, those who live tend to be congratulated for being fighters and for their strong will to live, while those who die may be blamed for giving up or for lacking in willpower. Both congratulation and blame may be misplaced, and both demonstrate our tendency to psychologize death—that is, to overemphasize the power of psychological processes and to underemphasize the power of biological processes. In the case of Albert Kerestes, other considerations besides willpower—social supports, medical treatments and other health care, divine intervention, or the capriciousness of the disease—could be credited with prolonging his life. The reasons for the remission of Kerestes's cancer are not a particular concern of the filmmakers. Rather, the documentary shows that, while living with cancer and a terminal diagnosis brings pain and sorrow, living with dying can also have many meaningful and pleasurable moments.

Another NFB documentary, *My Healing Journey: Seven Years with Cancer* (Viszmeg 1998), reinforces this point. Joe Viszmeg was in his mid-thirties when he was diagnosed with cancer and told that he would likely die within a year. Seven years later he wrote, directed, and edited a documentary describing his experience. The documentary shows him in 1991, a filmmaker and single parent raising a daughter, newly diagnosed with terminal cancer. Saying that his first reaction was disbelief, he speaks of feeling cheated because of the anticipated shortness of his life. He tells his daughter that he has a tumour but does not mention cancer. A risky surgery goes well and a large tumour is removed. A year later Viszmeg marries, and the year after that he and his wife, Rachel, become parents to a baby boy.

Following his initial diagnosis and surgery, Viszmeg speaks of the many things he tried in an attempt to promote his health—Indigenous healing practices, spirituality, macrobiotics, transcendental meditation, yoga, and shark cartilage. Nevertheless, many tumours grew back, and by 1993 he once again expected that he did not have long to live. He treated his extra time as a gift and concentrated on the moment. The new baby, in particular, brought much joy.

Then, unexpectedly, the cancer went into remission, which lasted for several years. In 1997, Viszmeg had surgery again and almost died. His recovery was slow, and he wondered how much time the surgery had bought. Acknowledging these difficulties, he said that sometimes he thought that it would have been better to do nothing.

Finally, Viszmeg tried the chemotherapy treatment that he had previously resisted because of its harsh side effects. At that point, he knew there was almost no chance of a cure, but he hoped for relief from his constant pain. Initially his newly diagnosed cancer had seemed like a novelty; seven years later, it had become "a drag." He said he was bored with it, bored with the pain and nausea and weakness. He wanted the cancer to end. This did not mean that he wanted his life to end—he liked his life and wanted more, he just wanted the cancer to end. At the end of the documentary, Viszmeg spoke of the importance of loving and of the wonderful events and people in his life. He died the following year, in 1999.

The stories of Albert Kerestes and Joe Viszmeg emphasize that living and dying are not mutually exclusive. A person can have a meaningful life while dying. Sometimes death comes quickly following a terminal diagnosis; however, many with terminal illnesses spend years of meaningful life with family before their death. Joe Viszmeg saw his daughter grow up. He remarried and had a baby, and he enjoyed good times with his wife and children before his death. Similarly, Nissim et al. (2012) found that people experiencing prolonged dying from advanced terminal cancer set goals to live as long, well,

and meaningfully as possible while dying. These dying individuals emphasized maximizing the quality of their remaining time, valuing their present
life, and leaving a legacy.

PREPARING FOR DEATH

In the year before her death in 2014, the first author's mother had an accidental
fall and was hospitalized. I had been designated as a contact person, and soon
after her hospitalization I received a call from the hospital. Did my mother
have an advance directive indicating her end-of-life care preferences? Had
she designated someone to make health care decisions for her if she could not
do so for herself? No, I said. The person on the phone then told me that we
"should" get formal documents drawn up. I was irritated by the prescriptive
and pushy verb "should." I thought my mother might live for years yet—
certainly that was her plan. My mother had indicated in many conversations
that she wanted to stay alive as long as possible and did not want to give up on
life or have her death hastened. So, I did not see the need for creating formal
documentation to facilitate the decision making that the person on the phone
anticipated regarding the end of her life. I ignored her advice. One of my
brothers, however, did not. He took our mother to a lawyer, and together they
drew up papers indicating her preferences for end-of-life care and designating
who her decision makers would be in the circumstance that she was unable
to make her own decisions. Formally, these constituted a personal directive
and an enduring power of attorney. To my surprise, my mother indicated in
her personal directive that she did not want us to subject her to aggressive
health care if that care was deemed futile. Less than eight months later, after a
series of small strokes, Mom was confused and aphasic (she could not put her
thoughts into words). A declaration of incapacity to make decisions about a
personal matter was enacted. Four months later, her family and physician consulted her personal directive and her enduring power of attorney and made the
decision she had asked us to make: to allow her to die without futile treatments
having been used. Her physician and a family member she had designated as
her decision maker stood by her hospital bed and decided to designate her care
as terminal palliative care. Her death occurred three days later.

This experience was highly instructive. I now believe it is important
for each of us to prepare in advance for death. We "should" create formal
documentation, including a will, personal directive, and power of attorney

(Howlett et al. 2010). I know I should, though I haven't yet. I will . . . someday. I am not quite sure why I keep putting it off; I suppose I want to believe that I have lots of time left.

EXPERIENCING END-OF-LIFE CARE: THE PERCEPTIONS OF DYING INDIVIDUALS AND THEIR FAMILY MEMBERS

A lawyer told this story. She said that a client's wife called her. Three years earlier, the lawyer had done the client's will. The wife reminded the lawyer that they "knew then [three years ago] that he was dying." Three years later the client's wife admitted, "I didn't know dying was so messy. I thought you just closed your eyes and kind of went to sleep. But dying has been kind of gruesome." She mentioned that her husband had had his leg amputated, was on dialysis, got a staph infection that almost killed him, but still "hung on long past how long people thought would be possible in his circumstances." The wife told the lawyer that even though doctors told her that her husband was no longer capable of making decisions, she did not want to be the one to make decisions that would end his life. So, she asked her husband if he wanted to stop dialysis. He said that he had been thinking about it. She took this as a lucid moment and as a "yes" and stopped treatment. He was expected to die within the week. The wife added that she was also caring for her husband's father and mother. Her father-in-law had early signs of dementia, was legally blind, legally deaf, and, she added, legally stubborn. Her mother-in-law had advanced Alzheimer's disease, wore adult diapers for incontinence, fell a couple of months ago and broke her pelvis, and was now in a care facility. The woman said that she "felt like she has been caring for three 3-year-olds." She was very emotional as she described her situation to the lawyer.

Stories like this provide a point of view that can be missing in textbook generalizations and academic discussions that distance us from the real world of real people and their "messy" stories. Narratives like this recall the title of an article by Evans et al. (1989): "The Long Good-Bye." The point is that death is seldom quick these days. For most, the process of dying takes many months and often years. And it is often "messy."

There is a widespread perception that the dying often do not get the deaths they prefer. For example, a person may wish to die at home surrounded by loving and caring family members but instead dies in the hospital or nursing home. The dying may wish to remain in control of decision making regarding their care but instead lose control to health care professionals and health care institutions and die while enduring unnecessary, futile, and unwanted medical intervention. These scenarios are critical of the medicalization and institutionalization of dying and death and express widely shared fears about how each of us might die. Nevertheless, what do the dying and their family caregivers say about their actual experiences of dying in Canada in the early twenty-first century?

Although the usual argument is that health care workers and health care institutions can frustrate the dying person's wish for a "good" death, in some cases family members frustrate the health care professionals' efforts to achieve a good death for their patients. Tan and Manca (2013) interviewed family physicians in Edmonton about conflicts they had experienced during discussions with family decision makers about end-of-life care for dying patients. The authors noted that the physicians desired a good death for their patients. They noted that it was important for family physicians (and other health care workers) and family decision makers to find "common ground" to make decisions about end-of-life care to achieve a good death and to avoid conflict that might result in poor care decisions and a bad death. Tan and Manca (2013) described finding common ground as a three-step process involving building mutual trust and rapport, understanding each other, and making informed and shared decisions. Failure to find common ground could result in mistrust, miscommunication, frustration, and conflict. Sources of difficulty included family members' denial of the impending death, unrealistic expectations for a cure, and a lack of advance planning by the patient and family for the death. The authors noted that it takes time for family members to come to terms with the impending death but that the dying process may not allow sufficient time to do so and frustrates efforts to find common ground.

Stajduhar et al. (2011) interviewed family members who had recently experienced the end-of-life care and death of a family member in institutional health care settings in Western Canada. The authors asked the family members about their experiences and assessments of the end-of-life care. The family members appreciated timely diagnoses, effective symptom management, caring and competent staff, psychosocial and emotional support for their dying family member, and were impressed when staff made exceptions to meet the particular needs of the dying patient. Family members noted the importance of being kept informed. Complaints focused on occasional instances of poor communication or conflicting information from different personnel or an abrasive or impatient staff member. Family members valued clean and quiet accommodations, privacy, and pleasant roommates. Complaints mentioned situations involving a lack of privacy and dignity. Family members appreciated being able to leave their dying family members in the institution and feeling that they were in good hands. When family members did not have this feeling, they were reluctant to leave and experienced increased frustration, anxiety, guilt, anger, and dissatisfaction.

Thompson et al. (2008) conducted focus groups with bereaved family members who were more satisfied or less satisfied with the end-of-life care that their dying family members had received in nursing homes in Central Canada. The authors noted that participants who were less satisfied "described experiences that clearly demonstrated staff members' failure to recognize and acknowledge that the resident was entering the terminal phase of life" (40). This undermined family members' confidence in the nursing home staff and resulted in perceptions of inadequate treatment, including ineffective pain management. In contrast, "those who had been satisfied with care felt that staff members not only acknowledged that the resident was dying and thus the plan of care was altered, but that they also engaged family members in discussions on what to expect at the end of life" (40). This allowed family members to discuss the residents' preferences for their end-of-life care. A common complaint was that communication with the nursing home physician was limited and inadequate, and that decisions about the care of the dying family member were not always communicated consistently among all levels of staff and between staff working on different shifts. Dissatisfied family members "expressed a strong sense of regret, anger, and frustration over the care their relative had received in the last month of life. Family members felt that they had let the resident down by not facilitating the kind of death the resident would have wanted. Often, this meant feeling that the resident had not achieved a good death" (41). Nevertheless, it is notable that satisfied family members far outnumbered the dissatisfied.

Brazil et al. (2012) surveyed family caregivers of deceased family members who had been designated as palliative care patients and had received formal home care services in Ontario. The focus of this study was on family members' assessments of patient-centred end-of-life care. This patient-centred model of care emphasizes a partnership among the patient, their health care practitioners, and their family members. The family caregivers in this survey had used a variety of formal services during their family member's last month of life including home nursing care, contact with family physicians, and personal care workers assisting in the home. Most family caregivers indicated that they knew what services to contact and that care was accessible and effective. Nevertheless, some reported difficulties getting help when needed, though most family caregivers positively assessed the help they received. In this model of care, the patient and family members who care for the dying person are central, and formal health care services are mobilized to support the dying person and their family in caring for the dying person at home.

Similarly, a survey of bereaved family members in British Columbia asked about the care their deceased family members had received in institutional care facilities during the last 48 hours of life (Gallagher and Krawczyk 2013). Overall, family members were mainly positive in their ratings of the care their loved one received immediately preceding death; only one in six indicated that they were not satisfied. The great majority (90 per cent) said that doctors, nurses, and other health care staff respected patient wishes, and 88 per cent said that symptoms were controlled adequately. While some family members identified specific shortcomings—for example, some would have preferred better communication and more information—the overall picture was one of general satisfaction.

Another survey contacted bereaved family members about the end-of-life care their loved ones had received in a major Canadian hospital during the month before their deaths (Sadler et al. 2014). The survey found that two in every three family members were very satisfied or completely satisfied with the care their family members had received. Nevertheless, while almost half of all deaths had occurred in the intensive care unit, family members of half of these patients believed that their family members would have preferred to die elsewhere. Family members who believed that their loved ones died where they preferred to die were more likely to be satisfied with the care that their family members had received.

Widger and Picot (2008) contacted parents whose babies or young children had died in a major health centre in Eastern Canada. The authors wrote that 85 per cent of parents "reported being very satisfied with the care provided by the health center. . . . However, nearly all parents also described specific incidents in great detail that had a negative impact on their experience. These incidents related to miscommunication or interactions with particular health professionals who were described as abrupt or unfeeling or who did not listen to concerns raised by parents" (56).

Sankaran, Hedin, and Hodgson-Viden (2016) interviewed parents in Saskatchewan whose babies had died shortly after birth. The babies had a gestational age at birth of 22 to 41 weeks and were born with severe health conditions incompatible with survival. End-of-life decision making, in particular the decision to initiate palliative care, involved several conversations between health care staff and parents. First Nations and Catholic parents required more consultation, and First Nations parents required more time to decide. Most parents (90 per cent) were satisfied with the decision-making process and two-thirds returned to the hospital to bring thank-you cards and gifts for the staff. Parents said that they appreciated having a quiet, private space in the hospital to grieve and being able to hold their baby when it died.

Caron, Griffith, and Arcand (2005) interviewed family caregivers who were helping care for family members who had late-stage dementia and had been placed in a nursing home. A frequent complaint concerned the limited interaction and communication about end-of-life care decision making between the family caregiver and the health care workers in these long-term care facilities. Family caregivers indicated the importance of being able to trust the health care staff. The authors noted that trust could be pre-existing and blind or acquired over time. The authors wrote: "A number of elements facilitate establishing trust: (a) regular contact with the family, (b) providing pertinent information on the progression of the disease as well as on treatments to control symptoms, (c) advising families of changes in the loved one's condition, (d) establishing a personalized approach, and (e) considering the family as a partner in the care of the patient" (242).

Heyland et al. (2009) interviewed terminally ill patients and their family caregivers in Kingston, Ontario. The authors found that, out of a maximum possible score of 100, the average satisfaction with care score was 69 (scores ranged from 25 to 99) for patients and 62 (ranging from 25 to 95) for caregivers. The authors re-interviewed the patients and caregivers every two months during the dying process for up to a total of four interviews. They determined that satisfaction scores for both groups tended to be stable or increase over time. Patients interviewed at home tended to report higher satisfaction than patients interviewed in hospital or long-term care. There was some indication that patients tended to feel more socially isolated as they approached death and that family caregivers found meaning and purpose in caring for their dying family members. Nevertheless, family caregivers tended to experience a letdown after the death of their family member, leading to existential and spiritual concerns for some.

Several authors have noted the importance of considering the needs of specific populations; for example, veterans dying in veterans' health care facilities (Gibson and Gorman 2010), African Canadians in Nova Scotia (Maddalena et al. 2013), and the families of children who have a progressive neurodegenerative illness (Rallison and Raffin-Bouchal 2012). The African-Canadian community emphasizes caring for a dying family member at home; however, Maddalena et al. (2013) noted that they often had limited knowledge of the services available to help them care for a dying person at home. Rallison and Raffin-Bouchal (2012) observed that progressive neuro-degenerative illnesses sometimes unfold over years in a child's life before resulting in death and, accordingly, require that palliative care be not only adapted for children but also be designed as a long-term strategy instead of a fairly short end-of-life initiative.

Researchers have explored patients' experiences with chronic and life-threatening illnesses such as kidney disease (Molzahn et al. 2019; Sheilds et al. 2015; Schick-Makaroff, Sheilds, and Molzahn 2013; Molzahn, Bruce, and Sheilds 2008), heart failure (Molzahn et al. 2020), and cancer and HIV/AIDS (Sheilds et al. 2015). This interrelated set of studies focused on the unpredictability of the illness trajectories associated with these illnesses. This unpredictability led to a sense of uncertainty. Uncertainty tended to bring doubt and a "delicate balance between *a focus on living their lives and an awareness of death*" (Sheilds et al. 2015, 210, italics in the original). In this context of uncertainty, some patients and their family members found it difficult to discuss the possibility and eventuality of dying and death. Indeed, some things remained unsaid or "unsayable" (Schick-Makaroff, Sheilds, and Molzahn 2013). Patients and their family members typically "wanted frank, open conversations with their healthcare providers that both acknowledged that they were at end of life but did not remove all hope" (Molzahn et al. 2020, 1). Nevertheless, Nouvet et al. (2016) reported that physicians and nurses in Canadian hospitals generally delayed having conversations about dying and death until death was imminent. Reasons for this delay included discomfort discussing dying and death, the unpredictability and uncertainty of the timing of death, professional ethics, along with patient and family expectations that efforts be made to extend life as long as possible, and a death-denying culture both in the hospital and in the broader society.

Molzahn, Bruce, and Sheilds (2008) noted that patients facing the uncertainty of life-threatening illnesses were "liminal," as they experienced ambiguity and paradox. For example, they were caught between the possibility of dying and the promise that treatment would preserve life, the experience of living while dying, and the "fine line between living and not living" (16).

They felt simultaneously independent and at the same time constrained by their illness and treatment. They struggled to maintain a normal life while dealing with disease and treatment that were not normal. Some observed that they were both worse off and better off, finding both good and bad in their present circumstances. Patients spoke of feeling alone with their illness while also feeling supported by family members and health care providers.

The COVID-19 pandemic that started in late 2019 and quickly spread around the world created an unusual experience for the dying, their caregivers, and their family members. The first confirmed case appeared in Canada in mid-January of 2020. It soon became apparent that not everyone who contracted the virus showed symptoms, not everyone who had symptoms was admitted to hospital, not everyone who was admitted to hospital was treated in the Intensive Care Unit (ICU), and not everyone who went to hospital or the ICU died—although many did. These statistics allowed many people, especially younger ones, to feel that they were unlikely to get sick or to die.

Canada was relatively successful in "flattening the curve," that is, in reducing the spread of the infection, through social isolation at home; social distancing when in public and the wearing of masks in public spaces; and the temporary closing of public venues such as schools and universities, restaurants and bars, sport and concert venues, airports, and cruise ships. Plexiglass barriers were installed in many places of business such as stores and banks to separate the public from the staff. Curbside pickup of groceries and deliveries from stores to homes increased. A search for vaccines involved medical science laboratories around the world.

Despite these measures, however, by 28 June 2020 over 8,500 Canadians had died from COVID-19 (Government of Canada 2020c; Estabrooks et al. 2020). Many of these deaths were frail older people residing in long-term care facilities (81 per cent). Of all reported deaths, 72 per cent comprised persons 80 years of age and older, and another 25 per cent were persons 60 to 79 years of age. Only 3 per cent of reported deaths were among people under 60 years of age. Females comprised over half of the deaths (54.3 per cent), reflecting the larger number of women in older age groups.

The COVID-19 pandemic changed the usual experience of dying in Canada. Many of those who were infected were in nursing homes, which were closed to visitors as the pandemic spread. Interactions between family members and residents was limited to phone conversations and visual contact through closed windows. Moreover, many of those who died were isolated in nursing homes or hospital ICUs, largely without family contact. The ideals of family coming together and providing support to their loved one and mutual support for each other at the end of a loved one's life were frustrated. It is thought that deaths like these heighten the various emotions that are associated with death and loss, including distress, anger, grief, and regret.

Assessing satisfaction with health care and assessing the quality of care received is a complicated endeavour (Northcott and Harvey 2012). Many studies have shown that, in general, ratings of health care tend to be very positive. Nevertheless, when asked about specific aspects of health care, respondents often identify shortcomings and room for improvement (Funk et al. 2012). The studies reviewed above reflect this general pattern. When asked about the end-of-life care that loved ones have received, family members tend to be positive in their assessments, although when given the opportunity to comment on specific aspects of care or on things that might be improved, they often voice criticisms and make suggestions for improvement. Nevertheless, the overall impression arising from studies of end-of-life care in Canada is that the family members of those who have died generally rate the quality of care and satisfaction with care in positive terms.

Most studies assessing end-of-life care do so from the points of view of family members and family caregivers or from the vantage point of professional health care workers. Researchers rarely ask the dying themselves to comment on the care they are receiving or wish to receive. Physicians, hospitals, and nursing homes, for example, tend to be reluctant to refer dying people to researchers, and research ethics boards tend to be reluctant to approve research that involves asking dying people to comment on their experiences with the dying process and with end-of-life care. This reluctance shows how we continue to dance around dying and death. Nevertheless, when given the opportunity, dying persons are generally quite willing and open about expressing their points of view (Clarke, Korotchenko, and Bundon 2012). Consequently, we need more research that gives voice to the dying themselves instead of proxy voices that speak for the dying or the dead.

MEDICAL ASSISTANCE IN DYING

The Government of Canada legalized Medical Assistance in Dying in June of 2016. Four interim reports covered the adoption of MAID during the first 28 months following its implementation, from June 2016 to October 2018

(Health Canada 2019). A new reporting system was designed subsequently, with a first report in July 2020 (Health Canada 2020).

During the period from June 2016 to December 2019, almost 14,000 persons died by MAID—2 per cent of all deaths in Canada in 2019 (Health Canada 2020). Almost all who were approved for and utilized MAID chose clinician-administered death. This meant that a physician (94 per cent) or nurse practitioner (6 per cent) administered a drug cocktail to cause death at the request of the patient. Only six deaths involved self-administered medications. Canada jumped to the forefront of the Right to Die/Death with Dignity movement by legalizing both self-administered and clinician-administered death.

Most MAID deaths in Canada from June 2016 to December 2019 took place either in hospital (36 per cent) or in the person's home (35 per cent). The average age of persons receiving MAID was 75 years and most (80 per cent) were 65 years of age or older. Males and females were equally likely to choose MAID. They were suffering from cancer (67 per cent), circulatory or respiratory diseases (21 per cent), or neurodegenerative diseases such as ALS (10 per cent).

Holmes et al. (2018) interviewed family and friends who supported a loved one who had chosen MAID in Vancouver in 2016. While some were initially opposed or conflicted about their loved one's decision to utilize MAID, all of the persons interviewed were supportive of their loved one's decision at the end. Because the timing of death was known in advance, the participants in this study said they valued the time spent with their loved one and the opportunity to say goodbye. They felt that MAID provided a more peaceful death than their loved one would have had otherwise. Andriessen et al. (2019) reviewed similar studies in Switzerland, the US, and the Netherlands. They concluded that a loved one's decision to die by legal euthanasia or assisted suicide did not increase the likelihood of adverse grief or mental health problems for the bereaved.

Beuthin et al. (2020) interviewed physicians in British Columbia about their experiences providing MAID during the first two years following its implementation in Canada. The physicians spoke about the satisfaction they received from providing compassionate care to dying patients and their families. They also spoke of certain risks and challenges including concerns about stigma; fear of reprisals; disagreements with colleagues, family, and friends; and concerns about workload, paperwork, and legalities. The physicians "shared stories that conveyed how the rewards of the practice outweighed the risks and burdens . . . in a way that was unexpectedly satisfying and meaningful, both professionally and personally" (7–8).

Beuthin, Bruce, and Scaia (2018) interviewed nurses in British Columbia about their experiences with MAID during the first six months following its implementation. Some nurses were unable to reconcile participating in MAID with their ethical, religious, and/or professional values, and they expressed concern that they might face professional sanctions (criticism, bullying, pressure, accusations of violating duty to care norms, etc.) for their moral distress and conscientious objections. Most nurses interviewed, however, were able to reconcile MAID with their professional and personal values. The authors concluded that "most nurses perceived assisted dying as an extension of their professional role of providing holistic care without judgment, advocating for patient choice, and supporting a new option for a good death" (519).

Some physicians and nurses prefer other strategies than MAID for end-of-life care. They may do this for reasons of conscience (ethical and/or religious objections to MAID) and/or for practical reasons. The following story told by a physician makes this point.

> I work mainly as a hospitalist—that is, I direct the care of hospitalized patients. Many of these patients are very sick, some die. The following story illustrates the difference between MAID (Medical Assistance in Dying) and palliative care.
>
> A while ago, as I took over the service's patient load, I noticed that one man in his mid-seventies had advanced, severe, terminal respiratory illness, but was still being treated very aggressively. I wondered if this was appropriate—if it was what the patient wanted. A few hours later I was called STAT to the ward. The patient had gone outside for a smoke but failed to turn off his oxygen and blew himself up. He had extensive second degree burns to his face, and there were obvious burns in his upper airway. This was very bad news. I knew that there was a high likelihood that he would develop respiratory distress and require ventilation. With his already advanced lung disease, I knew he would not survive. He was conscious and able to respond, so I asked him, "Were you trying to kill yourself, or was this just a mistake?" His brothers, who were gathered around the bed, chuckled a bit. He sheepishly confessed that this was just a stupid mistake, then added, "but I want you to kill me."
>
> "I don't do that," I replied, "but I can refer you to someone who will. But let me tell you about the process. First, you will require two doctors

to examine you and determine that you are suffering from a disease that will likely kill you within six months. Then a psychiatric evaluation will be required to ensure that you are of sound mind. Then the application will be reviewed by an ethics committee. If they approve, there will be a waiting period in case you change your mind. The process takes at least two weeks, and up to four. You don't have two weeks."

"So, what can I do?" he asked.

"I can offer you palliative care."

"What's the difference?"

"In palliative care, we withdraw all the treatments that are keeping you alive and treat to relieve pain and suffering. We can give you medications that will make you comfortable and take away your air hunger as your lungs fail. The medications are not given to purposefully end your life, but to give you comfort as your life ends due to your disease. We have palliative protocols in place. We do not need two physicians or a psychiatric evaluation. There is no need for an ethics committee review, and we can start today if you wish."

"OK. Let's do that!"

I turned to his brothers, "Do you all understand?"

"Yes."

"Do you all agree?"

"Yes," they responded, some with a few tears in their eyes. "It's what he wants."

So, I stopped all his medications and started him on hydromorphone and midazolam. He died peacefully about 30 hours later, with his family gathered around him.

One of the arguments that led to the adoption of MAID in Canada was that options of withdrawing and withholding care and/or offering palliative care do not always relieve suffering. MAID gave those patients who were enduring suffering an option. However, the bureaucratic restrictions and safeguards put in place to prevent abuse mean that MAID is not easily or quickly accessed, and it is not available to all. As the physician in the story above points out, in some circumstances hospice/palliative care is more accessible than MAID, and it is a practical, effective, and humane solution to suffering and end-of-life care. Furthermore, the physician makes a distinction between helping a patient to die and causing a patient's death. This distinction is important to health care providers who are uncomfortable with death hastening, but who still wish to provide their patients with a good death, or at least as good a death as possible under the circumstances.

Note that the physician in this story is an effective communicator. He is clear and concise in describing options, makes sure all involved in the decision understand the options, encourages the patient and family members to decide together, and ascertains that all agree with the implementation of the patient's decision.

To qualify for MAID in Canada under the original guidelines, a person had to be an adult 18 years of age or older whose death was reasonably foreseeable, who was suffering and wished to die, and who was able to give consent at the time of death. This meant that persons with advanced dementia, for example, who can no longer give consent, were ineligible, even if they had previously written an advance directive approving MAID. Further, mature minors under 18 years of age were excluded, as were persons who were suffering but not dying, for example, those with chronic mental illness or painful but non-terminal conditions.

The Department of Justice Canada (2020) reported in early 2020 that there had been extensive consultations about MAID with "experts, practitioners, stakeholders, Indigenous groups, provinces and territories, and an online questionnaire that received over 300,000 responses" (see also Department of Justice Canada 2021a, 2021b). Based on these consultations, the Government of Canada in 2020 began considering extending eligibility for MAID to allow persons who had previously given consent, but who could no longer do so, to receive MAID through a "waiver of final consent." This would reduce pressure on individuals to choose MAID prematurely fearing they might lose capacity to consent if they waited too long. The Government of Canada also planned to remove the requirement that a person's death be "reasonably foreseeable." Other issues under consideration included the eligibility for MAID for persons with mental illness and mature minors. In March of 2021 (Government of Canada 2021; Department of Justice Canada 2021a, 2021b), legislation was passed to remove the requirement that death be reasonably foreseeable and to allow for a waiver of final consent for persons who had consented previously for MAID but had subsequently lost the capacity to consent. Finally, the Government of Canada announced that persons suffering solely from mental illness could apply for MAID beginning in March of 2023. The two-year delay was designed to give legislators and health care providers time to develop and implement appropriate guidelines and safeguards.

SUMMARY

Death inevitably raises questions about meaning—the meaning of life and the meaning to be found in both dying and death. Proximity to death because of a chronic or life-threatening illness, old age, or a "brush with death" tends to motivate an individual to reflect on the meaning of life and death.

A century ago, death was expected more often and earlier in life than it is today. Now, in the twenty-first century, death is not expected except in advanced old age. The premature death of a child, a young adult, or a middle-aged person has become almost entirely unexpected and thus often extremely difficult to accept.

While individuals generally do not wish to die, some deaths are preferred over others. The ideal death occurs in old age following a life lived to its fullest extent and happens suddenly or after a brief illness, without pain, in a familiar setting where final goodbyes can be said. People tend to fear the process of dying, with its potential losses, indignities, and suffering, more than they fear death itself. People facing death often express more concern for the loved ones they will leave behind than they do for themselves.

The dying and their family caregivers generally assess their experiences with end-of-life care in positive terms. Most express satisfaction with the care received and indicate that they have received quality care. Nevertheless, some express dissatisfaction and most, when pressed, can identify elements of care that they feel could have been better and that they believe could have helped achieve a good or better death. Health care workers also wish to provide their dying patients with a good death and sometimes complain that family members make this difficult when they deny that their loved one is dying and demand futile care, for example. Just the same, most family members judge the end-of-life care received by their dying family members in positive if not glowing terms in Canada in the early twenty-first century. There are still improvements to be made, but in general Canadians evaluate the end of life care provided positively and appreciate the concern and efforts made to support the dying and facilitate as good a death as possible.

The COVID-19 pandemic that started in Canada in 2020 revealed shortcomings in the care of frail elderly Canadians, many of whom died in nursing homes while isolated from their loved ones. These deaths are resulting in a reassessment of nursing homes and institutional end-of-life care. Another significant change unfolding in Canada concerns the ongoing implementation of MAID and the preference for clinician-administered rather than self-administered lethal medications. MAID is transforming the experience of death for many Canadians, their families, and their health care providers, not just through the opportunity to get or provide MAID, but also by opening up a major social dialogue about dying and death.

This chapter has primarily focused on perceptions of dying and death from the point of view of the people facing death. In the next chapter the focus will shift to the perceptions of those who lose a loved one to death—that is, survivor perceptions of dying and death.

QUESTIONS FOR REVIEW

1. Discuss death and the "problem of meaning." Refer to Becker's denial of death thesis, terror management theory, existentialism, and spirituality. With reference to death anxiety/fear of death, what are people afraid of (in addition to death itself) and how do they deal with their fears?
2. How can an understanding of death develop over the life course? What are the consequences of open versus closed family orientations to dying and death for personal perceptions and behaviours?
3. Examine the concept of the ideal versus the less than ideal death, including preferred, better, good, good enough, bad, least worst, and shameful deaths. What is the relationship between the "good patient," as judged by the health care professional, and the concept of the good death, and what is the relationship between the "bad patient" and the bad death? What effects do these social constructions and normative prescriptions have on dying people?
4. Discuss cultural variations or preferences around openly discussing terminal illness, the dying process, and death. What are the implications of this for end-of-life care and for family and formal caregivers?
5. Why do some people engage in voluntary risk taking that involves the possibility of death? In particular, compare the edgework and centre work interpretations of voluntary risk taking.

6. While most people seek to avoid death, some actively choose death. Explore the motivations for suicide, death associated with refusing usual or conventional care, and Medical Assistance in Dying (MAID).

7. The end of life is impacted by decisions made by the dying, their family members, and their physicians and other health care workers. Discuss this decision-making dynamic in contemporary end-of-life care. What is the importance of and difficulties involved in finding "common ground" among all of those involved?

8. How satisfied are the dying (and their family members and health care providers) with end-of-life care? What are the determinants of satisfaction and dissatisfaction?

9. Discuss the various ways in which death can be "messy."

10. Describe the initiation, social acceptance, and increased uptake of MAID in Canada since its inception in 2016. What are your thoughts about extending MAID to mature minors, the mentally ill, and to persons who cannot give consent at the time MAID is to be performed?

KEY TERMS

edgework – Exploring the limits of safety, social convention, and so on. Usually associated with voluntary risk taking. (p. 159)

generativity – Making meaningful contributions to others and to society. Gerotranscendence is a related concept referring to generativity in old age. (p. 155)

near-death experience (NDE) – Unusual experiences associated with almost dying that are remembered when the person recovers. May include perceptions of experiences that seem to occur out of one's body; hence the term "out-of-body" experience. (p. 157)

CHAPTER SIX

Survivor Perspectives on Dying and Death

This chapter examines perspectives on dying and death from the point of view of family and friends who grieve the death of a loved one. Health care workers' perspectives on dying and death are discussed in chapter 7.

GRIEF AND BEREAVEMENT

A vocabulary has developed to describe the reactions to the death of a close friend or family member. People who lose a loved one are often referred to as the **bereaved** and are said to go through a period of **bereavement**. The bereaved typically experience **grief**—that is, acute suffering—and go through a process of grieving. Bereaved individuals who display their grief publicly are often referred to as mourners and are said to mourn or to be in **mourning**. If a distinction is to be made between grieving and mourning, it is that grieving is personal and spontaneous while mourning tends to conform to social and cultural norms (Counts and Counts 1991; Howarth 2007; Kastenbaum 2012).

People may suppress emotions that they feel; others may express emotions that they do not feel. In other words, there is not a one-to-one relationship between private and public grieving. Cultural rules describe what emotions can and should be expressed, and when and where they are to be expressed. These rules shape the grieving process and can both facilitate and impede grieving. Although cultural rules can legitimate feelings and their expression, these rules also define what is appropriate, and the person who grieves too long or too intensely (or not enough) tends to be defined as abnormal, deviant, pathological, or a danger to self or others (Counts and Counts 1991; Howarth 2007; Kastenbaum 2012).

While individuals may be moved emotionally, although momentarily, by the evening news with its frequent accounts of tragedies around the world, the death of strangers is typically not associated with grief, mourning, or bereavement. It is the death of a significant other, a person with whom one has a meaningful personal relationship, that is much more distressing. In one sense, death ends the relationship; in another sense, it transforms the relationship. While the deceased is no longer physically present, the relationship continues, although in an altered form, as evident in survivor memories, thoughts, feelings, conversations, behaviours, and even dreams or imaginings.

Several factors influence the extent of grief and the course of grieving. The timing of death can influence grieving—whether death is sudden and unexpected or if it occurs at the end of a long dying trajectory. Grieving is also influenced by the nature of the death. Death from suicide, accident, or homicide may be seen as preventable, senseless, and tragic; death from cancer or Alzheimer's disease may be seen as unpreventable and perhaps even a "blessing" that brings an end to suffering (Aiken 2001; Hadad 2009; Marshall 1986). The severity and length of grieving is also based on the survivor's perception of how good or bad the dying process was (Wilson, Cohen, et al. 2018).

Grieving is also influenced by certain characteristics of the deceased, such as age. It is generally more difficult to lose a loved one who is young than to lose a loved one who is very old (Marshall 1986; Morris, Fletcher, and Goldstein 2019). Furthermore, grieving is influenced by the characteristics, personality, and experiences of the survivor. Someone who has never experienced the loss of a loved one may have more difficulty than a person who has experienced such a loss, although multiple losses can also be very difficult (Norris 1994). Males may grieve differently than females (Hadad 2009; Martin 1998), and the young may grieve differently than the old (Hadad 2009; Kastenbaum 2012).

Finally, grieving is influenced by the relationship the survivor had with the deceased. Grieving may differ for a parent who loses a young child, an adult who loses an aged parent, a wife who loses her beloved husband, a husband who loses his senile wife, or an adult who loses a best friend. Furthermore,

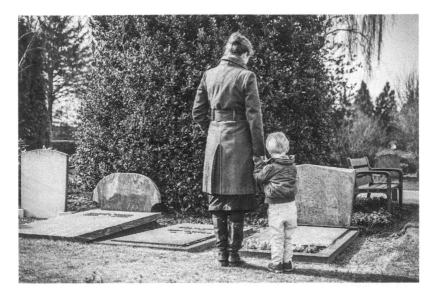

Image 6.1. There is no one-size-fits-all grieving process. People grieve differently depending on the circumstances of the deceased person's death, the age of the griever, and many other factors
Source: Twin Design/Shutterstock.

while it may be very difficult to lose someone with whom one had a good relationship, it may also be very difficult to lose someone with whom relations were strained, given that feelings of regret and guilt tend to exist and persist. In the context of the family, the loss of a loved one results in a change in social status and social roles. A wife who loses a husband becomes a **widow**, a husband who loses a wife becomes a **widower**, a child who loses a parent becomes fatherless or motherless, while a child who loses both parents becomes an **orphan**. These changes in status and role imply changed relationships, changed circumstances, and alterations in personal and social identity. Adjustments following the death of a loved one involve coming to terms not only with the loss of the loved one but also with all of the associated disruptions to the survivor's life, identity, and social relationships (van den Hoonaard 2001, 2010).

While grief tends to become less intense and less disruptive over time, grief may persist in various forms and to varying degrees. Early descriptions and models of grief tended to focus on gradual dissipation over time and assumed that a point was reached when grief was no longer felt. These early models tended to be linear, showing a sequence of stages leading to a resolution of grief. More recent models recognize that grief waxes and wanes, or comes and goes, and returns again. It follows that more recent models tend to be nonlinear and are not temporally bound or limited (Hadad 2009; Leming and Dickinson 2016).

The early models of the grief process tended to become normative expectations for grieving that were imposed on the bereaved. When the bereaved did not conform to these expectations they were made to feel as if they were deviant, and their grief was defined as complicated or pathologic. One student spoke of the death of her mother that had occurred some years ago. The student said that she had never gotten over her loss and that social expectations to recover had made her grieving all the more difficult. She had been made to feel that she had "failed grief," as she put it. In other words, she had failed to get over her mother's death, as society made her feel she should. She was angry that her mother was dead, and she was angry and hurt that society had made her feel deviant for not grieving "properly."

MODELS OF GRIEF

Granek (2010) pointed out that before the twentieth century, grief as a reaction to the death of a loved one was considered to be a natural, normal experience with support coming from family, community, and church. In the twentieth century, with the rise of psychoanalysis, psychiatry, and psychology, grief was reconstructed as a disruptive, or at least potentially dangerous pathology requiring the therapeutic intervention of a range of professionals from family doctors and psychiatrists to counselling psychologists and social workers (Granek 2017). Even medical examiners and funeral directors could play a role in assisting the grieving.

Grief began to be viewed as something that had to be worked through (Howarth 2007). According to dominant models of thinking, successful grief work involved a series of stages or phases and a set of tasks that led in a reasonably short time to a dissipation of disruptive emotions, the re-establishment of normal functioning, and reintegration into society. Grieving was work, and the goal was the end of grief. Failure to accomplish this work in a reasonable amount of time constituted pathology and was variously labelled as abnormal, chronic, prolonged, complicated, or delayed and required therapeutic intervention. Even "normal" grief could potentially benefit from professional intervention and support. Note that the bereaved could grieve too intensely or not intensely enough, for too long or start too late (delayed grief), or they might fail to grieve at all (Rando et al. 2012). The bereaved were expected to grieve normally and to follow a course in their grieving that brought them to the end or resolution of grief and returned them to normal social functioning. Deviation from the prescribed course constituted pathology. Harris (2009–10) argued that the pathologization of grief oppressed grievers, forcing them to constrain and deny their grief to be productive members and consumers in a capitalistic society. Harris argued that grief needed to be depathologized and renormalized so that the bereaved could grieve in the many ways in which they might be inclined. Regardless, the DSM-5 (*Diagnostic and Statistical Manual of Mental Disorders*, 5th ed.), a commonly used psychiatric manual last published in 2013, continues to pathologize grief, with prolonged initial grief still considered problematic and needing treatment.

Granek (2017) observed that grief used to be normal, expressed in public, and supported by the community. Since the late twentieth century, grief has been pathologized and medicalized and is to be expressed in a therapist's office and endured in private. Granek noted that a countercultural movement has developed in the twenty-first century that involves spontaneous public shrines, both real and virtual, and collective expressions of grief in public spaces, either physical or online. This shows that the public may be reclaiming the right to grieve collectively, publicly, and on their own terms, resisting the prescriptions and proscriptions of experts who have medicalized, pathologized, privatized, and monetized grief.

Further, by the end of the twentieth century, the earlier linear and time-limited models of grief had become more flexible (Howarth 2007). It was increasingly recognized then that the process of grieving is not a series of linear steps and that grief does not necessarily end (Hadad 2009). Grief may evolve over time and come and go, often at unexpected times. Furthermore, grief does not necessarily result in the living separating themselves or distancing themselves from the dead; indeed, the living often maintain bonds and relationships with the dead. Increasingly, grieving is viewed as a process of meaning-making as the bereaved attempt to integrate the death of loved ones into their lives by constructing stories and memories of the deceased (Howarth 2007). Howarth warns that while ongoing remembrance of the dead is common, we have to be careful that this does not become a new prescriptive orthodoxy resulting in the bereaved being counselled to remember, create memorials and legacies, and so on, and being sanctioned if they are not inclined to do so.

To illustrate diversity in patterns of grieving, Clark (1993) studied six people from Alberta who were having difficulty with their grieving. The subjects of this study were a young woman who had lost her 16-year-old sister in a motor vehicle accident, a man who had lost his 79-year-old father in a motor vehicle accident, a man who had lost his wife at the age of 52 to breast cancer, a woman who had lost her daughter at the age of 34 to a diabetic coma, a woman who had lost her mother at the age of 77 to complications following surgery, and a man whose 16-year-old son had been murdered. The death of most of the loved ones had occurred from one to three years before the study; in one case the death had occurred seven years earlier.

Difficulties with their grieving arose for various reasons. One subject had difficulty coming to terms with her loss of connection with her sister. She also experienced the loss of her sense of security because of the nature of her sister's sudden, unexpected, and horrifying death. A son had difficulty because his love for his father was intertwined with resentment toward the man who had never made him feel loved or respected. A husband suffered intensely following the loss of his beloved wife and the life that they had shared. A mother felt that there must have been something she could have done to save her daughter. A daughter felt that there were things health care professionals could have done to save her mother, or to at least give her mother more dignity in dying. A father remained confused about how to deal with the emotions he felt regarding his son's death.

The subjects expressed various emotions including intense sorrow, anguish, depression, bitterness, anger, rage, regret, self-blame, guilt, loneliness, pessimism, hopelessness, despair, confusion, emptiness, and numbness. They experienced fatigue, lack of motivation, low self-esteem, feelings of failure, a sense of personal vulnerability, loss of faith, loss of meaning, and loss of purpose. Alienation from other surviving family members was not uncommon. Some turned to thoughts of suicide, looked forward to their own death, or displayed inappropriate behaviour. Clark (1993) pointed out that each person's grieving is, to a degree, personal and unique as it reflects the particular circumstances of the bereaved person's life, their relationship with the deceased, the circumstances of the death, and the survivor's coping style and resources. In a sense, each person follows his or her own path in the course of grieving.

Martin and Elder (1993) titled their article on grief "Pathways through Grief." The use of the plural, "pathways," emphasizes the uniqueness and the individuality of grief. Martin and Elder suggest that each person tends to grieve in a unique way and thus has their own pathway through grief. They acknowledge that, while there are commonalities among individuals, there are always differences as well.

Despite Martin and Elder's phrase "pathways through grief," the authors argue that grief is not a process with a beginning, an ending, and well-defined steps between the two. A person does not necessarily ever get "through" grief, in the sense of being done with it or getting beyond it. Instead, Martin and Elder proposed a figure-eight model of grief. In this model there is no end point, and an individual can return to a "place" where they have been before. The "places" in the model include protest, despair, and detachment in one-half of the figure eight, and exploration (of ways to rebuild a disrupted life), hope, and investment in new relationships in the other half.

At the intersection of the two circles, Martin and Elder located meaning, their central concept. Meaning refers to interpretations or "frames" that individuals use in their attempts to define and make sense of their loss and of their lives. Frames of meaning can be religious, philosophical, cultural, literary, and so on. Individuals may choose different meanings, and the meanings taken influence the pathway that an individual then follows.

Accordingly, intense grief may dissipate and return, rise and fall. Martin and Elder's model allows for the cyclical nature of grief. It also acknowledges that some people follow better, or perhaps more positive and adaptive, pathways than others. Regardless of the pathway, however, grief is never truly over.

POST-DEATH ENCOUNTERS

Bereaved individuals sometimes report encounters with their deceased loved ones, usually soon after the occurrence of their deaths (Nowatzki and Grant Kalischuk 2009). These encounters most commonly involve hearing, seeing, or feeling the presence of the deceased, and they are experienced as real and therefore are consequential. Most encounters are experienced positively and are associated with feelings of warmth, love, peace, and connection with the deceased. Those who experience post-death encounters usually find them comforting. Further, post-death encounters often involve a sense of communication with the deceased who provide messages of reassurance or instruction. People experiencing post-death encounters with loved ones often report them as life changing and leading to positive changes in attitudes, values, and beliefs. For example, some report that they are more compassionate, less fearful, or more certain of a life after death. For the most part, post-death encounters have a therapeutic healing effect. They promote a sense of connection and facilitate an ongoing bond and continuing relationship with the deceased.

A woman in her early thirties reflected on the death of her grandfather some 15 years earlier:

> I have almost never dreamed of Papa. And when I do he just grins at me
> and walks away. I try and get him to talk, but he never does . . . he just
> gives that closed mouth grin and leaves! Except one time he didn't walk
> away . . . it was before my wedding. I dreamed he was sitting at the table
> at my reception. He stood up and applauded. He was proud of me . . .
> [There have been] two other times I would say I felt his presence—those
> two times felt real. Once the day of his funeral—he was comforting
> me—and once hiking [in the mountains]—he was enjoying the meadow
> of flowers with me.

Grandfather and granddaughter shared a deep meaningful bond that endured after his death. When he died, the granddaughter was distraught that because of final exams at school and great distance she could not attend his funeral. On the day of his funeral, she felt his presence, and this comforted and reassured her. Later, she felt his presence when hiking in the mountains, something they used to do together before his death. Over the years that followed, she occasionally dreamed of him. The dreams kept their special relationship alive and reassured her of their continuing bond.

DEATHS OF LOVED ONES

The nature of the relationship between the deceased and the griever affects the grieving process. Here we will discuss the death of specific loved ones and how these particular relationships might affect survivor grief and the grieving process.

Death of a Child

In the past, the death of a child was a frequent and expected event. However, throughout much of the twentieth century the death of a child became an increasingly rare event in Canada (Marshall 1986). Today, children are expected to grow old. Indeed, the death of a child at any age has come to be largely unexpected, and parents assume that they will predecease their children (Fry 1997). Partly because of the unexpected nature and timing of the event, it is particularly difficult for a parent to accept the death of a child (Martin 1998; Morris, Fletcher, and Goldstein 2019).

The death of a fetus before birth can also be problematic given that society tends to minimize this loss and disenfranchise the parents' grief (Lang et al. 2011; Watson et al. 2019). Lang and her co-authors studied parents who had been treated in Montreal hospitals after they had experienced the death of preterm babies (fetal death). The parents had experienced ambiguity about the viability of the pregnancy (whether the fetus would live or not), unanswered questions about the physical process of losing the fetus (when will the fetus be delivered, how, and what to do with the fetus?), and uncertainty about who to tell and what to tell them. Furthermore, the parents typically had different coping styles, with the mothers needing to talk more or longer than the fathers, leading to marital tension. The men tended to cope by avoiding emotional discussions and focusing on instrumental activities. This tended to leave their partners feeling unsupported emotionally. To further complicate grieving following fetal death, health care professionals tended to treat it as a medical event rather than the loss of a baby and were perceived by the parents as insensitive and unsupportive. Health care professionals, friends, and family members tended to discount fetal death, denying the parents the opportunity to grieve and mourn and to receive social support. This social invalidation of their loss disenfranchised their grief and made their grieving more difficult.

Watson et al. (2019) reported an online survey of 596 parents who had experienced the loss of a pregnancy (miscarriage or stillbirth) or infant death in Ontario. The authors noted that the parents' loss was commonly unacknowledged or minimized. Respondents to the survey highlighted feelings of isolation, exclusion, and stigmatization. They often faced silence, insensitivity, and lack of support from their employers, co-workers, and others. Further, while some reported that health care professionals were sensitive, caring, and supportive, others complained that health care professionals were insensitive and unsupportive. Respondents commented that while their loss might be routine or trivial to health care professionals, it was very significant to them. Social conventions continue to exist that minimize the loss of a pregnancy and undermine the significance of this loss to the expecting parents.

The following account reports the experience of a woman who had a miscarriage and spoke openly about it with the first author:

> I knew the numbers. I knew that women over 35 and under 40 (such as I was) had around a 20 per cent chance of a miscarriage, and additionally I knew that when the father was over 40 (such as my husband was), that the miscarriage risk was significantly compounded, though studies were unclear as to how much. Still, when it happened to me, in my first pregnancy, a pregnancy I so very much wanted and had looked forward to my whole life, I was completely unprepared.
>
> I was unprepared because a person rarely thinks that they will be the one to be so unlucky, but also because I had no real information about what the process of miscarriage was like and what the physical and emotional recovery could entail. Other than hearing passing references to a deceased grandmother who had a miscarriage, or maybe two, I did not know anyone who had a miscarriage—or so I thought. My grandmother, like so many women today, had been taught that this is not something you discuss. Consequently, no one seemed to know how many miscarriages she had and there had never been any discussion of the impact it had on her. When I lost my baby, I was amazed at how many friends and family members suddenly came forward with stories of their losses. I was heartbroken for them, but while grateful for their support and understanding I was also bewildered. How could this not have been something we discussed before? The more stories I heard, especially as I kept hearing the recurring use of the word "trauma" in relation to the experience, the more I found myself becoming a little angry. It would have helped me during my miscarriage to have known their stories, and I could have helped them deal with their loss had they not felt it was something you just do not talk about.
>
> I had often been told you really "shouldn't" share that you are pregnant until at least the second trimester because "what if you lose the baby?" This always seemed odd to me—if I lost the baby, then why wouldn't the very same people who I wanted to rejoice with me and share in my joy of having a child be the same people who I wanted to comfort me and share in my sorrow at losing that child?
>
> Having no idea anything was amiss with my pregnancy, one day I noticed the tiniest blood clot in the toilet, and while noting that was unusual and planning to mention it to my doctor, I still did not suspect

a miscarriage was in the works. Two days later, however, I began to feel some cramping and experienced very light bleeding. At that point I called my doctor's after-hours support line and was informed what I already knew: that this could be nothing, or it could be a miscarriage. I was given the choice to go to the hospital if I wanted immediate attention, or to come in to the doctor's office for an ultrasound first thing in the morning. I wish that I went into the hospital, because then I would have had an ultrasound in time to capture a picture of my baby. Instead, my cramping and the bleeding worsened at home through the night. I lay awake for hours thinking this was probably bad news, yet telling myself to have hope and praying that I was wrong. Still, I told my husband to see if he could get permission to miss work because I suspected this ultrasound might be his only chance to see the baby.

We got to the doctor's waiting room the next morning and suddenly the cramping became extreme. I could barely sit still I hurt so badly. I became nauseated and was shaking. I was trying very hard not to draw attention to myself in the waiting room but so desperately wanted to curl up in a ball. I could tell the bleeding was becoming intense and I started looking around the room wondering where the bathroom was and how I was going to get to it being in so much pain. I was just about to beg my husband to ask the receptionist for help when I was finally called back to a room.

They asked me to change into a gown and I was horrified to find my extra absorbent pad, underwear and pants soaked with blood. I began crying at this point, from pain, from fear, from the reluctant acknowledgment that this had to mean I was losing the baby . . . but also from embarrassment. That last admission still makes me angry. To think that I was losing my baby and yet I had room in my mind and heart to feel embarrassed that I was getting blood on the floor initially made me wonder what was wrong with me to waste time on that—but as time has passed also makes me wonder what was/is wrong with our society that shaped me to feel embarrassed of a natural, albeit horrible, process.

The ultrasound technician was kind and somber. She told me she needed to do a vaginal ultrasound instead of an abdominal one and as such I needed to go to the bathroom down the hall to empty my bladder. As I relaxed my muscles to urinate I felt a rush of blood and felt something substantial fall out of me. Hysterical, I stood up, turned and saw a fist-sized clump of tissue in the toilet along with so much blood. Feeling horror, but also feeling like I had no other option, I flushed the toilet. This haunts me. I have since heard how it is very common for women to lose their baby in the toilet and take the same action I did. One friend told me how she was at a birthday party, lost the baby, flushed it, and went back to the party without telling anyone, because she did not want to disrupt the party.

In the moment, I was so very traumatized, and yet again feeling embarrassed. I realized I was getting blood all over the floor. Sobbing and shaking, almost in a panic, I starting cleaning [the floor] as best I could with paper towels. I finally made my way back down the hall to the ultrasound room and through my sobs tried to tell my husband and the technician what had happened. I kept apologizing for messing up the bathroom.

Eventually the doctor came in to confirm what I already knew. She started talking about how I still needed to pass more pregnancy remnants over the next few hours or days and that if I did not do this naturally they could give me medicine to help things along or that they would surgically remove the remaining tissue. I was genuinely confused when I was offered pain medication, not comprehending and having not been told explicitly how painful the muscle contractions could be that would help expel the rest of the tissue. I quickly came to understand this later that day while curled up over the edge of my bathtub, throwing up from pain. For me, only the first day was horrifically painful, but I was surprised at how much pain there was for many days to come and I was surprised that the physical process took days.

I was not surprised that the emotional healing was going to be a long journey, as I was not a total stranger to loss due to death. Still, this loss was different than any other loss I had experienced before. While I have never bought in to the idea that one should keep these kinds of losses to oneself, I still found myself careful about who I talked with in depth. I did not wish to encounter the types of non-helpful responses a friend of mine incurred after losing her baby six months into her pregnancy including "well it was not a real baby" (that may be their belief, but certainly was not my friend's belief, nor mine, and as such very unhelpful to us in managing our grief) and "well people miscarry all the time" (Why is it okay to say this about a baby? You do not hear someone say, "my mother just died," and have people answer, "yah, well mothers die all the time").

My husband said that he could not believe how much he could miss someone he never knew. My father, the baby's grandpa, said that he was grieving the loss of possibilities. I shared both sentiments for days, waking at night crying and replaying the pregnancy and miscarriage, wondering what I could or should have done differently. Soon however, I found myself eager to try again to have a baby, and while not totally surprised at how much fear I felt this time, I was surprised at the guilt. I did not want to forget about my first baby, and I did not want it to look, or feel like, my little one was replaceable.

Unlike many women, I was lucky enough to be buoyed up through my grief by very supportive family and friends who listened to me, let me cry, and sometimes just sat with me in silence. My experience made me 100 per cent sure that if I were lucky enough to get pregnant again, I would once again tell those I cared about as soon as I could.

I continue to share my miscarriage story without hesitation so others will have the information I wish that I had and also to combat the idea that this is something a woman has to go through alone. While it does seem that there are changes coming slowly to the social barriers regarding sharing stories about miscarriage, it still seems that it is okay to share only if you are a celebrity with a blog and not just an ordinary woman. This has got to change.

This account illustrates a social expectation (rule) that expectant parents wait before announcing that they are pregnant. Waiting until the end of the first trimester to announce a pregnancy provided time to be sure that the pregnancy was viable. But this practice also tacitly acknowledged the widespread idea that a miscarriage early in the pregnancy was not a significant loss and, as a result, any grief felt was "disenfranchised"—unrecognized and unsupported. The person telling her story above had rejected the social convention of hiding her pregnancy for the first months and had announced her pregnancy from its beginning. Consequently, when she experienced a miscarriage, she was able to draw on the support of others.

Nevertheless, her story focused on the normative conspiracy of silence surrounding miscarriage. The storyteller noted that women are expected to suffer in silence, and because most do not share their stories with each other, they remain unprepared, unsupported, embarrassed, and silenced. This is in contrast to childbirth. Stories of childbirth are told and retold and serve to prepare, guide, legitimize, and support (and sometimes irritate) the expectant mother.

In a separate correspondence, the storyteller noted that "the earlier the loss, the less sympathy you get and the less grief you are allowed to have." She observed that toward the end of a pregnancy the baby is recognized and that the death of the baby is acknowledged and the mother's grief supported. In the early months of the pregnancy, however, the baby and its death are less likely to be acknowledged. She pointed out that in the middle of the pregnancy, the mother is in a liminal space between the early months when miscarriage is associated with menstruation and the later months when the death of the baby is acknowledged. Finally, the storyteller highlighted the need to bring miscarriage into open conversation and noted the role that celebrities play as opinion leaders who are increasingly defying convention by telling their stories on social media.

The internet has led to the emergence of several virtual online support groups designed to help parents who have experienced a **perinatal death**; that is, the death of a baby before or soon after birth (Davidson and Letherby 2014). On these sites, parents and occasionally grandparents and others can share their stories, provide emotional support and advice, and validate the experience of grief that is otherwise minimized and disenfranchised. On the negative side, mean-spirited people may engage in internet trolling and criticize and demean the bereaved online, undermining their attempt to find a sympathetic and understanding audience to share and support their grief.

Braun (1992) interviewed 10 Canadian mothers who had each lost a child. At the time of their death, the deceased children ranged from 5 months gestation (note that most babies born at 20 weeks gestation will survive) to 25 years of age. Braun wanted to understand how bereaved parents developed an understanding of their child's death by focusing on the parents' existing "meaning structure" at the time of their child's death (62–3). Meaning structure refers to a person's understanding of the nature of life, including their beliefs and assumptions—a construction of reality that gives life meaning and purpose. For some parents, their existing construction of reality was able to provide a meaningful explanation of the death of their child. Other parents experienced disorientation when their meaning structures could not provide an adequate explanation. Disorientation took the form of a deconstruction of existing beliefs. Adjustment involved a process of reconstructing meaning. Braun (1992, 89) pointed out that parents who ask "why?" are indicating that they do not have a readily accessible meaning structure in place that they can use to make sense of their child's death.

A person who believes that whatever happens is a manifestation of God's plan has an explanation for a child's death, while a person who believes that God should be looking out for the innocent has a problem. Similarly, a person who believes that there are no guarantees in life has an explanation of a sort, while a person who believes that being a good parent will protect a child has a problem. A child's death can raise questions about whether there is a caring God and whether life is just, fair, safe, meaningful, manageable, predictable, purposeful, and ordered. Furthermore, because a child can give a parent's life meaning and purpose, the loss of that child can be particularly difficult. According to Braun, loss of meaning resulting from a child's death is associated with guilt, anger, incomprehension, feeling disconnected from the world, placing blame, a wish for the parent's own death, thoughts of suicide, loss of a sense of security, lack of hope for the future, loss of motivation, and lack of interest, as well as loss of a sense of personal control and purpose. The process of adjustment then involves searching for an explanation for the child's death and searching for a new sense of meaning and purpose in life.

Martin (1998) also studied the reactions of Canadian parents to the death of their child. In Martin's study, the children all died as a result of sudden infant death syndrome (SIDS). In this situation, parental grief tends to be particularly intense because SIDS takes the life of a healthy baby, occurs suddenly without warning, has no known cause, and is investigated by legal authorities that include the police and the medical examiner.

Reviewing the existing research on SIDS, Martin noted that bereaved parents manifest a wide range of individual grief reactions, including emotional manifestations such as shock, numbness, sorrow, depression, anxiety, anger, and fear. Cognitive reactions include "flashbacks" to the moment of discovering the deceased baby, obsessive reviewing of the circumstances before the baby's death, preoccupation, difficulty concentrating, dreams about the baby, self-reproach, guilt, and difficulty controlling thoughts. Physical reactions include problems sleeping, headaches, stomach problems, fatigue, dizziness, chest pain, and loss of appetite. Regarding spiritual reactions, some parents rely on their faith while others question or lose faith. For some, life loses meaning and purpose. Behavioural reactions include crying, restlessness, moving to a new residence, losing interest in social activities, difficulties at work, ineffective functioning, taking medications, and increased smoking or drinking. Some consider or attempt ending their own life.

The studies that Martin reviewed also showed that spousal relationships are affected by the loss of an infant to SIDS. The husband and wife may grieve in different ways, and their grieving may follow different timelines. These differences can be a source of marital strain. Yet, while some couples experience increased marital difficulties including divorce, other marriages are strengthened (Albuquerque, Pereira, and Narciso 2016).

When there are other children in the family, SIDS takes a baby away from both its parents and its siblings. The other children may feel guilt that they are somehow responsible for the baby's death. They may show anger or anxiety, have nightmares, ask repeated questions, regress behaviourally, or exhibit problematic behaviours. The loss of the baby also affects the relationships among the surviving children and their parents. Both the parents and the surviving children are changed because of their grief and loss. The siblings have to cope with a changed relationship with their grieving parents, and the parents have to cope with their children who are also grieving, each child in their own way. Sometimes children become angry with their parents. Parents can become distant from their children or, alternatively, can become overly protective.

In reviewing the wide range of reactions of individual parents to the loss of their baby, Martin (1998) concluded that underlying these various individual reactions was the undermining of the foundation upon which the parents had built their lives. The baby's death abruptly and substantially altered each parent's life. Not only was the baby suddenly gone, but also the seeming randomness of SIDS undermined each parent's sense that the world is ordered, comprehensible, predictable, manageable, just, and meaningful. Accordingly, the baby's death led to a "search for reason" in an attempt to find the cause and meaning of the baby's death. Parents sought to make sense not only of their baby's death but also of their own lives once again.

Grieving for a deceased baby involves major emotional pain. Similarly, searching for the reason for the baby's death involves cognitive, intellectual, and spiritual pain (Martin 1998). At a cognitive level, Martin observed that some parents were able to reconcile the loss of their baby with their previous worldview. Other parents constructed a new worldview, some for the better and some for the worse. Still others were unable to make any sense of their baby's death. The perspective that parents took "made the difference between eventual healing or continual hell" (Martin 1998, 219).

Additionally, Martin described five phases of the grief process. Parents who had lost a baby spoke of the loving attachment that had developed before the baby's death. They then spoke of being devastated, trying to carry on while struggling for control, learning to let go, and being changed. Martin argued that being changed does not necessarily imply recovery, resolution, or healing. Indeed, she challenged the myth that people can ever fully recover. According to Martin (1998, 232), "Since some people improve and some people never function well again, I propose that we stop using the word 'recovery' to describe the goal of the grief process. We need to start talking about how traumatic experiences can change survivors. My study clearly shows that the death of a child changed the parents, some negatively and some positively." She concluded by commenting on the power and potential of the human mind to construct interpretations of devastating events such as the death of a child, constructions that often helped the bereaved deal with their grief.

The following is a written account provided to the first author by a father who experienced the unthinkable—the unexpected loss of two of his four children in separate fatal accidents:

> "When a loved one dies, a part of you also dies." This cliché, is in fact, true. The moment someone close to you dies, you are a changed person. Instantaneously. Your whole being transforms the moment a close one departs from his or her earthly existence. They exit, and in reality, your being as you knew it also exits. You immediately become a different person. Whether you like it or not, or wish to acknowledge it, it's true. If you don't believe it, a perception check of those immediately around you should make you aware of this fact. The world's perception of you changes. This truism is all the more pronounced when one loses a close one tragically. Instantaneously. One second a loved one is here. A second later gone. Your total world goes numb. You hope that it is just a bad dream, a nightmare, which you will awake from and get on with normal living. Deep down you know this is only wishful thinking. Your world, as you knew it, has changed forever. You walk around in a daze, put up a brave front, and proceed to do all the normal things like nothing has happened. Pick up the mail, wash the dishes, all the while fighting a deep depression that totally engulfs your whole being, from the tips of your toes to the bristling hairs on your head. You reflect on how life was a few moments ago, a few days ago, and yearn for the clock to be turned back just enough to bypass the tragedy you are now faced with. But in your heart, you know you have to somehow muster the strength to deal with the situation at hand, impossible and unreal as it might seem.
>
> No one has prepared you for this moment. You read about it happening to other people; the sudden loss of a child—it sent shivers down your

spine, made you feel totally uncomfortable and vulnerable. Something to quickly forget. A parent's worst nightmare; sudden death of a child. Now it has happened to you. Not once, but twice, in the matter of a couple of years. Moments earlier, your daughter was healthy and alive. Now the policeman, in your living room, at three o'clock in the morning, tells you she is dead. How can this be possible? Two years later, one o'clock in the morning. Two policemen on your back step. Your son has been in an accident, they're working on him, we'll drive you to the hospital. Body language and the words of the police tell me that our son is indeed dead. We drive to the hospital and meet reality face to face. Another child suddenly departed. Without warning. How does one cope; where is one's statute of limitations on grief and pain? Numbness, depression, a longing for moving the clock back, just a couple of hours.

Years earlier, the phone rang at approximately five o'clock on a Saturday afternoon in early February. A relative is on the other end. "There's been an accident, your mother is dead." I was introduced into the real world of grief, pain, and coping with loss. Anxiety, depression, and sense of loss. Ongoing. How to muster enough energy to get through a day; this was an ongoing battle. Now two children dead in the short span of just over two years. When does one's reservoir run dry? I remember, at this time, using the quote attributed to William Irwin Thompson: "The future is beyond knowing, but the present is beyond belief."

When our daughter died, I felt that I was regressing in grief and despondency. After six months I felt worse than after the first week. I was fortunate that a counsellor gave me some materials on "coping with loss." I then recognized the grief cycle I was going through; first six months, a year, and so on. It didn't make it easier, but at least I became aware that there are some usually predictable happenings in the grief cycle, and one usually has to go through the full grief cycle before one can return to cope with a "normal" life again. Not dealing effectively with grief can leave one stranded in "grief limbo," endlessly fighting a futile battle until the end of one's mortal existence.

What coping mechanism worked for me? I have no magic answer. Daily, I have to deal with memories, an enormous sense of loss. However, I feel that part of our difficulty in dealing with the death of close ones, and those others in our immediate environment, is that it puts us in direct touch with our own mortality. Realizing this, one has to acknowledge the minute shortness of time one has on earth. To live to 80, or 8, the time spent on earth in comparison to eternity is minuscule. I look around, and death is continuous. A close friend, a neighbour, a relative. Everyone dies a mortal death. Thus, it makes it all the more important that we make the most of the few minutes we do have on earth. We should not become a victim of a close death; by martyring oneself to the memory of a departed close one, we in fact also become a victim of the initial death. However, it is much easier said than done. Our emotions, our sense of loss can be overwhelming.

A close friend of mine passed away, shortly after my daughter's death. A couple of years ago I saw his widow on the street. I asked her how she was doing. She said, "It's okay to remember, but not to dwell."

I found that co-workers, friends, neighbours, and acquaintances have difficulty acknowledging your dilemma. We are all good at sending cards, flowers, and attending the immediate functions such as the funeral and luncheons. Then it is over. You are on your own, to grieve your loss in a vacuum. Very few want to enter this domain. It becomes your own personal battleground. Everyone gets back to their life, their worries, their concerns. You feel isolated, despondent, abandoned. The pain of loss is usually too much for "outsiders" to comprehend. It is better to stay a safe distance away. Most everyone wants to be "associated" with someone whom "lady luck" shines down on—the sweepstakes winner, the person who visibly is on a positive track in life. The opposite holds true for those perceived to be "down on their luck." Whether we like it or not, there is a general perception that we are in control of our destiny; we reap what we sow. Death is not where it's at. Avoidance of the situation is most prudent for most concerned. I have no problem with that—when I was younger I tried to avoid thinking of death—a casket was cause for concern. However, the reality is that death is a major part of life. No one can escape it. We must all someday face death head on.

Personally, I sincerely believe that on earth we are but travellers, passing through a transition period. A very short trip in an eternal spectrum. But a very important trip. We are not human beings having a spiritual experience. We are spiritual beings having a human experience. In my mind, this belief brings reason to an otherwise meaningless existence.

How does one really cope with extreme grief? With great difficulty. I found that some very close friendships can add some comfort, family pets, physical activity such as weights and tennis, walking, a strong belief in the "hereafter," a loving wife, a sense of humour, and most of all the avoidance of the word "why?" As other individuals played significant roles in the demise of our two children, I was initially adamant that these said parties formally acknowledge responsibility for their actions. In both cases, neither party was willing to do so. I have accepted this as something I have no control over, and life must go on. However, I think it indicates a common significant human factor in coping with the sudden death of a loved one; someone or something is perceived to be totally or partially responsible for the tragic sudden ending. Surely it is more than just "chance."

Also, I found that in the cases of all three deaths [mother, daughter, son], I felt a strong urgency to have their memories live on. It seems that the moment a person dies, he or she becomes a nonentity to the rest of the earthly living population, with the exception of the immediate loved ones. Therefore, any dedication to their memory was and is most important to me. I find that most people have trouble talking about the "dead." . . . It is like a pretense that they never existed. I find this disheartening. These departed individuals are still family. The fact that they have departed earth a few minutes before me does not change their status. They are still loved ones, my family members.

Death, tragic or otherwise, of loved ones, weighs heavily on the minds and souls of those left behind. Coping is an ongoing process. And like a member of Alcoholics Anonymous, the survivor must take one day at a time. Grief can overtake one instantaneously, if one leaves the door open. Honour those that have gone before you, and fill your remaining days on earth with good works.

This father's story of the deaths of his daughter and son contains four themes: change, personal feelings of grief, personal coping, and social reactions. The father notes that the loss of each child brings change. He feels that part of him has died, his world as he knows it has changed forever, he feels different, and he believes that others see him differently. Yearning for life as it was before tragedy struck, for his normal life, he nevertheless recognizes that his previous life is irretrievable. For friends and neighbours, disruption is temporary. The father's life, however, is permanently altered. There is no going back, and going forward involves coping with grief.

The second theme is personal feelings of grief. The grieving parent experiences a range of emotions including numbness and feeling dazed, yearning and longing, depression and despondency, isolation and abandonment, pain and a sense of loss. He writes of feeling worse months after the initial tragedy and of going through the motions of daily living while fighting deep depression. Keeping the memories of his deceased children alive becomes a goal. He suggests that one never fully recovers from grief, for it can intrude again in an instant.

With regard to the third theme, this parent describes coping as an ongoing process. He writes about putting on a brave front, mustering strength and energy to deal with immediate situations, and *acting* normal as if nothing has happened. His coping is facilitated by his wife, some close friends, his pets, physical activity, and a sense of humour. Although he notes that going through the "full grief cycle" helps one to cope, at the same time he observes that grief is ongoing and can surface and overwhelm at any moment "if one leaves the door open."

In the process of coping, he is initially adamant that the people who were directly involved in the tragedies acknowledge the part they played and accept responsibility for their actions. Otherwise, he explicitly avoids asking "why?" Indeed, he adds, "I have always felt that it is pointless to pose the question 'why' when a death occurs—I feel strongly that part of my survival gear for coping is to never let 'Why did this happen?' be part of my repertoire." Instead, he finds assurance in his beliefs in spiritual existence and eternal life. From his beliefs, he gains a sense that human life and, therefore, human events ultimately happen for a reason and have meaning.

In addition, this parent uses an intellectual strategy to normalize death. He comments on the pervasiveness of death: sooner or later everyone dies. He himself has experienced the death of loved ones; he knows others who have lost loved ones; he acknowledges his own mortality. This normalization of death, tied to his beliefs in eternal life, renders death more acceptable.

Finally, this parent comments on the social reactions to his family's losses. He makes three points, all of which relate to the concept of stigma. First, he notes that the world's perception of him has changed. He is now seen as one of the unlucky, one of the unfortunate. In this new social status, he receives sympathy but also blame, reflecting the tendency for people to assume that the unfortunate are in some way responsible for their misfortune. This social reaction is both victim blaming and stigmatizing, and supports the argument of Posner (1976), discussed in chapter 4, that people associated with death are stigmatized because death itself is stigmatized. The father acknowledges this lack of social acceptance when he notes that people avoid the unlucky and unfortunate.

Second, the father recollects a widow saying to him, "It's okay to remember, but not to dwell." He interpreted this comment positively. He understood her to mean that "it is important and okay to remember a dearly departed one, but one should not dwell on the memory to a point that one gets depressed and regresses into deep depression." The widow's comment conveys encouragement and advice and reflects society's rules for the bereaved. The widow encourages him to remember but also to be careful not to wallow in self-pity.

Third, the father observes that, after the initial events of the tragedy and funeral, others go back to their normal lives and distance themselves from the grieving family. These people have difficulty acknowledging or participating in the family's grieving. Indeed, avoidance is the typical response. On this point the father says, "I find that most people have trouble talking about the 'dead.'. . . It is like a pretense that they never existed." This avoidance indicates social stigma. When people are faced with social stigma, they experience discomfort, distance themselves, use avoidance, and act as if nothing is wrong. The father finds this social response disappointing and unsupportive.

Years later, the father added an epilogue to his story that he shared with the first author:

> Twenty years [have] now elapsed since our last tragic loss. In those 20 years, I have gone from a mortal man of 50 to an old mortal man of 70. The loss of our children is still very real and sad. We (my wife and I) just in the last couple of weeks cleaned up the gravesite (our daughter and son are buried side by side in the cemetery). The wreath was replaced with the latest edition. This is regular protocol each time we go to our cabin at [the lake]. Our itinerary always includes visits to the gravesite. A couple of years ago we had the base of the headstones redone because our son's headstone seemed to be slightly tilting. Both headstones now rest on one main base.
>
> As time passes, it becomes more evident that old age is now a real item. Each day we are reminded in many ways (physically, mentally) that our own days on earth are rapidly dwindling. Therefore, the gap between our children's deaths and our own impending mortal deaths is getting smaller with each passing day. This message is hammered home on a regular basis when we hear of the deaths of friends, neighbours, and acquaintances. The reality of life is that our days on earth are relatively short. I think I mentioned in my previous dissertation that as part of our grief in the loss of someone close to us, we are also dealing with the

reality of our own mortality and impending death. At the time of a loss, we might not consciously recognize this fact, but it registers in the subconscious mind. At this time, with old age now being a reality, the aspect of grief is now succinctly transformed into a hope of soon reuniting with our children.

After 20 years the parents continue to grieve and mourn. Their loss "is still very real and sad." Their deceased daughter and son are remembered and memorialized in the regular ritual of visiting and caring for their children's graves. In addition, this parent reminds us that we are all mortal and that as we age we get closer and closer to the dead. In our mind's eye it is easy to visualize a reunion with the dead as we anticipate our own transition from life to death and as we anticipate leaving the living and joining those who have died before us.

At the time of writing the latest edition of this book, the father was asked if he had any final words to add. He said that telling his story about grief many years ago "was very therapeutic." One of the ways people make sense of loss is by telling their stories and having those stories heard (Frank 2013). And the stories can be very instructive for the listeners and readers as well. As it so happens, the storyteller's wife, the mother of the deceased children, emailed the following to the first author in 2020, years after the deaths of her two children:

> I know that [my husband] has been the chief correspondent for the family but I thought I would like to share this. Perhaps you are familiar with this passage from George Orwell's *1984*. It is part of a song sung from the distant memory of a woman who is hanging her washing on the line. In the book it is in dialect but I have written it in regular English:
>
> They say that time heals all things,
>
> They say you can always forget;
>
> But the smiles and the tears across the years
>
> They twist my heart strings yet!
>
> I particularly like the choice of the word "twist," not touch, pull or tug at, but the violence of a twist.
>
> For me the grief journey has been linear but also circular and a spiral as well. I am not in the place that I was. I have a life different from the one I hoped for. I am happy with my life but am always conscious at some level that it is not of my choosing. I am reconciled to my loss

but continue to have difficulty with reconciliation to what my children have not been able to experience in this life. It challenges but does not overcome my faith.

Twenty-seven years later I forgot to notice when the calendar turned over to the day [my daughter] died. I always remember her birthday but this date crept past me. What does that mean? However, the body does seem to remember. Oh, that is why I felt so crumby that day.

As a family, we [father, mother, and two surviving children] do not talk at any depth about our response to the deaths. In the early days, I was not capable of the conversation and, as time went on, it became part of history and not current conversation. I think that is not the best way to go. Perhaps we will come to it at some point. I admire those families where there is more sharing.

The garage still holds the boxes of the kids' stuff that was packed away. The bag [my daughter] was carrying when she died and her Walkman and headphones are sitting in the closet in the computer room. We have not "cleaned out" the remnants of our children.

I still feel angry about the way [the city] handled the death scene [where my daughter died], the [institution's] response to us, and the court experience, if I let myself really think about it. So, the feelings are still there although muted by time and the rational conclusion that there is nothing I can do about any of it.

I think that the trauma haunts me as much as the grief.

So where would you put me on a scale of "recovery"? I am occasionally very sad. Is that not part of the general mortal condition or is it particular to me?

I don't think that the experience has made me more compassionate. It is often said that this experience results in a more compassionate person. I think sometimes that the opposite is true. The things that many people are moaning about do not meet my scale of trouble.

I do love my life and the good things in it. I am so grateful for the children and grandchildren I have, for the things I have been able to do, for my place in the world. What more can anyone ask?

Her story demonstrates that young people look to the future, while people as they age look increasingly to the past. Young parents have a future that is lost when their children die. Parents grieve the loss of their children and the loss of the future that they could have shared. This mother looks back over the years and reflects on the deaths of her children and on her life as it unfolded since those tragic events. Her reflection can be read as a life review including two central themes: (1) loss, trauma, and grief; and (2) the existential challenge of dealing with life's complex dualities including life and death, living and dying, happiness and sadness, celebration and grieving, remembering and forgetting, satisfaction and regret, resignation and resistance, acceptance and despair, choice and contingency, and gratitude overall despite not having the life of her own choosing.

Regarding loss, trauma, and grief, this mother comments on models of grief that emphasize the temporality of grief and its shape over time. She observes, paradoxically, that for her, grief is linear but also circular, a spiral, muted by time, yet also an ongoing violent twisting of her metaphorical heart strings. While her grief has lessened with time, the trauma of her children's deaths "haunts" her still.

Regarding the existential dualities, this mother notes that she is happy with her life, loves her life, is grateful for the good things in her life, and is reconciled to her loss and accepting of what cannot be changed; at the same time, she notes that she also is sometimes very sad, is angry still about the circumstances of her children's deaths, and has regrets about living a life that has not been entirely of her choosing, a life different from the one she had hoped for. Erikson (1959) similarly explored life's dualities. He argued that the challenge at the end of life was to achieve what he called "ego integrity" and avoid despair. This mother's life review summarizes her life's existential complexities. Her life review is a story of "smiles and tears across the years" with an emphasis in the end on the positive aspects of her life.

Marchenski (2004) compared parents in Manitoba who had experienced the death of a child from either sudden, violent, accidental injury or previously diagnosed life-threatening illness. She distinguished the symptoms that comprise grief from the symptoms that indicate post-traumatic stress. Marchenski noted that the bereaved parents experienced grief as a reaction to the death of their child, and that some parents also experienced post-traumatic stress as a reaction to the *nature* of their child's death. She noted that the death of a child, especially from sudden, violent, accidental injury, tended to result in elevated levels of post-traumatic stress. Marchenski concluded that her "research adds to the evidence that the death of a child is a traumatic experience for parents. It suggests the importance . . . of assessing posttraumatic stress in all bereaved parents [and] especially parents of children who die at a young age or as a result of injury" (ix).

Woodgate (2006) interviewed parents in a Western Canadian city who had experienced the death of a child. The children had died at ages ranging from 3 days to 28 years, and their deaths had occurred recently for some parents and years ago for others. Regardless of how recently or long ago their child had died, the parents indicated that they had not experienced a sense of closure, nor did they want to. They equated closure with forgetting their deceased child, something they did not want to do. In this sense, parents do not "get over" the death of a child; instead, parents live with their loss for the rest of their life.

Barrera et al. (2009) interviewed parents (18 mothers and 13 fathers) six months after the death of their child from cancer. Those parents that were identified as adjusting well were able to accept the death of their child, maintain a spiritual bond with the deceased child, and remain connected to their surviving children and the child's other parent and a supportive social network. They were able to redefine themselves, restructure their lives, and find new purpose in life. Some parents had more difficulty than others adjusting in the initial six months following the death of their child. These parents tended to still have difficulty 18 months after the death of their child (O'Connor and Barrera 2014). Furthermore, some parents who seemed to be adjusting well after 6 and 12 months reported difficulties 18 months after the death of their child. Despite the common assumption that grief dissipates with time, some parents felt worse as time passed. This shows that grief can ebb and flow, come and go, and return again.

At both 6 months and 18 months after the death of their child, a study by Alam et al. (2012) found that fathers tended to be more task-focused and involved in work while mothers were more focused on family life and the surviving children. Mothers initially showed their emotions more openly than fathers, who preferred to grieve privately. Over time the mothers experienced less pain and greater control over their emotions, while fathers became somewhat more comfortable showing their grief. Mothers were more successful than fathers in connecting with surviving children. Spousal relationships improved for some parents and deteriorated for others. Support from extended family tended to be greater six months after the child's death but declined over the following year. These and other researchers suggested that the differences in parental grieving reflect gender socialization that encourages men to control their emotions and focus on instrumental tasks while encouraging women to be more open emotionally and focused on nurturing children (Alam et al. 2012; Barrera et al. 2009; O'Connor and Barrera 2014).

Nicholas et al. (2016) studied Canadian fathers who had children with a life-limiting illness. The fathers reported that the stereotypical social expectation that they be unemotional providers and problem-solvers conflicted with the emotional realities of nurturing and caring for their sick and dying children. And at times these stereotypes were maintained by others such as employers and some health care providers, who downplayed the nurturing caretaking roles in which the fathers engaged. As a result, some fathers felt unsupported and marginalized.

Like natural parents who grieve the death of a child, there is also evidence that foster parents tend to grieve deeply when a child placed in their care dies. Schormans (2004) interviewed foster parents in Ontario who had experienced one or more deaths of disabled foster children placed in their permanent care. The author noted that the foster parents thought of themselves as parents having a parent–child relationship with their disabled foster children. They viewed their foster children as family members and reported that they experienced the death of their disabled foster children as being as difficult as the death of a birth child. Despite the grief they experienced, these foster parents reported that their grief was not always recognized or legitimated but was often disenfranchised and unsupported.

When parents lose a child, grandparents also lose a grandchild. Fry (1997) studied grandparents in Alberta who had lost a grandchild in the previous three years. Fry found that grandparents often reported survivor guilt—that is, they felt that it was their turn to die and that the grandchild should not have died. Furthermore, the grandparents grieved not only for the deceased grandchild but also for their own child who was now a grieving parent. Nevertheless, despite the grief, pain, and guilt that grandparents experience when a grandchild dies, their grief tends to be disenfranchised and overlooked in the emphasis on the grieving parents (Fry 1997; Tatterton and Walshe 2019).

Davidson (2018) made a similar observation about the siblings of a deceased brother or sister: "Bereaved siblings are forgotten mourners" (129) who carry "the double burden of their parents' grief" (130) together with their own grief, which tends to be disenfranchised.

Bolton et al. (2016) studied over 7,000 siblings who were under 18 years of age when their brother or sister died in Manitoba during the 25-year period from 1984 to 2009. The researchers found that the death of a sibling resulted in elevated rates of a wide variety of mental disorders including depression, anxiety, alcohol use, drug use, attention deficit, and suicide attempts in the surviving siblings over the two years following the death of their brother or sister. While a child's death affects families across the social class spectrum, this study in Manitoba also indicated that poverty increased the likelihood that a child would die and that siblings would be more greatly impacted.

There are numerous studies that focus on family members who have experienced the death of a child in the family. These studies explore the grieving of mothers, fathers, siblings, and grandparents. Bartel (2020) pointed out that very few of these studies focus on the family dynamic; that is, on how the family grieves together as a whole unit rather than as individuals grieving separately within a family. For example, Bartel studied several families in the Greater Vancouver area and observed that the family together may develop rituals and mechanisms by which family members collectively share their emotions with each other and maintain an ongoing relationship with their deceased family member. Further, family members collectively may develop or share a frame of meaning that helps them cope with their loss. In a family, members may grieve both separately and together, each individual and each family in its own way.

Death of a Partner

Many marriages end with the death of one of the partners. In heterosexual marriages, the husband is more likely to die before his wife, leaving her a widow. This happens because women have a longer life expectancy than men and tend to be younger than their male partners. Indeed, in Canada in 2019 there were nearly four widows for every widower (Statistics Canada 2020k). Widowhood typically occurs in the older years, and the likelihood of being a widow or widower increases with age (Novak, Northcott, and Kobayashi 2021).

The death of a partner tends to be experienced as a particularly stressful event. Indeed, widowhood increases the likelihood of dying—an effect that is more pronounced for widowers than widows and for younger widowed persons than older widowed persons (Shor et al. 2012). Ennis and Majid (2019) refer to the increased risk of mortality following spousal loss as the "widowhood effect." In some cases, however, a widowed person may view the death of a spouse as a positive thing, as in the case of a death following a long terminal illness, or the death of an alcoholic, abusive, or mentally-ill spouse (Martin Matthews 1991; Watford 2008).

Waskowic and Chartier (2003) showed that the nature of the spousal relationship before the death of a partner affects the experience of grief for the surviving partner. In particular, people who had been securely attached to their

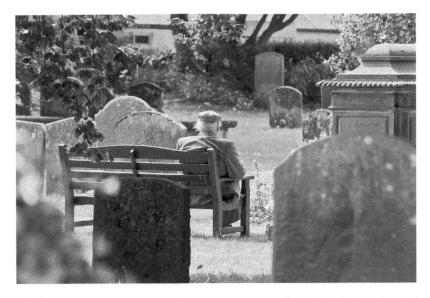

Image 6.2. Many widows and widowers go to cemeteries with their thoughts and memories
Source: Leadinglights/iStock.com.

partner before their partner's death experienced more moderate symptoms of grief, were better able to resolve their grief, and maintained a better ongoing relationship with the deceased. Interestingly, Belicki et al. (2003) suggested that dreaming about the deceased partner may express and help to maintain the ongoing relationship between the surviving partner and the deceased.

Widowhood is more expected later in life than early in life, although widowhood is now somewhat less common at any age than it was several decades ago (Martin Matthews 1987, 1991, 2011). There is a complicated relationship between the timing of widowhood (i.e., early or late in life), the anticipation of the partner's death (i.e., whether widowhood is expected or not), the intensity of grief, and the resolution of the grieving process. Some evidence indicates that widowhood is most stressful when it is unexpected and occurs early in life (Martin Matthews 1991). Further, women who are widowed when they are older may find that widowhood is less disruptive to their sense of identity and self-image in contrast to women who are widowed when they are younger (van den Hoonaard 1999). Nevertheless, the death of a partner in old age can jeopardize a life that depends on two people cohabitating and assisting each other in managing life in old age.

In marriage, partners tend to develop a shared identity and a shared life. The loss of a partner undermines this shared identity and transforms the life of the surviving partner (Lowe and McClement 2010–11). Furthermore, the social status of the surviving partner is devalued, even stigmatized to a degree. Widowhood may be psychologically and socially disorienting. Adjustment for many widowed people—both male and female—tends to occur within several years. Some see widowhood as an opportunity for growth and also a time for autonomy, independence, and freedom (Gee and Kimball 1987; Martin Matthews 1991, 2011; van den Hoonaard 2001).

Many older partners will become caregivers for their aging partners while they deal with cancer, for example. Many of these same family caregivers will also experience the death of their partners and will have to adjust to being alone. Studies of older widowed individuals in Saskatchewan who had been caregivers for their spouses dying from cancer have shown that widowed people face several challenges during the first year of bereavement (Holtslander, Bally, and Steeves 2011; Holtslander and Duggleby 2009, 2010). These challenges include personal, relationship, and social issues such as grief, exhaustion, and loneliness; adjusting to life alone, relying on social support, and dealing with difficult relationships; finding a new identity and role as a widowed person; and dealing with housing and financial concerns. The widowed people spoke about "losing a part of yourself," "striking out alone," and needing to "find [their] way." These widowed individuals were concerned about losing control and losing hope and attempted to gain a sense of balance by "walking a fine line" between positive and negative emotions, hope and despair. The ultimate challenge was to find meaning and purpose again.

Widowhood may affect men and women differently. Women are more likely than men to be economically disadvantaged by the loss of their partner. Further, men and women often have different coping strategies and tend to have different social support networks, which they access differently. Although it may be experienced somewhat differently, the loss of a partner may be equally difficult for both men and women (see Martin Matthews 1991, 89; Norris 1994). Nevertheless, Martin Matthews (2011) cautioned against the tendency to over-problematize widowhood. She noted that many adjust with relatively little difficulty to the death of their spouse.

Van den Hoonaard (1997) analyzed published autobiographical accounts of widowhood written by widows. Most of the widows in this study had experienced widowhood while still relatively young, and most of the authors lost their husbands after long illnesses. The stories of their marriages and the deaths of their husbands were integral parts of these stories of widowhood, indicating what was lost and how it was lost. Despite long dying trajectories and the anticipation of death, these women all experienced shock at the time of their husbands' deaths.

Because these accounts were written for an audience, mostly other widows, they are both descriptive and instructive. That is, the stories are descriptive personal accounts with which a reader can empathize, and at the same time they provide guidance for a reader who is seeking to know what to do in a similar situation.

Van den Hoonaard's (1997) analysis of these accounts of widowhood yields common themes relating to loss of identity and its reconstruction. In a process that van den Hoonaard calls **identity foreclosure**, the loss of the husband and of social interactions (including friendships) that depended on being a couple undermined the widow's sense of self. At the death of the husband, the old identity as a wife and as a couple became obsolete. The widows described themselves as neither knowing who they were nor how they fit into society. A new identity as a widow was thrust upon them, an identity that was not chosen, not welcomed, and that was perceived as a devalued social status. Being called a widow or filling out a form and having to select "widow" for one's marital status for the first time became **identifying moments** in which the wife's new status as a widow was often shockingly and painfully driven home. In these moments, the widows came to know that their identity had been transformed and that they were viewed differently by society. They were made to feel that they were different, and they were treated differently in a couples-oriented society.

According to van den Hoonaard (1997), the transformation of identity is a process in which the individual's previous identity as a wife is lost and replaced with the socially imposed identity of a widow. The loss of the old identity is disorienting, and the imposition of the new identity is distressing. In time, however, a new and positive identity is created. The authors of these stories tend to describe themselves as becoming "new women" with new characteristics, such as greater self-reliance and increased independence.

Women who are widowed when they are older may be less likely to experience identity foreclosure and may find widowhood less threatening to their self-image, according to van den Hoonaard (1999, 2001), who interviewed widows over 50 years of age in New Brunswick whose husbands had died within the past five years. Van den Hoonaard (1999, 69) noted that these older widows readily volunteered to tell their husbands' death stories and that these stories and the telling of them seemed to provide comfort and meaning regarding "their sense of themselves and their lives as widows." These women, in part through the telling of their husbands' death stories, were able to hold on to their identity as wives, maintain a positive self-image, and facilitate their transition into widowhood.

Van den Hoonaard (2010) followed her studies of widows in Atlantic Canada with a study of widowers. While a woman can expect to be widowed, a man expects to die before his wife. Widowerhood, then, is unexpected, relatively uncommon, and socially ambiguous. While the status and role of a widow is more clearly defined, van den Hoonaard argued that this is not the case for widowers. Van den Hoonaard points out that a woman might be known as John's wife before John's death and John's widow afterwards. In contrast, a man, even if identified as Mary's husband before Mary's death, is not defined as Mary's widower afterwards. It appears that widowerhood is a socially ambiguous status for both the widower and society.

Van den Hoonaard's (2010) accounts of the widowers she interviewed in Atlantic Canada emphasized the efforts these men made to claim and preserve their masculinity. The men described caring for their wives during their illnesses as "doing what needed to be done." This statement was a justification and explanation acknowledging that what they were doing as caregivers was outside of the traditional male role. They focused on what they did rather than what they felt. The stories they told of their wives' deaths were often brief and matter-of-fact (van den Hoonaard, Bennett, and Evans 2014). In widowerhood, the widowers minimized their new roles of cooking and cleaning ("women's work") and emphasized the masculine values of independence and self-reliance along with keeping busy and going out—strategies for avoiding loneliness and self-pity. One way of getting out of the house involved meeting other men regularly at the local Tim Horton's coffee shop. While the widowers spoke of repartnering, they also tended to be ambivalent about this. The loneliness of widowerhood had the advantage of freedom and independence, reflecting masculine ideals. Nevertheless, repartnering also spoke to masculine ideals, and these widowers often began new romantic relationships.

The widowers in van den Hoonaard's study had typically relied on their wives to mediate relationships with family members and friends. After the deaths of their wives, the widowers often found that they no longer fit comfortably in the social world of couples. Further, they found that they had to negotiate and redefine their relationships with their adult children.

Sometimes a spouse has a "brush with death" that leads the spouse's partner to contemplate the possibility of widowhood or widowerhood. For example, a woman in her thirties related to the first author her reaction to her husband's brush with death:

> I have been married to my husband for 15 years. My husband spends about 50 per cent of the year out of the country on business, leaving me and our three children alone to cope without a husband or a father. Needless to say, I have become a part-time single parent. I have gotten used to this over the years, but never did I think that part-time single parenting could potentially become full-time single parenting. Last week my husband had a brush with death that would have left me a widow and our three children without a father.
>
> My husband travels frequently to Taiwan on business, experiencing small earthquakes on almost all of his trips. So, I didn't get too hysterical when I was told of another earthquake in Taiwan, this time registering 7.6 on the Richter scale. My friend, who informed me of the most recent Taiwan earthquake, was surprised that I was so calm. She wondered if I was in a state of shock. But I knew that what you heard on the radio or saw on TV was the worst damage caused by the earthquake and that my husband was probably just fine. Meanwhile, my husband left a voicemail on our answering machine that he was alive and well.
>
> When I received his message, I returned his call immediately. I was relieved to hear that he was well but didn't really expect that I would hear any differently. My husband told me to call all our family to let them know that he was fine should they watch the evening news and panic. Being in the middle of the day, most of our family members were working, so I just left messages on their answering machines. My voice was cheerful and reassuring. But when I got a live person on the end of the phone, that's when my whole outlook changed.
>
> When I talked to my husband's sister, I fell apart. She started the conversation by asking (as she always does), "How are you?" That's when it happened. I fell apart. I could hardly get a word out. I was crying uncontrollably. I could hardly speak between sobs. I guess it was at that point in time that I realized I could have been a widow at a very young age. I wasn't prepared to be a widow and a single mother of three children. The possibility of becoming a widow was terrifying. I was used to being alone and a part-time single mother, but I always knew that this

was a temporary situation. In a few days or weeks, my husband would be arriving home and we would share the parenting role once more. It took about 10 minutes before I gained some sort of composure.

Within minutes another one of my friends phoned. Once again, my tears took me by surprise. So why was this happening now? I concluded that it must be because at the time I was talking to my husband, I was just grateful that he was all right. I didn't really think about the "what ifs?" I didn't really think about potentially becoming a widow until I started talking to more and more people.

This emotional period was short-lived. In the end, I realize that I have no time or energy to dwell on the "what ifs," and therefore my fleeting thoughts of widowhood were just that, fleeting.

At first, the storyteller cognitively assesses the odds of her husband being killed in the earthquake and concludes confidently and unemotionally that everything is most likely all right. Concern expressed by others, however, cues her and leads her to re-evaluate her own level of concern—to consider the "what ifs," as she puts it. This draws out an intense, although brief, emotional reaction.

Why did the "what ifs" upset her? A family is a set of relationships, roles, circumstances, and patterns, and all of these are disrupted by the death of one of its members. In this story, the person who might have been killed occupies the roles of husband and father, roles that would have been vacated and left unfilled by his death. The family's circumstances and patterns would have been disrupted, and the survivors' roles and social statuses would have been transformed—from wife to widow, from part of a parenting couple to a single parent, and from children with a father to fatherless children. These transformations were things that the storyteller had not really considered previously, was not prepared for, and found terrifying. Death is disruptive. While death is the final disruption of the life of the deceased, death also disrupts the lives of the surviving family members. The family, as it had been, no longer exists. The family is transformed, and the survivors have to adjust to a new life.

Death of a Parent

The preceding storyteller describes her husband's brush with death and her thoughts about being left a widow. The storyteller's two eldest daughters, aged 12 and 13, also described their reactions to the question "What if my dad had died?" Nina (name has been changed), aged 12, wrote:

> As my mom was explaining that my dad was in a near-death experience (Taiwan earthquake), the question "What if my dad were to die" flashed through my mind. Shortly after she was done talking and said that my dad was all right, I stopped thinking about it. I thought about the question for about one minute, and after that I thought about it a bit occasionally, but after I found out he was okay all the questions just slowly disappeared. Although I only thought about it a little while, I still cared just as much as someone who couldn't get their mind off it.

While the question "What if my dad were to die?" flashed into her mind, Nina was quickly reassured. Her dad was safe, so there was no reason to get upset. She did not dwell on what might have happened but instead focused only on what did happen. Her last comment suggests slight defensiveness, as if she felt that she might be criticized for her reaction. However, she saw no reason for concern, reminding the reader that this does not mean that she does not care.

This is a 12-year-old's honest report of her reaction and, at the same time, an acknowledgment of her awareness that others may have expectations about how she should react. As people age, it perhaps becomes increasingly difficult to distinguish one's unique personal reactions from one's socialized reactions that reflect one's understanding of society's expectations.

In contrast, Nina's 13-year-old sister, Mackenzie (name has been changed), also gave her thoughts on the question "What if my dad had died?" She wrote:

> A million questions went through my mind at that time. Such as, how big was this earthquake? How many lives did it take? I was relieved that my dad was all right but couldn't help but wonder how many kids had lost their dads. . . . I feel bad for people that lost someone close to them.
>
> "What if my dad had died?" That is a question that I thought about a little more than once. It was weird to think my dad wouldn't come home after work and say hello to all of us. Or that I would never get to spend time with him again or even talk with him because he would be gone. The last words that I said to my dad were to go away and turn off the lights. I said that because it was, like, 6:00 a.m. and I was half asleep. If my dad were to die, then I wouldn't want those to be my last words to him. That was probably what I thought about the most.

Mackenzie, like her sister, is quickly reassured that her dad is fine and sees no reason to get upset. Nevertheless, she identifies and sympathizes with children who did lose their fathers. She acknowledges that, if her dad had died, it would have been "weird"—her life would have been transformed by the loss of both her father and the familiar pattern of her relationship with him. She would also have regrets. For example, she would regret the last words that she said to him when he woke her early in the morning to say goodbye as he left for his business trip. Mackenzie recognizes that the loss of a loved one implies not only the loss of a relationship but also the loss of the familiar and the necessity of adjusting to a new and unanticipated life.

Silverman, Nickman, and Worden (1995) studied children who had recently lost a parent to death. They found that the children constructed connections to the deceased that helped them maintain a relationship with their dead parent. Five things helped in this process. First, the children tended to locate their dead parent, often in heaven. Second, they experienced the deceased in dreams or in feelings, for example, by feeling that the parent was watching them. Third, they reached out to the dead parent by visiting the cemetery or by speaking to the deceased. Fourth, they thought about and remembered the parent. Finally, they held on to certain objects that served as reminders of the deceased. The authors found that while the connection that the child constructs with the deceased parent tends to evolve over time, it does not end. They wrote, "Bereavement should not be viewed as a psychological state that ends or from which one recovers. The emphasis should be on negotiating and renegotiating the meaning of loss over time, rather than on letting go" (269).

Schultz (2007) interviewed young women in Western Canada whose mothers had died when they were 15–20 years of age. The loss of a mother in adolescence tended to redefine the daughter's life and influenced her sense of self. For example, the daughters in this study tended to demarcate their lives before and after their mothers' deaths: there was life before when one was cared for by one's mother and life after when one had to take care of oneself. Further, the daughters tended to report feeling different from their peers and had a sense of inferiority as a result. While these young women often formed attachments with mother substitutes (such as an aunt or a friend's mother), their memories of their deceased mothers also continued to shape their developing sense of self. They were defined, in part, by their mothers' lives and their mothers' deaths. That is, the lives and deaths of their mothers became both a part of their own life history and an integral part of their developing identity.

Apelian and Nesteruk (2017) interviewed young adults in Montreal and New Jersey who had experienced the death of a parent when they were teenagers. The young adults commented on the accumulation of stressors following their parent's death including financial issues, household responsibilities, and dealing with grief. They noted that their parent's death ended their childhood and forced them into adulthood. They spoke of the importance of social support from the surviving parent, siblings, extended family members, and friends. They coped by focusing on schoolwork, relying on friends, and isolating themselves at times when they felt the need to grieve privately. Despite the many and significant difficulties of losing a parent prematurely, the young adults generally reported that over time they had adapted positively.

Most often, though, the death of a parent occurs when the child has grown into an adult or even into old age. Note that if a parent dies at 75 years of age, their child may be in their fifties. If a parent dies at 95 years of age, their child may be in their seventies. The loss of a parent, and in particular the death of the last parent, can have profound meaning for children who are middle-aged or older. The buffer between them and death is no longer there (Colarusso 1999; Hadad 2009; Moss, Resch, and Moss 1997). As such, the death of a parent has additional meanings and implications beyond the grief that is experienced for the deceased parent. To this point, the first author of this book recalls the funeral of his father-in-law's mother. His father-in-law had said that his mother's funeral was particularly difficult for him, given that his father had died previously and now his mother was dead and, as he put it, "Now I am next."

A former student of the first author wrote about her mother's and grandmother's deaths in Alberta. She said:

> Mom's and Gran's deaths were two of the most profound experiences of my life.
>
> My mom let us know in early May that her prognosis wasn't good in her three-year battle with ovarian cancer. We thought we had months, like at least the summer, but it turned out to be less. I got to spend a couple of precious weeks with my mom in palliative care in the hospital in [city]. She passed on June 1st and we were privileged to be able to get so much time with her in hospital during a pandemic [COVID-19].
>
> We were faced with care directives and working towards the provision of a "good death"; or what we considered a "good death" with my mother's wishes as the driving force. We stayed overnight with her, made sure she wasn't alone, advocated for her care wishes, read books, played music, had family members say goodbye via iPhone. . . .
>
> I spent six straight nights in hospital with my mom leading up to her death and my sister was with us for the final three nights. The last night

that Mom was on this earth we smuggled in home-popped popcorn and drinks for a late-night "Happy Hour." My sister brought a tiny travel bottle of Moscato which was my Mom's favourite wine, dipped one of the mouth care sponges in it and popped it in her mouth to suck.

My dad had tagged me off for dinner. A half hour later, she passed while he held her hand and happily chatted away about the latest family communications and what her cats were up to.

I will never stop missing my mom and I will never be able to fill the void her death has created in my life, but I am able to turn my perspectives to appreciation and gratitude.

The same student also described the death of her grandmother that had occurred years previously. She wrote:

My devout Catholic grandma died in the presence of her daughters, daughter-in-law, granddaughters and great granddaughters all around her bedside with hands on her as a chaplain sang *Ave Maria* in the [name of] Hospital.

The student concluded that "a good death is possible in certain circumstances."

Death of a Grandparent

Ens and Bond (2005) surveyed 226 adolescents in Manitoba who were 11–18 years of age. The authors found that 61 per cent had experienced the death of one or more family members (1 mother, 6 fathers, 7 siblings, and 183 grandparents), including 55 per cent who had experienced only the death of one or more grandparents and no other family members. This study determined that adolescents who reported grief brought on by the death of a grandparent reported higher levels of anxiety about death compared to adolescents who had not experienced the death of a family member. It would appear that an experience with death in the family may raise fears among young people about death.

Death of a Friend

A young adult woman was asked by the first author if she had had any experience with dying and death. She answered with the following account about the death of a school acquaintance:

When you first asked if I had experienced death in my life, I initially thought of family situations, of which I have no close experiences. It surprised me when I remembered that a friend, Joyce, died when I was in high school. For all the time that I had known her she had leukemia. We met in junior high school when her family moved [to the city] to be closer to the hospitals for her sake. She never really seemed sick. Except for the initial rumours that circulated when she first came to our school, none of us really thought about it much.

I got to know her well in high school as we had English class together. We talked about a lot of things, including her illness. I remember her being a lot of fun and very strong willed. During that same year her cancer started to progress. I don't really know all of the medical things that were happening to her. Some friends and I went to visit her in the hospital; she seemed in great spirits. We never really thought that anything bad was really happening. We all got sick; we all got better.

Things progressed pretty quickly. She slipped into a coma and was put into intensive care. Then we arrived at school one day and her closest friend came up to us in tears and we knew that she had died. The first class I had that day was English. During the announcements they informed us that she had died, and we had a moment of silence. One girl in the class started sobbing, and I remember a guy in the back saying something like, "I don't know why she's crying, she didn't even know her." I didn't cry. I remember wondering why since I had known her pretty well. I continued going to classes through the day until someone told me that people who had known Joyce were in the guidance counsellor's office. I went because I wanted to make sure that some of my other friends were okay. A number of them met me in the hall because they had been looking for me. Many were crying, but I still wasn't.

It was very surreal. None of us really knew what to do. We decided that we should go to the funeral home. So, the night before the funeral, we decided to go together. One thing that sticks out clearly in my mind was that we did not know what we were supposed to do. It was strange because Joyce's mom was the one that took us under her wing and led us into the room where the casket was laying.

The casket was closed because she had wasted [away] a great deal and the family thought it would be better. As we stood around the casket, I was wishing that the casket was open so that I could really believe that she was gone. It was difficult to really believe it. I stared at the picture of Joyce on the casket and thought over and over again how it was her lying inside, that we would not see her again. That was when the tears started to come. It was overwhelming. I don't think I had ever really sobbed in my life, but I was right there in front of a bunch of strangers, but I wasn't thinking about that at all. My crying touched off the rest, so the five or six of us stood there sobbing our hearts out for a good long time. Joyce's mom and aunt were comforting us. They seemed to want to take care of us.

One of our friends had experienced death in her family a great deal more than the rest of us. We looked to her for guidance. There was a kneeling bench in front of the casket, so I whispered to ask her if it was for praying. I knelt and prayed for Joyce's family and for us. After our tears had dried up, we went to the lounge and talked together. I think everyone felt very badly for us. We decided to go back to my house together because my parents were away. We just wanted to be together for a while. We just talked, watched some TV, and played Twister. I think we wanted to laugh. We talked about Joyce a bit but mostly we chatted about nothing.

The next day was the funeral. I had a lot of anxiety because the only nice clothes I had were light colours and I thought that was sacrilegious, but I wore them anyway. I remember a lot of detail from that day even though it was seven years ago. I remember Joyce's mother, brother, and sisters coming in along with Joyce's boyfriend. I remember the minister's eulogy, how we laughed at Joyce's aggressive basketball skills but also reminisced about her tender concern for others. Everything about the funeral was new to me. I think it was the very first funeral I had ever been to. Again, I didn't cry. I think that [may have been seen] as a sign that I didn't really care but it was more that I don't cry very often. The outpouring at the funeral home was a great shock to me.

The reception seemed strange to me. To be sitting around eating, laughing, joking, chitchatting while Joyce was dead. It was awkward for me. After the funeral we talked about Joyce less and less. I would think of her in English class, wishing she was there so we could gossip in the back row, but life went back to normal quickly for us. When there was a write-up about Joyce in our graduating yearbook, two years after she died, I wondered why it was there. Nobody seemed to remember her. She would have accomplished a lot in her life; she had accomplished a lot by the time she died at 15. I suppose some of that came from knowing that she had a terminal illness.

I'm not sure how much of my grief was for Joyce and how much was over the fact that someone my age was dead. Her opportunities were over. As I think about all this now I am wondering "what if." What if she had lived to be 23 years old, as I have? What would she be doing now? Would she be proud of me? Have I used the years wisely that she didn't have? It's hard to think about those things; perhaps that was why she was so far from my consciousness when we discussed my experience with death.

The storyteller, who faced dying and death for the first time in her relatively young life, speaks of the strangeness of dying and death. At first the schoolmate who died is not perceived to be sick, despite her terminal illness, and the storyteller indicates that nobody really thought of the possibility of her dying. Even when the girl is obviously sick in the hospital, her schoolmates still assume that she will recover. Death is neither known nor understood; it is a stranger to these young people.

When death does come, the storyteller describes the situation as surreal, as dreamlike and without context. Accordingly, Joyce's schoolmates did not know what to do. Once again, death is described in terms of its strangeness. Those who were not experienced looked for guidance to the one schoolmate who had experience with death.

The storyteller speaks of her and her friends' intense, though brief, outpouring of grief at the funeral home, the night before the funeral. She notes that this was out of character for her and that she was shocked at her emotional display. Leming and Dickinson (2007, 346–7) similarly observed that funeral rituals "become **rites of intensification** whereby feelings and emotional states are intensified by ritual participation. . . . Oftentimes the function of death rituals is to intensify feelings and emotions and then provide a means by which individuals can express their sentiments." This seems to have been the case for Joyce's friends as they gathered at the funeral home. Furthermore, while the grief expressed was because of Joyce's death, it seems to have also been occasioned by a loss of naivety—by the realization that a young person can die and that so much unlived life can be lost. The moral taken from the story focuses on the value of life and the importance of living life wisely.

Finally, the salience of another's death tends to recede from active consciousness as survivors get on with the business of everyday life. While the story of Joyce is not a memory that the storyteller visits every day, it was nevertheless a significant event, a socializing event in the sense of providing instruction about dying and death, and a memory that the storyteller calls upon when she thinks of dying and death and their meaning for her.

Young men tend to react to the death of a friend differently than young women. Social constructions of femininity and masculinity shape and constrain young women's and young men's reactions to the death of a friend. Creighton et al. (2013) interviewed young men in Vancouver who had experienced the death of male friends to motor vehicle accidents, drug overdoses, sports injuries, or fighting. They found that experiences and expressions of male grief were influenced by ethnocultural and socioeconomic backgrounds. For example, young men socialized in Euro-Canadian culture tended to focus on ideals of masculinity that emphasized stoicism and emotional restraint to a greater degree than did young men socialized in immigrant cultures. Nevertheless, masculine ideals tended to cut across cultures and classes. The young men often reported a feeling of emptiness when learning of the death of their friends and tended to withdraw and isolate themselves to avoid social situations that might trigger un-masculine emotional responses like crying. In contrast, anger was one of the few emotions that men were allowed to express. For some, their friend's deaths were a wake-up call and led them to focus on living up to masculine ideals of being strong, caring, and responsible. For other young men, the deaths led to a fatalistic response and continued risk taking.

Creighton et al. (2016) noted that following a friend's death, young men in Vancouver and Whistler often used alcohol to deal with their grief. Soon after learning of their friend's death, young men often drank to excess, with a goal of getting drunk. They did this to "dull the pain" but paradoxically at the same time to express their sorrow. Drinking together allowed them to express their feelings in a manner that did not undermine their masculinity. Getting drunk in public with friends was deemed more therapeutic than meeting formally with trained professionals. Some continued to use alcohol on an ongoing basis to manage their emotions. While drinking helped to bond survivors together in the short term, drinking to suppress feelings over the long term was isolating and undermined the drinkers' ability to cope.

TRAUMATIC DEATH

Sudden and unexpected death can have a different impact on survivors compared to anticipated death that comes at the end of a protracted illness (Leming and Dickinson 2016, 511; Marchenski 2004). DeSpelder and Strickland

(2011, 361) noted that "how a person dies affects a survivor's grief." They observed that accidental death, death from natural disaster, and death by suicide or homicide tend to have different effects on survivors than death from cancer or Alzheimer's disease; that is, sudden death tends to be more shocking and tends to heighten the grief reaction. Furthermore, survivors of the sudden **traumatic death** of a significant other often find it harder to make sense of the death of their loved one. Similarly, experiencing terrorism, war, genocide, or death caused by a pandemic disease (such as COVID-19) can lead to post-traumatic stress and survivor guilt.

Traumatic death undermines survivors' confidence that the world is safe and meaningful (Kastenbaum 2009). Hadad (2009, 151) noted that sudden, unexpected, or violent death leaves "the survivors not only with grief but also with a shock to their entire sense of reality and world view." A recurring theme focuses on the problem of finding meaning in life and making death at the end of life meaningful. From an existential point of view, the fundamental problem concerns how one makes sense of what seems inherently senseless. Traumatic death to a greater degree than expected death undermines a person's sense that life is meaningful. The following is a brief discussion of the impact of traumatic death, including accidental death; natural disaster; suicide; homicide; terrorism, war, and genocide; and death during a **pandemic**.

Accidental Death

The most common accidental causes of death include motor vehicle accidents, falls, drowning, and poisoning. Accidents may result from individual human error; for example, when a person fails to stop for a red traffic light or falls while mountain climbing. Accidents may also constitute a human-made disaster affecting numerous individuals simultaneously, as in the mine disaster discussed below.

A Mine Disaster. The Westray mine disaster in 1992 in Nova Scotia resulted in the death of 26 men. Eight years later, Davis, Harasymchuk, and Wohl (2012) interviewed family members of 16 of the men who were killed in the explosion. The authors noted that coping with traumatic events is both an individual and a social process. In particular, family members often constructed shared stories and interpretations. Family members searched for meaning both individually and collectively. Moreover, family members who interpreted the mine disaster and the deaths of their family members in similar fashion tended to report less depression and better adjustment, indicating the importance of social support and shared perspectives in coping with traumatic death.

Workplace Death. Matthews, Quinlan, and Bohle (2019) surveyed surviving family members after the traumatic workplace death of a family member. These researchers found that family members had high rates of post-traumatic stress disorder, major depressive disorder, and prolonged grief disorder, especially if they felt they could not obtain adequate information about the death and felt that there was a lack of support for the bereaved family.

A Train Derailment Tragedy. In 2013, a train derailed in Lac-Mégantic, Quebec, causing 47 deaths and destroying much of the town. Généreux et al. (2019) reported two surveys done one year and two years later. They concluded that there were substantial ongoing psychosocial effects in the community including relatively high rates of psychological distress, depression, anxiety disorders, and post-traumatic stress symptoms.

Motor Vehicle Collision. Bolton et al. (2014) examined the health care records of parents who had experienced the death of a child in a motor vehicle collision (MVC) in Manitoba from 1996 to 2008. A total of 801 deaths were identified. The average age at death was 27 years, with about one in four dying before the age of 19 years. The average age of the bereaved parents was 55 years. The authors compared illness rates for the bereaved parents two years before the death of their offspring and two years after. In addition, the authors compared the bereaved parents to other parents who had not experienced the death of a child in an MVC. In the two years following the death of their child, the bereaved parents had higher rates of depression, anxiety, and marital breakup compared to the two years before the death of their child, as well as higher rates compared to parents who had not experienced the death of a child in an MVC. Following their child's death, 31 per cent of parents were diagnosed with depression and 22 per cent with anxiety. Note that these statistics report formal clinical diagnoses and indicate that psychological distress rises considerably for parents following the death of a child of any age in an MVC.

Death from Natural Disaster

Natural disasters include earthquakes, landslides, tsunamis, floods, storms, hurricanes, tornados, volcanic eruptions, and forest fires. DeSpelder and Strickland (2011) observed that survivors of natural disasters tend to experience survivor guilt, wondering why they survived when others died. Survivor guilt indicates that the survivors are struggling to make sense of a world that now seems capricious and malevolent.

Burton et al. (2016) reviewed studies of the health effects of flooding in Canada. They found that there was a wide variety of effects including post-traumatic stress disorder (PTSD), anxiety, and depression. These results indicate the vulnerability of individuals and communities to psychological distress when their sense of security is disrupted by seemingly capricious natural events. Fulton and Drolet (2018) pointed out that the effects of a major flood in Southern Alberta in 2013 affected individuals, families, and communities and that an adequate response focused on both individual and community. Natural disasters create trauma at both the individual and collective levels (Erikson 1976). Individual suffering is compounded when a supportive community is also disrupted.

On 31 July 1987, an F5 tornado hit Edmonton, killing 27 people and injuring over 300 more. On its 10-year anniversary, this event, known as Black Friday, was noted in the media, which offered a review of the events of that day in 1987, reflections on the cataclysmic event and its aftermath, and education about how to prepare for and deal with future events (Blanchard-Boehm and Cook 2004, 2015). Similarly, in 2020 the news media in Alberta recalled the F3 tornado that ripped through a campground at the Pine Lake recreation area in central Alberta 20 years previously on 14 July 2000, killing 12 people and injuring over 130 others (Sookram et al. 2001). These events become part of the collective memory of the respective communities and are recalled from time to time, in particular, on anniversary dates. They serve as a reminder of the vulnerability, losses, and strengths of a community in dealing with cataclysmic events and mass deaths.

Suicide

In contrast to an expected death from natural causes, the loved ones of a person who has died by suicide may blame themselves, wondering if they could have done more to prevent the suicide. Furthermore, others may blame the loved ones of a person who has died by suicide (DeSpelder and Strickland 2011, 363). For example, others may blame a husband whose wife has died by suicide or blame the parents of a child who has died by suicide. Grief, guilt, and anger become intertwined in the survivors' response to suicide.

Powell and Matthys (2013) observed that uncertainty tends to surround suicide and makes grieving more difficult for survivors. These authors interviewed the brothers and sisters of people who had died by suicide. For some, the reason their sibling had killed themself was known. Knowing "why" meant less uncertainty and reduced the tendency for survivors to blame themselves and have feelings of guilt. These survivors seemed to manage their grief more effectively. For other siblings, the suicide was unexpected, unexplained, and came as a shock. This high level of uncertainty tended to drive the survivors to seek information to reduce uncertainty, in part to determine if they could have prevented the suicide. Gaining an understanding of the reasons "why" reduced uncertainty, guilt, and anger, and facilitated grieving. However, some survivors recognized that they would never be able to answer all of the questions surrounding particular suicides. These survivors tended to experience high levels of uncertainty or varying levels of uncertainty from day to day and vacillated between acceptance on the one hand and guilt and anger on the other. A few found the question "why" distressing and avoided it altogether, preferring uncertainty instead of the challenges involved in seeking answers.

While it seems to be the case that parents never completely recover from the suicide of a child, Grant Kalischuk and Hayes (2003) suggested that a degree of "healing" is possible, even in the case of a youthful family member's suicide. Healing was defined in their study as "letting go of the negative impact of the suicide and achieving a sense of health and well being" (59). These authors interviewed parents and other family members of nine males who had died by suicide between the ages of 14 and 19 and of another two males who had died by suicide at the ages of 24 and 29. The families lived in rural and small urban communities in three Western Canadian provinces. Most of the suicides had occurred from six months to four years previously, although one suicide had occurred six years before and another 12 years before. Parents and family members spoke of being wounded by the suicide of their relatively young family member and of wishing to regain a sense of normalcy and wholeness. This healing process—or "journeying toward wholeness," as the authors labelled it—was facilitated by letting go of the question "why" regarding the deceased's motivations for committing suicide, releasing the survivors from responsibility for their family member's suicide, and believing that healing was possible and making a conscious decision to move toward healing.

Homicide

DeSpelder and Strickland (2011) observed that the loved ones of a homicide victim tend to have difficulty making sense of a world that has been made to seem chaotic, dangerous, unjust, and senseless. Furthermore, police homicide investigations and criminal justice proceedings tend to last a long time and make it difficult for loved ones to achieve a resolution for their grief. Indeed, grief precipitated by homicide and other trauma may be more intense and longer lasting and may never be fully resolved.

Yet Hadad (2009) noted that survivors have someone to blame when a loved one dies because of the actions of another, as in the case of homicide. This is a contrast to both expected and unexpected deaths from natural causes where there is no one that can be held responsible. Traumatic deaths caused by others who can be held culpable are especially difficult for survivors. Hadad (2009, 152) asked "how much harder might it be when we know that the person we loved did not have to die, that his or her life was taken by someone else, suddenly, unexpectedly, and maybe arbitrarily?" The survivors have to deal with traumatic loss, the undermining of their view that the world is relatively safe and just, the media that may sensationalize and misrepresent the death, and the justice system that may seem ineffective (Hadad 2009). As a result, the survivors tend to experience heightened distress and grief, including anger, depression, a sense of meaninglessness, and ironically self-blame (guilt) when survivors wonder if there isn't something they could have done to keep their loved one safe.

Terrorism, War, and Genocide

The 2008 Canadian movie *Passchendaele* captures the horrors of war and the capricious nature of death in war. The Battle of Passchendaele, in which thousands of Canadians were wounded or killed, is illustrative of the wholesale slaughter of the First World War.

DeSpelder and Strickland (2011, 497) stated that the reaction of survivors to war, terrorism, and genocide include "such symptoms as numbness, irritability, depression, relationship problems, and survivor's guilt," all of which signify post-traumatic stress disorder. In the context of twentieth-century wars, this pattern of symptoms had been previously labelled "battle fatigue" and "shell-shock." However, PTSD can affect not only military combatants, but also nonmilitary survivors of terrorism, war, and genocide.

Perhaps the most famous case of PTSD in Canada is the experience of General Roméo Dallaire (see Dallaire 2003). General Dallaire was the commander of the United Nations (UN) mission in Rwanda when civil war broke out in 1994, resulting in the genocide of 800,000 Rwandans in the short span

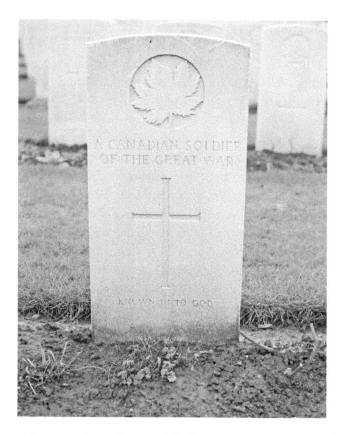

Image 6.3. The grave of an unknown soldier from a Canadian regiment who died in the First World War, fighting in Belgium
Source: Mark2481/Shutterstock.

of 100 days. Following the war, General Dallaire suffered very publicly from PTSD, devastated by the horrors he had witnessed and by the failure of the UN mission to prevent or stop the genocide. Dallaire wrote that after his return to Canada from Rwanda in 1994, he "plunged into a disastrous mental health spiral that led me to suicide attempts, a medical release from the Armed Forces, the diagnosis of PTSD, and dozens upon dozens of therapy sessions and extensive medication . . . It took me seven years to finally have the desire, the willpower and the stamina to begin to describe in detail the events of that year in Rwanda" (5).

It is common to refer to the "horrors" of war. The horrors are many, including mutilation, death, the stench of decay, and so much more. The very term "horror" implies trauma, a disturbing experience beyond the ordinary, a disturbance so great that it has the potential to overwhelm and destabilize. Not everyone who experiences the traumatic death of another person or persons (whether in war or in life more generally) experiences PTSD, but it is certainly understandable that many do. There is a lesson in this. Most of us are more vulnerable than we care to admit. Death, especially traumatic death, points to our vulnerability, a vulnerability that is emotional and existential. Death has the potential to undermine systems of meaning in which we find a sense of security. Senseless traumatic death can make the world seem senseless and undermine our feelings of security and confidence. These emotional and cognitive wounds can have consequences that are as great as or greater than the physical wounds that soldiers and civilians may have experienced.

Canada has not been immune to terrorism. On 23 June 1985, Air India Flight 182 from Toronto to Delhi was blown out of the air over the Atlantic Ocean near the coast of Ireland killing all 329 persons on board, including 280 Canadian citizens, most of Indian ancestry. Over a third of the dead were children and entire families were lost (Failler 2009; Ribkoff 2012). This is the largest mass murder in Canadian history. Eventually a man from British Columbia was convicted of the crime of creating the suitcase bomb that eventually made its way onto Flight 182. The bomber was possibly motivated by involvement in a separatist movement seeking an independent Sikh state in India (Failler 2009). A Government of Canada inquiry began 21 years later! And 22 years later, public memorials were created in Toronto and Vancouver.

Failler (2009) asked why this horrendous tragedy had been largely overlooked in Canada for so long. One might speculate that it did not find a place in the national imagination because it involved Canada's South Asian community, or because it involved distant politics in India (and tensions between Hindus and Sikhs there), even if the crime originated in British Columbia. Perhaps this tragedy slipped from public consciousness because it took so long (18 years) for anyone to be held responsible. Although there were a number of suspects, only one person was ever convicted. The victims' families and communities suffered individual and collective trauma, enhanced in part because of a sense of lasting injustice because the criminal investigation took so many years and provided little if any resolution, and in part because of a lack of recognition and support from the Canadian government. Failler (2009) suggested that this is a case of "historical trauma." The meaning and impact of this tragedy continued to be salient over the years for the victims, their families, and the wider South Asian community in Canada, although it was largely forgotten and unsupported by the rest of Canada. It was not remembered as a *Canadian* loss, nor as a national tragedy (Failler 2009).

Chakraborty, Dean, and Failler (2017) noted that while the Air India bombing was initially framed as a "foreign event," decades later it is being reframed as a Canadian example of domestic terrorism. These authors explored the concept of "official frames of remembering" and commented on how these frames change while continuing to serve governmental agendas. They noted that in 1985 Canada distanced itself from its involvement in a terrorist act, preserving an image of Canada's innocence. Decades later, when terrorism had become a recognized and imminent threat, the Air India tragedy was reframed and claimed as a justification for concern about the threat of contemporary terrorism and efforts to deal with that threat. In terms we have used earlier in this book, grief and public mourning following the Air India bombing of 1985 were largely disenfranchised. Only decades later has this collective trauma begun to be recognized.

In contrast, the downing of Ukraine International Airlines Flight PS752 on 8 January 2020 by a surface-to-air missile in Iran was treated as a Canadian tragedy and brought an immediate collective outpouring of grief. All 176 persons on that flight were killed, including 55 Canadian citizens and 30 permanent residents of Canada. The Canadian government announced: "This is a national tragedy and the whole country is grieving together." The government offered $25,000 per victim to the victims' families "to assist with their immediate needs" (Government of Canada 2020d). Memorial services were held, including one in Edmonton on a bitterly cold day on 12 January 2020, four days after the tragedy, in a sports arena with several thousand in attendance. Speakers included the mayor of Edmonton, the president of the University of Alberta, the premier of Alberta, and the prime minister of Canada.

Epidemic and Pandemic Death

Although the COVID-19 pandemic that began in late 2019 had global impact, probably the most infamous pandemic is the bubonic plague, or "Black Death," a bacterial infection that devastated Europe in the 1300s. In the six years from 1346 to 1352, one-third of Europeans are thought to have perished, and subsequent waves of the disease continued to claim lives over the following three centuries (Hammond 2020). Other epidemics and pandemics that have had catastrophic effects include smallpox, yellow fever, cholera, tuberculosis, malaria, influenza, and HIV/AIDS. The most impactful pandemics in Canada's history include the misnamed Spanish flu of 1918–20 and the coronavirus (COVID-19) disease beginning in 2020.

The Spanish flu of 1918–20 was a viral influenza pandemic that followed in the wake of the First World War (1914–18). It is thought that at least 50 million people died worldwide, including 50,000 in Canada, over an 18-month period—more than had died during the war. This disease killed young adults disproportionately, and poor and Indigenous communities were especially vulnerable (Hammond 2020).

COVID-19 made its way to Canada in early 2020. By mid-March 2020 there were concerns that the pandemic might overwhelm hospitals and intensive care units (ICUs) in particular. There were concerns that there might not be enough beds, respirators for seriously ill patients, or personal protective equipment (PPE) for hospital staff. Health care workers were concerned about catching the virus themselves or taking it home to their families. There was a concern that if the health care system were overwhelmed, health care personnel would have to engage in triage and rationing, facing difficult decisions about who to treat and therefore who lives and who dies.

While Canada was relatively successful during the first wave of the pandemic in "flattening the curve" and containing the spread of the virus, the interests of public health were pitted against the interests of the economy (businesses, employers, employees, and government revenues and expenditures). Furthermore, there were many concerning manifestations of ageism, sexism, and racism across the country. For example, because most deaths in the first four months of the pandemic were older adults residing in long-term care facilities (81 per cent), the egregious term "boomer remover" was coined (even though the "baby boomers"—born from 1946 to 1964—were under the age of 75 at the time, so many of the dead were actually the parents of the baby boomer generation). Moreover, most long-term care workers were poorly paid immigrant and visible minority women, and because of the believed origin of the virus in Wuhan, China, many Chinese Canadians were "blamed" for the pandemic, and scapegoating and conspiracy theories circulated. Canada also saw its military mobilized to work in selected long-term care facilities experiencing outbreaks of the disease, bodies often had to be stacked in refrigerated trucks while waiting for removal, and local funeral homes were overwhelmed. Funeral services were delayed or minimized.

The experience of dying during the pandemic was fundamentally transformed from non-pandemic circumstances. Families were often not allowed to visit their dying family members, who consequently died alone among strangers. Health care staff did their best to attend to the dying, on occasion by holding the hands of the dying, even as this added to their own distress. Families noted that there was no chance to say goodbye and also no funeral rituals later to support them in their grief. There was speculation that in these circumstances grief was changed, complicated by feelings of regret and frustration at the circumstances of the deaths of their loved ones. Finally, the pandemic identified a crisis in the long-term care of the frail and very old (Estabrooks et al. 2020). At the time of writing in early 2021 it remains to be seen how this pandemic will play itself out and what lasting effects it will have on Canadians and Canadian society.

ONLINE GRIEVING, MOURNING, AND MEMORIALIZATION

Death has always been a social event. Grief is shared, and mourning involves public gatherings and rituals. Following death, family, friends, and community are notified. In the past, this was done by letter mail or landline telephone. Today, family, friends, and community members often learn of a death by email, text, or social media. Announcements of death tend to be immediate and far-reaching given mobile phones. Furthermore, following a death in the past, family often provided a general notice to the community. For example, an announcement was made at work or church or school. The family often paid a local newspaper to publish an obituary to announce the death to the general public. The obituary functions as both an announcement of death and an overview or memorial of the life of the deceased. Today, social media sites announce death and memorialize the life of the deceased (McEwen and Scheaffer 2013; Granek 2017). The functions of these notices of death are to invite the community to share in supporting the bereaved, to mourn collectively, and to honour and remember the dead. Family, friends, and others then gather at a church or funeral home, the site of death, or some other venue to engage in rituals of public mourning. In the digital age, mourners can also gather online.

McEwen and Scheaffer (2013) examined the role that Facebook plays in virtual mourning and memory construction. Facebook and other such online sites facilitate social connection and identity construction. In life, a person on

Facebook creates a digital identity. In death, there are questions about what should be done with that digital identity. McEwen and Scheaffer argue that a deceased person's Facebook page is a digital asset that the deceased should be able to control after death. For example, the deceased could stipulate in a will that their digital identity be removed, preserved, or that control be passed on to a designated person who would then continue to develop the digital archive. When a Facebook profile remains active, the deceased can appear to send messages to the living (automated birthday greetings, for example), and the living can post messages for the deceased. In this sense, Facebook and other such social media sites facilitate a continuing bond and relationship between the living and the dead.

McEwen and Scheaffer (2013) noted that there are negative aspects to online grieving, mourning, and memorialization. First, the deceased lose control of their digital identity and memory when others take over the ongoing creation of their profile. Second, while Facebook can provide a vehicle for the collective expression of grief and support, it can also become a place where survivors feel coerced into participating and where a competition develops: a "war over who loved the deceased more" (70). Third, keeping a Facebook profile active after death allows for the possibility of identity theft after death.

Mitchell et al. (2012) examined virtual online memorials created by bereaved parents who had experienced the death of a child. The parents created virtual memorials by filling out templates offered by online memorial hosting sites that charged a fee for their services. These authors noted that virtual memorials create a digital immortality, an online afterlife, and facilitate an ongoing relationship between the living and the dead. On the negative side, they noted that the businesspeople providing these commercial online spaces have a vested interest in turning bereaved parents into paying customers and in extending the parents' mourning indefinitely. It follows, then, that these sites may both help bereaved parents grieve but may also perpetuate their grief.

Mitchell et al. (2012) observed that parents create these online sites not only to memorialize their dead child but also to show their dedication as parents who will never forget their beloved child. The child, along with the parent–child relationship, is often idealized in these online creations. And once the child exists online, there is an imperative to maintain that online presence. Furthermore, once online the child can have a relationship with a variety of social others, including siblings, grandparents, other family members, friends, and even strangers. While this ongoing relationship with a social network can be supportive for the bereaved parent, it also obligates the parent to maintain the online presence of the dead child. While this ongoing online presence may maintain parental grief, it also connects the parent and child in an ongoing relationship. Imaginings of a life after death and a place where the dead reside continue in this technologically enhanced virtual reality. Mitchell et al. (2012) pointed out that the dead live on digitally in an online afterworld and online afterlife. Parental grief is expressed, managed, relieved, and perpetuated in this online, ongoing virtual presence and relationship.

Gilbert (2017) discussed virtual connections between the living and the dead. She noted that a person's "digital persona" might be uploaded in the future after the person's death in "robotic or holographic form, which would interact as if it is an actual human form" (303). She then asked: "What are the implications for grief and mourning if the continuing presence of a loved one is not in our mind's eye but facing and chatting with us on a screen or transferred into a robotic body?" (303). Note that a South Korean mother in 2020 wearing a virtual reality headset and touch-sensitive gloves has been able to "see," "talk with," and "touch" her deceased daughter who died in 2016. The daughter had been brought back to (virtual) life through motion capture technology (Aljazeera 2020).

THIRD-PERSON ACCOUNTS OF DYING

Personal stories of the death of a loved one include third-person accounts. For example, a wife's account of her husband's dying is her version of how she experienced the dying and death of her husband. Sometimes the wife's story is then retold by a third person. This third person's account may be a more or less accurate representation of the wife's experience. Accurate or not, the third person's account reveals a subjective understanding and often an evaluation of the wife's experience. Consider the following third-person account provided to the first author by a young woman:

> I am really concerned about my aunt. My uncle is dying with stomach cancer. It was a great shock when he was diagnosed last year and the doctor determined that he would not survive. Over the year he has been in and out of hospital a great deal undergoing a number of surgeries to

relieve some of his pain and to help his digestive system. I have been pretty removed from the whole situation; even though I was living very close to my aunt and uncle, I only saw my uncle once since he was diagnosed and saw my aunt only a few more times than that.

My aunt has spent a lot of time trying to deny the fact that her husband is dying. She didn't tell their children for a time after she found out that his cancer was terminal. Each time my uncle has had to return to the hospital, it serves as a reminder that he is dying, but then when he is again released it seems that she tries to forget the end prospect. She has done very little planning for a future without him; I recently found out that a will has not even been signed. When I think of the difficulties that she has been dealing with and will have to deal with, I wonder how she will get out of bed every day.

She is my father's sister and is relying on him for a great deal. Any time she has a crisis he is the first one she calls. When I speak with him on the phone, I notice the toll it is taking. My aunt is expecting when my uncle dies that my father will make all of the funeral arrangements and bail her out of the difficulties of not having a will, etc. All this time I think that my father is facing his own fears of death. I think that for him cancer is very frightening, and stomach cancer the most frightening of all. His grandfather died of stomach cancer; he fears that he is in line as cancer can be hereditary. Watching the suffering of my uncle is no doubt bringing back memories as well as touching on a great fear for his own health.

While this woman's account of her aunt's reaction to her husband's dying is empathetic, it is also critical. The storyteller indicates her concern for her aunt. However, while acknowledging her aunt's distress, shock, and denial and her difficulty facing the dying and impending death of her husband, the storyteller is also critical of her aunt. She feels that her aunt should face reality, plan more adequately, cope better, and be more self-reliant. The aunt is portrayed as overly reliant on her brother (the storyteller's father). Finally, the storyteller is concerned for her father, whom she perceives to be overly burdened by his sister's difficulties and distressed by concerns for his own health, which are exacerbated by his brother-in-law's dying of a feared disease.

Accounts, such as the one above, are both descriptive and prescriptive. On the one hand, they describe the storyteller's perception of the facts of the situation. At the same time, in describing the difficulties a distressed spouse is having in the face of her husband's dying and the problems that inadequate coping brings, the storyteller prescribes how the distressed person *should* respond. The telling of such stories serves as more than the simple communication of a person's perceptions of a distressing situation; it also creates and reinforces collective norms about how one should cope with the dying of a loved one.

SUMMARY

It is hard to lose a loved one to death. While, in one sense, death ends the relationship with the loved one, in another sense it transforms the relationship, which continues in the survivor's memories, thoughts, feelings, conversations, and behaviours. Because the relationship continues, albeit in a transformed way, grieving for the presence of the deceased is ongoing. While the intensity of grief tends to wane over time, grief does not completely disappear. It comes and goes and returns again.

To the extent that our lives are made up of our relationships with others, the death of a loved one transforms our own life. Part of us dies with the deceased. Life is never completely the same again. We grieve for the deceased and we grieve for ourselves—for what we have lost of ourselves. Nevertheless, out of loss and despair many find meaning, purpose, and hope. To paraphrase the father who lost two children to unexpected and premature deaths, we can remember the dead and honour them, we can accept our own mortality as the natural order of things, and we can do good works while we are among the living.

QUESTIONS FOR REVIEW

1. Define the following terms: bereavement, grief, and mourning. In what ways is bereavement disruptive? What are the personal and social gains derived from mourning rituals? What are common social rules for mourning and grieving? How or when can a person "fail grief"?
2. Until recently, analyses of the experience of grieving have been dominated by linear and temporally limited grief recovery models. More recent models tend to be nonlinear and ongoing. Discuss these contrasting models of the grieving process.

3. Compare and contrast the following:
   a) Traumatic or unexpected death and expected or anticipated death.
   b) The survivor's experience of the death of a child versus the death of a parent, grandparent, partner, or friend.
   c) The survivor's experience of the death of a loved one from natural causes versus deaths due to accidents, natural disasters, suicide, homicide, war, genocide, terrorism, and pandemic.
4. In what ways do the dead live on? How do the living maintain an ongoing relationship with the dead? How has this relationship between the living and the dead been maintained and/or transformed in the contemporary digital age?

KEY TERMS

bereaved – People who experience the death of a loved one. (p. 189)
bereavement – The bereaved go through a period of bereavement. (p. 189)
grief – Intense suffering caused by the death of a loved one. (p. 189)
identifying moments – Experiences that make a person realize their current social status. (p. 219)
identity foreclosure – A change in social status (e.g., widowhood, retirement) resulting in the termination of one's former identity (e.g., as a wife, employee). (p. 219)
mourning – Public displays of grief conforming to social and cultural norms. (p. 189)
orphan – A child whose parents are dead. (p. 191)
pandemic – An infectious disease that is widely prevalent across multiple countries or that has spread worldwide, as contrasted with an epidemic, which is confined to one country or one region of a country. (p. 231)
perinatal death – The death of a baby before or soon after birth. (p. 202)
rites of intensification – Social rituals that intensify feelings and emotions and then provide a means by which individuals can express their sentiments. (p. 229)
traumatic death – A death that is out of the ordinary and may be particularly gruesome or disturbing. Includes unnatural and unexpected deaths such as some homicides, suicides, or motor vehicle accidents, for example. (p. 231)
widow – A woman whose husband has died. She experiences widowhood. (p. 191)
widower – A man whose wife has died. He experiences widowerhood. (p. 191)

CHAPTER SEVEN

Caregiver Perspectives: Caring for the Caregivers

Encounters with dying and death can be deeply disturbing not only for families and friends but also for health care professionals and other occupational group members that become involved with the dying and dead. Besides attempting interventions in dying and death situations, military personnel, police officers, firefighters, emergency medical technicians and paramedics, and nurses and doctors at times also have to cope with the risk of losing their own lives. Difficulties in personal coping with dying and death include **post-traumatic stress disorder (PTSD)** and other emotional and mental health issues such as depression, acute and chronic anxiety, anger, despair, moral distress, burnout, alcohol and substance abuse, relationship problems (e.g., spousal abuse and family violence), and suicidal ideation, planning, and suicide (Bradley 2015; Jeannette and Scoboria 2008). Attempts have been made in recent years to raise awareness of these emotional reactions, and programs have been designed to destigmatize and normalize these reactions. It is recognized now that people who work with the dying and with death may need time and support to deal with their emotions and maintain their mental health.

In chapters 5 and 6 we focused on people who were dying and their survivors—usually family members who grieve the death of their loved ones. In this chapter, we focus on strangers who become involved with the dying and the dead as first responders, health care workers, and death care workers. **First responders** include police officers, firefighters, emergency medical technicians (EMTs), paramedics, search-and-rescue and recovery workers, suicide distress line personnel, 911 operators and dispatchers, and others. **Health care workers** include nurses, doctors, respiratory technicians, rehabilitation therapists, nursing home staff, hospice staff and volunteers, social workers, and grief counsellors. **Death care workers** include medical examiners, funeral directors, and cemetery grounds and crematory facility workers. While family members' reactions to the death of a loved one are typically conceptualized as grief and mourning, the reactions of nonfamily members who are involved as first responders, health care workers, or death care workers are often conceptualized as work-related stress, more specifically as PTSD or emotional and mental health impacts.

This chapter provides an overview of PTSD and other emotional issues as experienced by first responders, health care workers, and death care workers. The overall thesis in this chapter is that dying and death can be disturbing and can lead to emotional, cognitive, and even behavioural difficulties. Death, and traumatic death in particular, can undermine a person's sense of security and belief that the world is meaningful, comprehensible, and controllable. The same applies to those who are exposed to threats to their own lives, as in the case of police officers, firefighters, nurses, and physicians. We noted previously that the idealized view of the world as meaningful, comprehensible, and controllable is what Antonovsky (1987) called a sense of coherence. PTSD, on the other hand, reflects a perception of the world as incoherent, incomprehensible, chaotic, hostile, arbitrary, and meaningless (Staniloiu and Feinstein 2017).

As we have noted frequently in this book, a central task for all people is making life and death meaningful when confronted with their own and with others' mortality. This book explores the following question: In the face of our own and others' mortality, and in particular when confronted by traumatic death, how do people find meaning, cope, and go on with life? In this chapter we ask how those who deal regularly with dying and death react, cope, or fail to cope, and how we can help those individuals who are having difficulty.

PTSD AND RELATED EMOTIONAL REACTIONS

The increasingly widespread acknowledgment in the early twenty-first century of post-traumatic stress disorder and related emotional reactions is part of a larger discussion that is attempting to destigmatize emotional

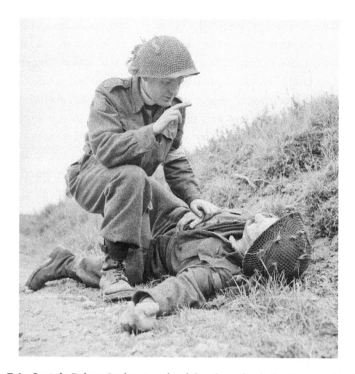

Image 7.1. Captain Robert Seaborn, a chaplain, gives absolution to an unidentified soldier of the 3rd Canadian Infantry Division near Caen, France, 15 July 1944
Source: Lieut. H. Gordon Aikman/Canadian Dept. of National Defence/Library and Archives Canada/PA-142245.

problems and mental illnesses. Previously, people who had difficulty coping with dying and death in the context of their occupations were often stigmatized and labelled weak and incompetent (Granek et al. 2012; Halpern et al. 2009a, 2009b; Knaak et al. 2019). Traditional male-dominated occupations such as soldier, police officer, firefighter, and physician have long been influenced by a masculinist culture that tends to deny the legitimacy of "disruptive" emotions. Individuals in these occupations and others have been expected to manage difficult situations and their emotions while continuing to function normally. The adoption of a culture of professionalism by these occupations has added to this notion, as professional cultures take the position that being emotional at work is unprofessional (Granek et al. 2012; Halpern et al. 2009b). It is expected that professionals keep their emotions under control or maintain emotional detachment to be able to perform their expected duties. Accordingly, many people working in occupations that deal with dying and death have long suffered in silence, unable to admit any emotional difficulties and unable to seek support (Conn and Butterfield 2013, 281; Halpern et al. 2009a). To illustrate this problem, a *CBC News* report claimed that "police officers, firefighters and paramedics are still reluctant to seek help with post-traumatic stress disorder because of the stigma attached to mental health issues within their occupations" (Gollom 2014).

Nevertheless, the contemporary discourse attempts to normalize PTSD and related emotional reactions as a common, expected, and acceptable response amenable to therapeutic intervention (Jeannette and Scoboria 2008). This discourse normalizes emotional responses to stressful events as legitimate psychological reactions. It also creates an environment in which people can acknowledge their difficulties in coping with dying and death, gain support from their co-workers, and seek help from professionals and programs designed to assist those suffering from emotional reactions.

The contemporary discourse tends to highlight PTSD and suggests that exposure to traumatic events puts people at risk for PTSD. However, the term is often used to encompass a wide variety of reactions to traumatic stressors. The clinical literature attempts to be more precise and restrictive in the definition of PTSD in order to distinguish PTSD from related mental health diagnoses such as anxiety, depression, burnout, and so on, with specific criteria developed for assessing these various problems (Stein et al. 2014). It is important to note that not all people who experience traumatic events have clinical symptoms leading to a diagnosis of PTSD, depression, or other mental health concerns; nevertheless, they may still suffer considerable distress during the traumatic event and afterwards.

Estimates of the prevalence of PTSD and other emotional problems following exposure to death vary (see Asmundson and Stapleton 2008; Jeannette and Scoboria 2008; Wagner, White, Fyfe, et al. 2020; Wagner, White, Randall, et al. 2020; Regehr et al. 2019). These estimates depend on the definitions chosen, the diagnostic tools used, and the timeframe of measurement—whether immediately or shortly after experiencing the traumatic event, or years later (Stein et al. 2014). As expected, reactions tend to be most intense at the time of and immediately following a death. For most, there is a return to baseline over time. For some, however, symptoms persist or worsen. These symptoms can become disruptive and lead to absenteeism from work, alcohol and substance abuse, difficulties in personal relationships, physiological problems, and suicide (Bradley 2015; Veterans Affairs Canada 2015).

The media have highlighted the high rate of suicide among first responders (see Canadian Press 2015). However, suicide is an extreme act and can be viewed as the "tip of the iceberg," indicating that many more first responders suffer to varying degrees and are easily overlooked.

Besides potentially traumatic events experienced at work, work-related stressors can also include the culture and conditions of work (Fraess-Phillips, Wagner, and Harris 2017). Shift work, interpersonal difficulties, sexual harassment, and a non-supportive or toxic work culture can lead to PTSD, depression, anxiety, alcohol or drug abuse, and suicide. A supportive work environment governed by camaraderie and a shared sense of purpose can reduce risk. In addition, non-work variables such as family conflict can also influence mental health. The point is, assessing PTSD and related mental health issues is complex, and estimates of the prevalence of these problems vary widely.

Stein and et al. (2014; see also Asmundson and Stapleton 2008) listed four categories of PTSD symptoms associated with the experience of a traumatic event: (1) re-experiencing (e.g., repeated unwanted memories, repeated unpleasant dreams, flashbacks), (2) avoidance (of reminders of the traumatic event), (3) emotional numbing, and (4) arousal (e.g., hypervigilance, easily startled, trouble concentrating, trouble sleeping, irritability). Yet PTSD has come to the attention of the public largely because of its association with interpersonal difficulties (e.g., family violence) and suicide (Bradley 2015; Canadian Press 2015; Gollom 2014). Nevertheless, PTSD is associated with other emotional and mental health issues. In Canada, the term "operational stress injury" is sometimes used to refer to this complex pattern including PTSD, anxiety, and depression when experienced by soldiers, police officers, and others in the line of duty (Veterans Affairs Canada 2015).

Although one might think that repeated exposure to death or frequent risks to life and limb would inoculate people against PTSD, the disorder may actually be more likely with repeated exposure. PTSD is also more likely when deaths or dying processes are particularly gruesome, when deaths involve personal connections, and when deaths are perceived as particularly tragic, such as the deaths of children. DeSpelder and Strickland (2011, 205–7) noted that it has become common to offer **critical incident stress management (CISM)** quickly to first responders following a traumatic death, although it is not clear how effective this program is (Jeannette and Scoboria 2008; Fraess-Phillips, Wagner, and Harris 2017). CISM typically involves giving first responders a chance to talk about their experiences, feelings, and reactions with co-workers and professional counsellors.

The COVID-19 pandemic that spread to Canada in early 2020 illustrates the exceptionally difficult circumstances that first responders, health care workers, and death care workers have to deal with from time to time. EMTs and paramedics were called on to transport persons sick with the coronavirus to hospitals. Physicians and nurses and others in the hospital dealt with the sick, some who needed intensive care and some who were dying. Funeral homes were challenged by the volume of dead bodies and their grieving families, as well as the need to prevent disease transmission through crowd control. Images from the evening news reporting on the pandemic elsewhere in the world raised the spectre of overcrowded hospitals and bodies stacked in refrigerated trucks in parking lots waiting transport to funeral homes that were unable to keep up. Health care workers were concerned that if they ran out of ICU beds they would have to turn some patients away, essentially deciding who lived and who died. Patients were isolated from family members who "visited" through closed windows or on cell phones. Patients died "alone" in the care of strangers.

Many of the first COVID-19 deaths involved frail elderly residents in long-term care facilities. It soon became apparent that the overworked and underpaid staff often worked in more than one facility, and that these long-term care homes were hotspots for the virus to cluster and spread. The military was called in to help in some of these homes. At the time of writing in early 2021, vaccines were being distributed in the hope that they would protect individuals, lead to "herd immunity," and prevent the rise of "variant" viruses that threatened new waves of infections. One can assume that the distress of health care workers and others directly involved in the pandemic will be substantial. Moral distress, including a concern for others but also for self and family, is expected. Burnout, compassion fatigue, frustration and anger, depression and anxiety, and PTSD are expected outcomes for many. Some may continue to show effects long after the pandemic ends.

FIRST RESPONDERS

Carleton et al. (2019, 2018a) surveyed paramedics, police officers, firefighters, correctional officers, and dispatchers in Canada about their work. They found that "public safety personnel are exposed to a diversity of potentially traumatic events more frequently than the general population" (2019, 48) and that exposure to potentially traumatic events, especially to sudden violent death, was associated with higher rates of mental disorders, including PTSD, depression, and anxiety disorders, in comparison to the general population. Further, they found evidence for "cumulative trauma," with more time in service and more exposure to potentially traumatic events resulting in an increase in mental disorders. Finally, Carleton et al. (2018b; see also Stanley, Hom, and Joiner 2016) found that public safety personnel reported higher levels of suicide ideation, planning, or attempts than the general population.

Police Officers

When a traumatic death occurs, police officers, firefighters, and EMTs or paramedics typically converge on the scene. In 2015, an individual living in Edmonton, Alberta, fired a high-powered rifle at police officers who had come to his door to arrest him. One officer was killed; another was wounded. The man then set his house on fire, which burned to the ground after he had shot and killed himself. Firefighters and EMTs mingled with the police at the scene. The medical examiner's office later received the bodies of the deceased.

What is remarkable about this story is how extensive the local and national media were in covering it, and how quickly and completely the community went into mourning for the police officer, Constable Daniel Woodall, who died. Across and outside of Edmonton, blue ribbons were tied to trees along roadways. A few days later, thousands of first responders gathered for the police officer's funeral and memorial service. This story echoes similar scenes that have occurred and continue to occur across the country when police officers die in the line of duty. The following is an account of the public response to this tragedy, written by the first author of this book on 17 June 2015:

> Ten days ago, a madman killed a police officer in the city in which I live. Today the officer, lying in a flag-draped casket in a white hearse, was transported from the Legislative Grounds to the Conference Centre. The city's downtown streets were closed to traffic as the parade passed by. People, grim-faced, lined the streets, many wearing blue. Blue ribbons lined the way.
>
> The parade was led by police officers on motorcycles, red and blue lights flashing. A white hearse followed. A pipe and drum band, with drummers keeping time and bagpipers playing a mournful tune, led wave

after wave of police officers wearing blue dress uniforms and marching eight abreast. More pipe and drum bands and more waves of officers in blue followed, including officers from around the province and country, and from the United States and the United Kingdom. Then came yet another pipe band leading officers from the Royal Canadian Mounted Police marching in their scarlet dress uniforms. The crowds were quiet, subdued, paying their respect, and perhaps with many individuals trying to keep their emotions under control. It was a solemn, sad occasion.

A funeral service, billed as a Celebration of Life, followed at the large Conference Centre. The mayor, police chief, police chaplain, and friends of the slain officer all spoke. A lone piper and a lone bugler played their parts in the ceremony. The deceased officer's parents and two young sons sat next to his widow in the front row. The flag draping the casket was folded ceremoniously and presented to the officer's widow along with the officer's cap.

Several things stand out for consideration in this account. First, the hearse was white, a major shift from traditional black. Second, the public gathering and ceremony at the Conference Centre was listed as a Celebration of Life, not a funeral service focused on death, although death was what brought everyone together at this time and place. Third, the parade involving several thousand police officers constituted a show of solidarity reinforced by the thousands of people who lined the route. Ultimately, the parade was a reaffirmation of the social contract that binds us all together and a visible show of recognition for the role that police officers play in maintaining a civil society through enforcing law and order. Fourth, this event constituted a brief moment—a temporary disruption of everyday life. That moment motivated sober reflection and moved many to tears, although most people returned to their regular lives shortly thereafter. Long term, we can expect that the family of the slain officer will grieve, the city will ultimately put up a memorial statue, the officer's sacrifice of life will be mentioned from time to time and the perpetrator's killing of another and himself will be a long-lasting lesson for many. Nevertheless, within hours, life in Edmonton and elsewhere returned to normal for most people, although some continued to be deeply affected by this senseless tragedy.

Research is beginning to show how deeply police officers are impacted by their work. A study of Royal Canadian Mounted Police officers found that male officers reported that the most stressful events they experienced

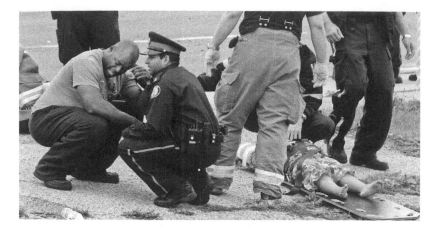

Image 7.2. Police officers are more likely than most to encounter violent and traumatic events that often lead to dying and death.
Source: David Cooper/ZUMA Press/Newscom.

were armed violent arrests (as in the story told above) and other threats to their own lives or the lives of family and friends. In contrast, female officers reported fatal motor vehicle collisions (MVCs) and other sudden deaths as most stressful (Goto 2006). Nevertheless, this study found that while officers frequently experienced stressors on the job, only a few experienced the symptoms of PTSD. It is possible that serendipity is a component here, as many police officers in Canada are never involved in a violent incident where they are shot at or need to shoot someone, although police are more likely to experience sudden and violent deaths involving accidents, homicides, and suicides.

A study of active and retired police officers in Montreal found that most reported having experienced at least one traumatic event at work during their career (Martin et al. 2009). When asked about their reactions to the most stressful event they had experienced, 8 per cent reported symptoms indicating they had experienced PTSD, and another 7 per cent reported having experienced symptoms consistent with partial PTSD. In all cases, the officers indicated that their symptoms had been temporary. Martin et al. noted that traumatic events tended to precipitate intense emotional and physiological reactions for most officers, and that receiving support from colleagues in the hours and days following the traumatic event helped officers cope and reduced or ameliorated symptoms.

Another study asked police officers in Quebec about a recent traumatic event they had experienced (Marchand et al. 2013). These officers were assessed for PTSD 5 to 15 days later, and again at 1 month, 3 month, and 12 month intervals. One month after the event, 3 per cent had experienced clinical PTSD and another 9 per cent had some symptoms (partial PTSD). Marchand et al. wrote, "The officers said that what particularly helped them after a TE [traumatic event] was to talk to colleagues about it, make use of support services and have time off" (iii). They also noted that "there seems to be a growing recognition among officers that they are not totally invincible and that it is acceptable to ask for help in the aftermath of a stressful event" (47).

Mishara and Martin (2012) evaluated a suicide prevention program for police officers in Montreal. While the suicide rate for police officers had been comparable to the general population previously, the program resulted in a dramatic reduction of the police suicide rate. Moreover, Knaak et al. (2019) described a workplace mental health training program for police organizations in Canada. They wrote about the importance of changing the stoic culture of police organizations. As one of the people interviewed said:

> When you are in a paramilitary organization it is very hard to change the culture. Ideas, beliefs, norms, values are entrenched in the culture. The idea is that you can take anything . . . there is a culture in policing that we are the cream of the crop, we can take anything, we are strong, we don't break down—that has been a prevailing stereotype for decades and moving past that kind of stereotype doesn't happen overnight. (32S)

Studies of police officers report a wide range of estimates of the prevalence of mental disorders including PTSD, depression, anxiety, and suicidal behaviours (ideation, planning, attempts) (Nota et al. 2020; Regehr et al. 2019; Wagner, White, Fyfe, et al. 2020). Responses vary depending on a wide variety of factors including the nature of the critical event (e.g., an automobile accident or a mass death event such as an airplane crash). Many officers appear to cope well, overall. While the numbers are hard to estimate, studies indicate that a minority experience various mental health issues including PTSD, depression, and anxiety.

Police officers may experience traumatic events directly (**primary trauma**), but more often have contact with others who have experienced traumatic events. For example, police officers may have to inform family members that a loved one has been murdered or killed in an accident. Police officers then tend to have frequent contact with family members during the long investigation of a missing or murdered person, or over the time it takes for a trial to occur. This ongoing exposure to the suffering of others can also be traumatizing. Conn and Butterfield (2013) referred to this as **secondary trauma**.

Firefighters

Firefighters are another group of workers who are at risk for PTSD and other emotional reactions as a result of potentially traumatic work-related experiences, although estimates of PTSD and other mental health disorders among them vary widely (Wagner, White, Randall, et al. 2020; Wagner and Pasca 2020; Fraess-Phillips, Wagner, and Harris 2017). Jeannette (a firefighter himself) and Scoboria (2008) asked firefighters in Windsor, Ontario, about their preferences for psychological intervention following traumatic events. The authors noted that "over time, firefighters may experience scenes of tragedy, destruction and horror that most people never see in their lifetime" and may, as a result, "be at risk of becoming 'hidden victims' of the tragedies that they encounter" (Jeannette and Scoboria 2008, 314). They observed that rapid critical incident stress debriefing (CISD) has become widely used since the 1980s, although its effectiveness remains unclear among firefighters and other first responders. CISD assumes that witnessing traumatic death may lead to PTSD for some firefighters and that talking about the traumatic incident can be preventative or therapeutic. In this study, the firefighters indicated that they welcomed social support and intervention in various forms including CISD, individual debriefing, and informal discussion among firefighters at the station where they worked. The outcomes of that support and intervention need to be investigated further, as it is not known how effective they are.

Firefighters are not only exposed to the traumatic deaths of victims of fires and accidents but also risk their own lives in attempting to save others and put out fires. One normally thinks that the risk involves dying in a fire, but the *Edmonton Journal* reported on the funeral for a retired fire captain who died at the age of 61 after 30 years of service (Zabjek 2015). He died of cancer three years after his retirement, with the journalist noting that "his illness was among 15 cancers officially recognized as linked to a firefighter's job." The president of the Edmonton Fire Fighter's Union was quoted as saying the following during the funeral service: "He died in the line of duty . . . he died as a result of fighting hundreds of fires over his career."

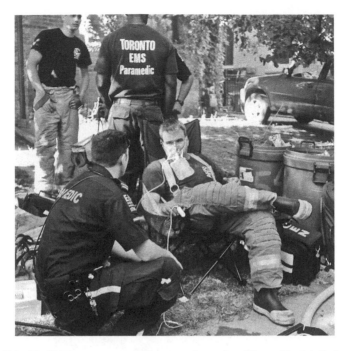

Image 7.3. Firefighters are exposed to many hazards while on the job that can affect their health over the long term
Source: Tibor Kelly/The Globe and Mail/The Canadian Press. All rights reserved.

Emergency Medical Technicians and Paramedics

Wagner, White, Regehr, et al. (2020) reviewed studies of ambulance personnel including paramedics and EMTs. They reported that ambulance personnel have higher rates of probable PTSD, depression, and anxiety compared to the general population. Hegg-Deloye et al. (2014) also reviewed the published literature examining the effects of work stress on paramedics. They noted that the literature suggests there is a relationship between work stressors, physiological arousal (e.g., elevated cortisol levels), anxiety, depression, PTSD symptoms, sleeping problems, obesity, and cardiovascular disease for paramedics. In January 2015, the news media carried the story of a paramedic who died by suicide at his workstation (Canadian Press 2015). He had been a paramedic for 16 years. The Paramedic Association of Canada noted that four paramedics in Canada died by suicide in January 2015, and 34 had done so in the previous eight months. An official noted that suicide statistics were

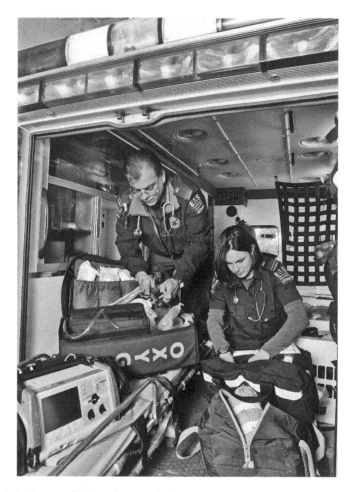

Image 7.4. Paramedic team in an ambulance
Source: Ron Bull/ZUMA Press/Newscom.

being collected and reported as "part of a national campaign to raise awareness about PTSD and first responder suicide" (Canadian Press 2015). Finally,
the news release observed that "many who need help may not seek it as the
public perception of first responders is they are heroes and some feel weak in
asking for assistance" (Canadian Press 2015).

Halpern et al. (2009a) interviewed EMTs in Ontario and noted that traumatic **critical incidents** were common and generated considerable concern
among EMTs. These EMTs commented on the importance of support, sympathy, and understanding from their supervisors. Nevertheless, the EMTs

expressed concerns about appearing weak and being stigmatized. The authors noted that there was "an organizational culture that stigmatizes emotional vulnerability" (144). Similarly, Regehr et al. (2002, 97) studied paramedics in Toronto and noted that "great cynicism often occurs within the organization toward paramedics who take time off for either physical or psychological injury." Halpern et al. (2009a) noted that concerns about stigma and confidentiality caused EMTs to be cautious about revealing their feelings because they needed to protect their reputations and appear strong and competent. They spoke, however, of the importance of a very brief timeout (30 to 60 minutes) immediately following a critical incident when peers could talk informally, decompress, and relax. The therapeutic benefit of these immediate timeouts was a reduction of "hyperarousal," a state of extreme emotional and physical readiness for action. During these breaks, the EMTs could calm down after experiencing a critical incident. It was thought that this therapeutic calming immediately after a critical incident helped prevent symptoms from persisting or developing over the long term. Nevertheless, Halpern et al. (2012) noted that 36 per cent of EMTs/ paramedics in Ontario reported having experienced a critical incident that had troubled them in the past, and 50 per cent reported an incident that was still troubling them.

The first author of this book asked a paramedic the following questions: (1) How do EMTs and paramedics who are exposed regularly to death in the course of their occupation deal with death? (2) How do EMTs/paramedics cope with everyday events? and (3) What events are most problematic and how do EMTs/paramedics cope with these critical incidents and traumatic events? He responded with the following:

First of all, let me give you some personal background. I was 29 when I began work as an EMT . . . in November of 1979. Training was given by distance learning from Southern Alberta Institute of Technology (SAIT). I did not grow up wanting to work on an ambulance. A nurse I was dating suggested I apply in my off-season when it became too cold to work as a bricklayer. The work was fun and challenging. Usually you never did the same call twice. Constant change was the norm. A few years later I enrolled in the paramedic program at Northern Alberta Institute of Technology (NAIT) and graduated in 1984.

Dealing with a death from cardiac arrest is what paramedics train for. That is, the challenge of performing a successful resuscitation was practised and evaluated as the final test of your licence and was evaluated every four years.

There is pressure to perform, but you worked with a partner and the fire department who did CPR. To initiate CPR, place and interpret the ECG, defibrillate if necessary, [suction the mouth, insert an endotracheal tube,] start the IV, and administer medication; all had to be performed in an accurate and timely manner. We all worked together and built solid friendships. If the resuscitation attempt failed, we knew we all did our best.

Sometimes we were able to visit someone a few days after the resuscitation. We would be respectful but used humour as we spoke to the patient. One of us would ask: "Does your throat hurt?" The patient would say yes and I would say that was my partner. We would ask: "Does your chest hurt?" My partner would say that was me. We would not spend long and would be back to work. The seriousness of the situation as well as looking into the eyes of the grateful patients emits gentle tears even as I write this piece. I cherish this gift of life and feel honoured to have been there at that moment in time.

Attending the suicide victims were always some of the saddest. [It was gruesome to witness the result of] people who blew the back of their heads off by placing a gun barrel in their mouth or overdose of pills. These experiences have taught me to observe the behaviour of others and be vigilant for signs of depression. I can name 10 or so EMTs/paramedics and a doctor who died tragically or killed themselves.

How to cope? Well I think the best way is to let it out. . . . A good cry at the appropriate time helps. I don't believe I have any behavioural issues as a result of dealing with death. Both my wife's and my parents have passed, and I do feel a sense of guilt that I did not make the most of the time we had together.

We had critical incident stress debriefing training and I taught this as well as one of our other courses in emergency medical services (EMS).

Faith [also] plays a part as I believe . . . in the next life.

This first responder's account contains four themes: (1) positive aspects of work, (2) an appreciation of life, (3) the most difficult aspects of work, and (4) coping mechanisms. While researchers and journalists tend to focus on the negative aspects of the work that first responders do, in particular on PTSD, depression, and suicide, it is important to note that the above account emphasizes the positive aspects of the work done by EMTs and paramedics. This work is described as fun, challenging, and interesting—"you never did the same call twice." He writes positively of the teamwork involving his immediate EMS partners and also firefighters and the resulting "solid friendships." He notes the satisfaction that came with knowing that the team "did [their] best" even when attempts at resuscitation failed. He mentions the satisfaction he feels to this day when he recalls "grateful patients." He looks back on his career with satisfaction, saying that he feels honoured to have been able to play a role in saving lives.

The second theme suggests that the work of first responders such as EMTs/paramedics can lead to a heightened appreciation of life. The writer indicates that he cherishes the gift of life and was honoured to participate in the saving of lives. He finds people who die by suicide the saddest aspect of his work experience. As an aside, he mentions the deaths of his parents and his wife's parents and wishes that he had had more time together with them when they were alive, again emphasizing an appreciation of the importance of life.

The third theme refers to the most distressing aspect of his work. He mentions calls involving people who had killed themselves and recalls colleagues who had done the same. The fourth theme highlights the coping mechanisms involved in dealing with stressful incidents. He states that "the best way is to let it out" and have "a good cry at the appropriate time." He also mentions that he taught the training course in critical incident stress debriefing, indicating that there was a procedure in place to help EMTs/paramedics cope with critical incidents. He notes that his faith in an afterlife was helpful for him. And it can be presumed that the positive aspects of the job, including the cohesive and supportive team environment and the satisfaction in a job done well and lives saved, also helped to sustain him through difficult times. Looking back, he indicates that he feels he was able to cope effectively with frequent exposure to imminent and actual death. Nevertheless, he notes that not all of his colleagues coped as well, and that he learned to watch for signs of depression in order to assist others when needed.

Journalists

Journalists often arrive on the scenes of tragedy. Some are sent around the world to report on wars, natural disasters, and human misery in all of its forms. Curt Petrovich reported for the CBC for three decades, always cool and professional. Then in 2013 he experienced the horror of rows of body bags containing the victims of a typhoon that devastated the Philippines causing some 6,000 deaths. This disaster affected him deeply and one has to wonder after all his years of reporting why this particular event "broke" him. Perhaps this is a case of "cumulative trauma" resulting from years of repeated exposure to traumatic events. Petrovich was diagnosed with PTSD in 2014 and told his story in a 2017 documentary film (Petrovich and Slinger 2017).

Petrovich said in the documentary: "Reporting on suffering, disaster, and death took its toll until finally one story broke me and left me trapped in the prison of post-traumatic stress disorder." Speaking to his wife, he said: "I carry around the guilt of having sort of brought this into our house. I just want to punch something." Petrovich came home from the Philippines disaster overwhelmed with PTSD, depression, anxiety, anger, guilt, emotional pain, and difficulty coping with everyday life. At one point, spiraling downwards, he said that he could not see a future for himself. Petrovich turned to running, researching and writing a story involving others who suffered from PTSD, and experimental treatments involving psychotherapy and psychedelic drugs. He had the support of his wife and daughter and son. The documentary shows the initial success of therapy, followed by a relapse, more experimental therapy, and ending with a hopeful but uncertain assessment of the future. He said: "I don't know if I will ever be released [from the prison of PTSD]. I can only hope that someday I will come home from the Philippines."

HEALTH CARE WORKERS

Dying and death generally take place in a social context involving both professional caregivers and family members. While the health care system tends to take control of dying and death, health care professionals are not always willing participants in the process of dying. As we discussed in chapter 3, doctors, who are generally trained to cure, tend to view death as a failure of treatment or medical care. Similarly, health care professionals of all kinds working in acute care hospitals typically work within a curative care model and so may not be equipped organizationally or even psychologically to deal with dying, palliative care, and death. Furthermore, Li et al. (2017) noted when implementing a hospital-based program in Toronto to administer Medical Assistance in Dying (MAID) shortly after its legalization in Canada that some hospital departments preferred not to be associated with the delivery of MAID. Reasons given included avoiding stigmatization (recall that anything and anybody associated with death tends to be stigmatized), maintaining their specialty's role and reputation for protecting life, and recognizing that some of their staff objected to MAID on grounds of conscience. Brooks (2019) reviewed studies of health care workers' experiences in other countries that had implemented MAID. She noted that physicians and nurses involved in the decision-making process and provision of MAID described it as an intense, complex, and difficult emotional process.

Health care workers, especially younger workers, may find caring for dying individuals and their distressed and grieving family members stressful. Some health care workers are threatened psychologically by death, particularly when they identify with the dying person, viewing them as similar to themself or to a family member. Those who choose to work with the dying— in palliative care units, for example—are often better suited to dealing with the dying, having more positive attitudes toward the dying process and the death of their patients.

There may be other issues with professional caregiving. For example, some health care workers may fear contamination and even death as a result of working with people dying from infectious diseases. Health care workers made up over 40 per cent of persons infected in Toronto in the 2003 SARS epidemic, with two nurses and one doctor among the dead (Health Canada 2003). Further, health care workers in hospitals and nursing homes during the COVID-19 pandemic risked their lives caring for the sick and dying and risked bringing the virus home to their families after work. Professional caregivers who work with dying individuals are reminded frequently, perhaps on a daily basis, of the mortality of others and presumably of their own mortality. Health care workers who care for the dying must therefore "come to terms" with dying and death if they are to provide quality care without undue personal distress.

Physicians

The first author of this book asked a medical doctor who had served as a rural family physician in Manitoba, and as a medical examiner, emergency department physician, and hospitalist (hospital medicine specialist or attending physician) in Alberta about his thoughts regarding dealing with the dying and the dead. He responded with the following stories. He noted that every health care worker is also a family member who must face the dying and death of their own grandparents, parents, and so on. Accordingly, he starts by telling

the stories of his parents' deaths. In these instances, the personal and professional intersect. After telling the stories of his parents' deaths, this physician
described death in the hospital emergency room (ER), death on the hospital
ward, and death as viewed by the medical examiner.

> I am happy to share some thoughts on dying and death. I find it easiest
> to express my opinion by telling stories.
>
> ### Dad
>
> Dad suffered a stroke at the age of 63, leaving him with serious disa-
> bilities. He had always said that "if I'm no good on the ground, put me
> under." He did not want to be useless. He lived to the age of 75, suffer-
> ing a series of strokes that left him more and more disabled. This was a
> source of great frustration to him, and a great trial for mom. When mom
> suffered a heart attack, then subsequently had open heart surgery, dad
> declined rapidly. I was a rural family doctor in Minnedosa, Manitoba, at
> the time. I made a trip into Winnipeg to see mom after her heart surgery.
> On the way in, I stopped to see dad in the Veteran's hospital. He was
> staring out the window and did not respond to me. It seemed to me that
> the dad I knew was not there; he was already gone. I wondered aloud,
> "How much longer does he have to live like this?"
>
> The next evening, back in Minnedosa, I received a call from the
> attending physician at the Veteran's hospital. Dad had suffered a res-
> piratory arrest. He was intubated and being ventilated, and was being
> transferred to ICU. What did I want him (the attending) to do? Now I
> was not dad's caregiver, not his power of attorney, and not his closest
> next of kin. But mom [had recently had heart surgery and] was in [the
> Coronary Care Unit], and I am a doctor. I guess that is why they called
> me. What a mix of emotions! I knew dad did not want to live like this. I
> knew that his chances of surviving resuscitation were slim. I knew that
> only one day earlier I wished he could be released from this life. But
> now was the moment of decision. I took a breath, told the attending to
> take out the tube, and called my two brothers who lived in Winnipeg.
> They came to the hospital with a family friend to administer to him (an
> ordinance equivalent to "last rites"). Dad passed peacefully within mo-
> ments after they administered.
>
> I was satisfied with the outcome—it seemed like the right thing. My
> brothers spoke of the peace they felt as they watched dad relax and take
> his last breath. Dad was released and I was happy for him, though I

grieved his death. But I never told mom that I had given the instruction to take out the tube. I don't know if anyone else [in the family knew] either. I'm not sure mom [w]ould have agreed if she had been competent at the time.

This scenario is not uncommon. When difficult situations arise requiring life and death decisions, if there is someone in the family in the health care professions caregivers often turn to that family member to guide their decisions. The assumption is that the nurse or doctor in the family will be able to make a more informed and objective decision regarding the care of their loved one. There may be some truth to this, but it is a burden. When dad was dying, I would have preferred to be his son, not his doctor.

Mom

Almost 27 years after dad died, my mother passed away. In her last years, she lived close to my wife and me, first in an assisted living facility, then in the hospital while waiting placement in a nursing home. My wife and I became her principal caregivers. We watched her as she declined, the inevitable result of diabetes, congestive heart failure, and atrial fibrillation. She suffered a number of small strokes, causing a step-wise loss of functions. At the end, she was noncommunicative and responded only by squeezing our hands. Our role included regular updates to the family on her activities and her health. I became closer to my mother during these last few years than ever before in my life.

It was, however, difficult to stay in the role of "son." I tried not to be her doctor, nor to interfere in the decisions the doctors made. But I did express to her doctors my expectations. I expected them to use medication to control symptoms and to improve quality of life. I wanted them to use as little medication as possible to achieve symptom control. I had no expectation of recovery or desire to prolong her life. At one point, her ventricular rate was poorly controlled as they tried to manage her pump failure. I suggested they use old-fashioned digitalis. Younger doctors are unfamiliar and often uncomfortable with its use, so I pushed a bit. The medication worked well, and mom had some relief of her symptoms. On the other hand, her doctor wanted her to be anticoagulated. At her advanced age, the risk of anticoagulation was significant, but the risk of stroke was also substantial. I preferred not to anticoagulate. I would rather that she died of her disease than from complications caused by the medications we were giving her.

She died after a series of strokes. Did I make the right choice? Would her last days have been different if I had consented to anticoagulation? It is not easy to be objective and clinical when the patient is your mother. Would I make the same decision if I was the doctor and the patient was someone else's mother?

Death in the ER

While death comes to each of us, death in the ER is usually sudden and unexpected. There has been trauma, or sudden collapse, which activates an emergency response. Every effort is made to save the life until it is [either] successful or obviously futile.

I recall a 31-year-old bull rider, brought in by EMS after he was thrown from the bull then stomped on. He was conscious, his eyes bugged out in panic as he gasped, "Help me Doc! I can't breathe!" He had obvious multiple rib fractures front and back on the right side—a flail chest. This is an emergency, but I could fix it, I thought. While the nurses were getting IVs started, I quickly inserted a chest tube on the right, and intubated the patient to provide positive pressure ventilation. While setting up for a chest tube on the left, his heart stopped. I started CPR and gave adrenalin. Nothing. I opened a pericardial window to relieve tamponade [compression of the heart by an accumulation of fluid in the pericardial sac]. Nothing. With the help of the trauma surgeon, we opened up his chest. His right lung was floating in a chest full of blood. It had been torn off the bronchus and was completely detached. The blood vessels on the right side of the heart were torn off the side of the heart. Blood was gushing into the chest cavity and there was no way to stop it. He was dead.

I paced the floor, hands on my head muttering to myself. Had I missed something? Did I do everything right? Could someone with more skill have saved him? One of the nurses touched me on the shoulder. "Are you all right?" she asked. Intellectually, I knew that there was nothing I could have done differently. The outcome was certain the moment a tonne of angry beef stomped on his right shoulder blade. But that was not how it felt.

I went out of the resuscitation room to tell his wife and six-year-old daughter that he was dead. His daughter said simply, "I don't want my daddy to die." Then I picked up a chart and went to see the next patient. No time to process. Just "who's next?"

I remember the details of that event like it was yesterday, but it was years ago. It is but one of many stories I could tell.

Death on the Ward

Death on the hospital ward is quite different. Often it is the expected outcome of what can be a long process. When death is inevitable, my main concern as a physician is for the patient's comfort and quality of life. At an appropriate time, I will usually have a conversation with the patient and the family about the dying process. I explain that I won't kill the patient on purpose, even if they request it, but I will help the patient through the dying process. I can offer pain control, relief from shortness of breath, relief from anxiety, and so on. I explain that they will be part of the team. They will help me evaluate if the management is adequate. I explain that if too much medicine is given, the patient will be unable to wake up, to respond, to interact with family. If not enough medicine is given, the patient will be in pain, or gasping for air, and so on, depending on the case. I explain that I will not prolong the dying process by giving medicines to sustain life. Generally, patients and family are very grateful to have this conversation, to know what is planned and what to expect.

I recall a 19-year-old boy who was dying from a brain tumour. All that could be done was done, but the tumour progressed relentlessly. Eventually, he could not speak, but could nod his head or squeeze a hand in response to questions. He could not eat or drink. He became weak and dehydrated, then acidotic. His breathing became rapid and irregular. His skin was breaking down. I asked him if he was suffering. He nodded yes. I asked if he wanted me to give him more medication. Yes. We started a small continuous dose of midazolam and hydromorphone to relieve his symptoms. He relaxed, went to sleep, and died peacefully before long. His family was grateful for the compassion and care he received.

The question is, did I kill him? I followed established protocols for what we call **terminal sedation**. It is accepted and legal. There is no intent to kill, but to relieve the symptoms associated with the dying process. So, no I didn't kill him. I simply allowed him to die in peace, the end result of his disease.

This is in contrast to assisted [death], where death is the result of substances administered with the intent to [cause death]. In assisted [death], it is not the disease process which kills the patient, but the drugs administered. I don't believe that I will participate in assisted [death]. It seems to violate one of the basic tenets of medicine, "first do no harm."

Medical Examiner's Perspective on Death

As a medical examiner for 14 years, my responsibility was to determine whether there was reasonable [natural] cause of death, or [if there] was any reason to suspect that the death was not natural. When a death could not be explained, an autopsy would be performed by a pathologist to determine cause of death. Most often, I would simply examine the body and perform some basic toxicology tests to determine cause of death. For example, whenever there was a death from a motor vehicle accident, I would view the body, determine if the injuries explained the death, and send blood, urine, and vitreous [from the eye] samples for alcohol and drug testing. It was my job to complete the certificate of death for all unnatural deaths.

This process was very academic, and often quite interesting. I rarely had any sort of emotional response, probably because the person was already dead by the time I was involved. On a few occasions, when I knew the deceased individual, I felt that my work as medical examiner was a final service I could offer the individual and their family.

These stories illustrate that health care workers experience death differently depending on their relationship with the deceased (who may be a family member, a patient they have come to know over time, or a patient they do not know at all) and depending on the role they play and the context in which they enact their role. In the story of his dad's death, the doctor notes that health care workers often turn to the health care worker in the family to negotiate difficult end-of-life decisions, assuming they will be able to make a "more informed and objective decision." It is also possible that in some cases health care workers assert their views. Other family members and the care team looking after the ill or dying person may accept this situation, since health care workers tend to share a common background and it is assumed that conversations and decisions can proceed more easily between the patient's professional caregivers and the family member who is presumed to speak for, or at least influence, the decisions of other family members. Despite being a physician and having an insider's perspective, the doctor in this story speaks of his "mix of emotions." He mentions the "burden" imposed on him to participate or take the lead in end-of-life decision making. When there is no health care worker in the family, decision making can be difficult for family members who similarly feel the burden of making life and death decisions. A double burden occurs, however, when the person has a health care background. The physician interviewed reflects on the role conflict he experienced by noting, "I would have preferred to be his son, not his doctor."

The doctor's story of his mother's death also refers to the role conflict that health care workers experience when they are both a family member and a health care professional. In this story the doctor was the family member primarily responsible for his mother's end-of-life decision making, but also a doctor who had considerable influence in the negotiation of her end-of-life care. He wondered not only about the role conflict but also the conflict of interest involved in this situation. He reflected on the tension between subjectivity (as a son) and objectivity (as a doctor) and wondered if he would make the same decisions for someone else's mother.

The doctor then contrasts his role and reactions to death in the ER, in a hospital ward, and as a medical examiner. In the ER, he notes that death is typically "sudden and unexpected," in contrast to the hospital ward where death is often the "expected" conclusion of a lengthy process. In the ER, every effort is made to save patient lives, but on the hospital ward the focus is on "the patient's comfort and quality of life" during the dying process when death is inevitable. The doctor tells the story of losing a patient he initially expected to save in the ER. When the patient died the doctor was distraught, wondering if he could have done something different to save the patient's life. Death in the ER tends to be viewed as failure, even when saving a patient is impossible. The expectation on the hospital ward and the doctor's reaction to expected death is different than in the ER. Death on the ward is more often accepted and usually can be managed more carefully by involving the patient and family in a conversation about how best to facilitate the dying process. With death in the ER, the family waits anxiously and is traumatized by bad news. On the hospital ward, the family is usually involved in the decision making and is often grateful for the care and compassion offered.

Death in the ER can be traumatic for health care workers. It can become a critical event, remembered long after its occurrence. "I remember the details of that event like it was yesterday," the doctor observed. Death on the hospital ward may also be remembered, but with some satisfaction that the process of dying was well managed and that the patient and family were appreciative. With death in the ER, there was often no time to immediately debrief, and thus reflect and recover. Other than the immediate support from a nurse, no therapy or intervention was offered to the ER doctor, who simply had to move on to the next patient in the queue. The event the doctor describes, like many other stories he could tell, is heartbreaking and frustrating, but not paralyzing.

He was expected to move on, and he did. With death on the hospital ward, in contrast to the ER, the doctor indicates a sense of satisfaction in doing his best for the patient and the family, alleviating suffering and facilitating as good a death as possible. There was no need for debriefing or intervention. The satisfaction the doctor experiences in doing his job well and in helping a dying person and his family is enough. The story told of death on the hospital ward is exemplary, a success story. In contrast, the story told of death in the ER, where death was unexpected, unwelcome, and distressing, is a story of frustration and disappointment. It is a story of how bad things can go, rather than a story of success.

In the physician's story of a sudden and tragic ER death, the nurse recognized and shared his grief. Nurses often grieve the death of patients they have come to know regardless of how short a time this is, and they have empathy for the families who will grieve hard over these deaths. Nurses often develop a relationship with the dying and their families through hours or days of hands-on direct care. This story is important in part because it demonstrates collective grieving. Many can grieve over a death, each in their own way and for many different reasons.

Finally, the doctor discusses his experience in dealing with death as a medical examiner. He describes the work as "academic, and often quite interesting" and notes that he "rarely had any sort of emotional response." He contrasts his experiences of working with the dead as opposed to working with the dying. In the ER and on the hospital ward, the patients are alive, at least initially; in the medical examiner's world, the patients are "already dead." This distinction gives him some emotional and cognitive distance as a medical examiner that is not possible when dealing with the living. For the most part he is able to avoid the emotional ups and downs that dealing with the dying can trigger. Even in the cases when he knew the deceased, he found satisfaction in providing "a final service" to the deceased and their family.

Kelly and Nisker (2010) asked final-year medical students at the University of Western Ontario if they had experienced the death of a patient in their care and if so to describe their first experience. The medical students who had experienced the death of one or more patients reported that they reacted differently to different kinds of death: "'Young' deaths were often perceived as tragedies that defied understanding and caused great emotional turmoil. 'Old' deaths were frequently experienced as so routine as to be dehumanizing. 'Unexpected' deaths often raised questions about how important control is to the professional role of doctor" (424). The medical students reported a tension between having an emotional concern for their dying patient and maintaining a professional detachment that they perceived was "expected of good doctors," and they described "the apparent paradox of being professionally detached and emotionally involved with a patient's death at the same time" (426). How they dealt with this tension was influenced by the kind of death they witnessed; their supervisor, who was viewed as a role model; and the support of supervisors and peers, including opportunities to debrief. The medical students coped by using rationalization, contemplation, and by focusing on lessons learned. "Young" deaths tended to cause "students to contemplate their life values" while "old" deaths tended to be rationalized and "unexpected" deaths were viewed as a learning experience. Debriefing with supervisors and peers helped students focus on lessons learned.

A study of oncologists (specialist physicians who treat cancer patients) working in three oncology centres in Ontario examined how they dealt with patient death (Granek et al. 2012). The oncologists in this study each experienced an average of four patient deaths per month. Oncologists are a unique set of physicians, as they, like palliative care physicians, are most likely to care for dying individuals. Cancer has become the leading cause of death in Canada. When asked what made some patient deaths more difficult than others, the oncologists in this study mentioned various aspects of their relationships with patients and their families, as well as aspects of physician culture. Factors that made the deaths of some patients difficult included close relationships with individuals and their families, younger patients, patients who had young children, patients with whom the physician identified, long-term patients, and unexpected deaths. In addition, deaths were made more difficult when patients or their families were unprepared and unaccepting of death, were demanding and had unrealistic expectations for cure and recovery, received or demanded futile treatment interventions, or when the oncologist was blamed for a death or for a bad dying process. Finally, dealing with patient deaths was made difficult by a physician culture that shared society's stigmatization of dying and death, emphasized cure rather than end-of-life care, and defined emotion as weak and unprofessional, especially for male oncologists. Female oncologists felt less constrained in showing their emotions regarding patient deaths. The authors suggested that the culture of physicians needs to change so that oncologist grief over patient loss could be acknowledged and normalized. They also argued that the discourse of cure (e.g., slogans such as "cancer can be beaten") needs to be downplayed so that patients, their families, and their physicians can have more open and realistic discussions about dying, death, and end-of-life care (see also Granek et al. 2013).

Granek et al. (2016) interviewed pediatric oncologists in Ontario who frequently experienced the deaths of children in their care. These physicians used a variety of coping strategies including relying on the support of family, friends, colleagues, and/or therapists; relying on faith/religion/spirituality; finding satisfaction, meaning, value, and purpose in providing the best possible end-of-life care for the dying child and their family; focusing on research and resulting improvements; taking breaks/vacations; engaging in exercise, entertainment, hobbies, and family activities; and recognizing the need to maintain emotional balance and mental well-being, at times through compartmentalization, distancing, and separation of professional and personal.

Nurses

Penz and Tipper (2019) asked, "Who cares for the caregiver?" They noted that nurses and other formal caregivers, especially those working in hospice/palliative or end-of-life care, may be at risk for occupational stress, burnout, compassion fatigue, vicarious trauma, PTSD, depression, and other mental health concerns. Stelnicki et al. (2020) surveyed a national sample of Canadian nurses and found that they reported higher rates of suicide ideation, plans, and attempts than the general population. Nevertheless, most nurses report high levels of job satisfaction despite the challenges of their work (Penz and Tipper 2019).

During the first decade of the AIDS epidemic in the 1980s, Reutter interviewed nurses who cared for people dying from AIDS in an active treatment hospital in Western Canada (Reutter and Northcott 1994). While the risk of contracting HIV/AIDS at work was small, the nurses expressed concern because of life-threatening consequences should they become infected with the disease. These nurses employed behavioural and cognitive strategies to gain a sense of control. They came to perceive risk as manageable by using precautions such as gloving and masking, reappraising risk as minimal or normal, and using distancing strategies, including denial and avoidance of threatening thoughts and situations. They also accepted risk through finding meaning in their work, by accepting the AIDS patient as a person who needed and deserved care, by finding work enjoyable and worthwhile, and by emphasizing professional commitment to care (Reutter and Northcott 1993). The notion of risk as meaningful and manageable gave the nurses a sense of security.

However, when they were exposed to HIV-infected blood or body fluids, their feelings of security dissolved (Reutter and Northcott 1995). They were instantly reminded of their own vulnerability and mortality.

Many of the same issues arose during the severe acute respiratory syndrome (SARS) epidemic beginning in early 2003, when nurses were once again exposed to infectious agents that placed them at considerable risk. In the next few months, 438 Canadians contracted SARS, and of these 44 people died, nearly half of whom were nurses. Nurses and other health care workers ultimately made up 43 per cent of the cases of infection in Canada from SARS in 2003. Some of the survivors suffered long-term effects. Some, especially health care workers who survived the epidemic, had PTSD (Branswell 2013). In short, nurses and other health care workers are exposed to deadly pathogens and other conditions in the course of their work that constitute a risk to their own lives and health, and also then to the life and health of their close family members.

In late 2019, another new virus (COVID-19) appeared and soon became a global pandemic, reaching Canada in early 2020. Once again, nurses and other health care workers found themselves on the front line caring for the sick and dying and risking their own health and the health of their family members.

In addition to physical risks, nurses are often impacted emotionally by the dying and death of their patients. Nurses frequently develop relationships with their dying patients and the patients' families. Nurses are involved in end-of-life decisions and they are sometimes forced to carry out difficult decisions, such as when family members demand futile treatment when they are not ready for the death of their loved one. In these cases, **moral distress** is common, as nurses have to take a direct role in creating or extending patient suffering (Austin et al. 2005). Moral distress and **burnout** are now commonly acknowledged in nursing, along with PTSD, as nurses work in ambulances, hospital emergency departments, battlefields, and other places where traumatic deaths and unsightly deaths or dying processes occur (Mealer et al. 2009).

Leung et al. (2012) interviewed registered nurses in Ontario who worked in bone marrow transplant units, a site where dying and death are common. The nurses said that they often found their work rewarding and frequently developed emotional attachments to the patients and families. Nevertheless, when confronted with the possibility and often inevitability of their patients' deaths, their work could be frightening, overwhelming, discouraging, disillusioning, and lacking in meaning. Possible outcomes included burnout and **compassion fatigue**. Nurses coped by acting professionally, maintaining a degree of distance, and balancing their professional and personal lives. The authors wrote, "Work-life 'balance' was the key to surviving the experience of so many patients' deaths. . . . Seasoned nurses reported that novice nurses were at risk of becoming 'unbalanced' with the emotional burden of work" (2181). In short, nurses learned to cope over time by finding a balance between their personal lives and the emotional demands of their work lives, and by maintaining some distance from their patients while at the same time providing empathetic care.

In contrast, Vachon, Fillion, and Achille (2012) interviewed nurses who worked in palliative care units in hospitals, hospices, and home care settings where there is no expectation of saving lives or curing diseases. One recurring theme was that the nurses "mentioned that dealing with suffering was actually harder than dealing with death on a daily basis" (161). Some nurses viewed suffering as meaningful; other nurses felt frustrated, powerless, helpless, fatigued, and exhausted. Some reported feeling guilt that they had not done enough or not been able to alleviate suffering. "Finally, almost all nurses mentioned having some kind of mechanism to ensure they were not personally too affected by the suffering they witnessed in their work. Whereas some of them mentioned that the transition between work and [personal] life was easy and did not require any special care or attention, the majority of nurses underscored the importance of having some time and space between work and home. They talked about their professional and personal lives as 'two different worlds'" (162). The nurses interviewed had chosen to continue to work with dying individuals and their families; many others who try working in palliative care may be unable to find this balance and move into different areas where death is less common.

Many of the palliative care nurses in the above study (Vachon, Fillion, and Achille 2012) mentioned positive aspects of working closely with death. They mentioned increased awareness of their own mortality and of the necessity of living a mindful and meaningful life. They noted that it was a privilege to assist the dying and that this gave them a sense of purpose. Nevertheless, these same nurses tended to find it difficult to deal with patients and family members who were negative, suffering, angry, hopeless, and despairing. "Intense suffering without meaning appeared to shake nurses' system of beliefs and put them in a state of helplessness and frustration" (166). Further, there was variation in the nurses' response to frequent exposure to death, with some coping better than others. Some found meaning and purpose, while others experienced distress and existential and spiritual crisis.

Health Care Aides

Health care aides have several related titles such as direct care workers, personal support workers (PSWs), residential care aides, and nurses' aides. Wiersma et al. (2019) studied the moral concerns of PSWs who cared for the dying in long-term care homes in Ontario. These PSWs felt "moral distress . . . because [they] identified the 'right action' to take but were often constrained from doing so" (272). They were concerned that dying residents receive adequate care and not die alone but often lacked the time and organizational support to provide needed care. They were caught between the dying resident and their family (although some of the dying had been abandoned by their family), and between the dying resident and the physicians, nurses, and managers in the organizational hierarchy. While the PSWs provided most of the direct care, they had little power or authority and often felt that they were unable to do what they considered to be right, important, and necessary. Some of the PSWs resisted and attempted to find ways to do what they felt necessary, while others gave in and accepted the constraints. Either way, the moral dilemmas led to distress, frustration, dissatisfaction, regret, guilt, and job turnover.

The COVID-19 pandemic identified long-term care facilities in Canada as high risk (hotspots), with many outbreaks occurring in these facilities along with a disproportionate number of deaths. Staff who were overworked and underpaid, themselves some of the more vulnerable elements of society (often immigrant women who are visible minorities), presumably experienced considerable distress as they attempted to care for their infected and dying residents, protect those residents who had not been infected, protect themselves and their own family members, and do so in minimal or inadequate organizational circumstances.

The COVID-19 crisis in long-term care facilities in 2020–1 was a crisis waiting to happen. Years prior, McClement et al. (2010) interviewed health care aides (HCAs) who worked with older adults in nursing homes. Although death is common among nursing home residents, these HCAs expressed frustration when dealing with residents who were dying. The HCAs highlighted their relationships with dying residents and the obligations they felt to alleviate suffering, maintain the dignity of the resident, provide care, and respect the patient's wishes. They complained that there was often inadequate pain control and that when they informed the nurses who were in charge too often nothing was done. (In the nurses' defence, physician medication orders are needed before any medication can be given, and long delays in contacting the resident's physician are common.) The HCAs noted that sometimes their own colleagues provided perfunctory care and did not show the concern for the dying person that they thought was warranted. The HCAs also complained that there were too few resources and too little time to properly care for the dying. Finally, the HCAs noted that frequently the dying person's wishes were overruled by other health care workers or by family members who visited infrequently. While some HCAs fought for their dying residents, others had retreated, given up, or been silenced. HCAs have the most contact with dying people in care homes and provide the bulk of care, but they have little status, limited influence on end-of-life care decisions, and are at risk of being silenced and alienated. High staff turnover is an outcome in part due to the frustration that HCAs experience in providing what they consider to be adequate care for dying residents.

Similar findings were reported in a study of residential care aides (RCAs) working in care facilities in Victoria (Funk, Waskiewich, and Stajduhar 2013–14). These RCAs frequently provided end-of-life care and reported feelings of distress, frustration, guilt, and helplessness in caring for dying residents. They wished they could do more to alleviate suffering and wished they could spend more time with the dying. At the same time, the RCAs spoke of the importance of being professional rather than emotional and maintaining a degree of detachment; nevertheless, some deaths were more difficult than others. The suffering of the dying and the attachment of RCAs to residents or their families made some deaths more difficult. Unexpected deaths tended to be difficult as well. Talking with colleagues about these deaths and the emotions they generated was helpful. These RCAs also tended to draw on "consoling refrains" such as "[death is] part of life," the resident is "better off," his or her death was a "blessing" or a "relief from suffering," the resident had lived a "good/full/long life," "I did what I could," and "I did my best." The RCAs also tended to emphasize the importance of what they do in helping residents die well and derived some satisfaction from that. For example, a common refrain was "It's an honour" to help the dying to die. Nevertheless, the RCAs complained that they had little opportunity to grieve or deal with their emotions at work or later, but simply had to "carry on." A related concern is that nursing home residents often have long or "dwindling" dying processes, where it is difficult to know if the person is actually dying or if they will recover and continue living (Cable-Williams and Wilson 2017).

Social Workers

Social workers can also be impacted by dying and death. Simons and Park-Lee (2009) surveyed bachelor's level and master's level social work students about their comfort with end-of-life care. They found that students who were older, had past personal experiences with death, had completed or would like to complete a hospice placement, and had less anxiety about death were more comfortable anticipating involvement in end-of-life care. In contrast, younger students and students who had no personal experience with dying and death were less comfortable with the possibility of providing end-of-life care or having contact with terminally ill clients and their families.

Muskat, Brownstone, and Greenblatt (2017) interviewed social workers employed in hospital pediatric acute care. They concluded that

> pediatric social workers caring for dying children in an acute care setting find their work rewarding and impactful. These social workers derive satisfaction from supporting families to experience their child's end of life . . . [however,] social workers often form close connections with patients and families which increase the feelings of loss and sadness in their work. This may result in experiencing challenging emotions that must be effectively managed in order to have healthy professional and personal lives and to provide the best possible care. (520)

Death Doulas

Death doulas are a newly emerging role designed to fill potential gaps in end-of-life care (Rawlings et al. 2019; Rawlings et al. 2020). The emerging role of the death doula, usually a woman, reflects the better-established role of the birth doula. Centuries ago, women as lay midwives attended birth, and as caregivers attended death. The concept of the doula in the twenty-first century reflects these earlier roles. At present, the role of death doula is not well-defined, and the relation of death doulas to other caregivers such as family members, palliative care physicians, hospital nurses, and nursing home health care aides is not clear. Doulas may act as advocates for the dying and their family members and may do so in either a volunteer or paid capacity. Presumably, death doulas self-select into this role and therefore may be well-suited in terms of temperament, education, and past life experiences. On the other hand, like other occupations exposed regularly to death, they may be at risk for PTSD and other mental health issues. Future research will be instructive.

DEATH CARE WORKERS

Death care (or death services) workers include persons who transport dead bodies, medical examiners and coroners, funeral directors, embalmers, and other funeral or memorial home workers. These personnel are exposed to death on a daily basis. Some deaths are more gruesome or unsettling than others. While many do cope with their employment, some may experience PTSD, depression, burnout, and other mental health issues (Brondolo et al. 2018; Pfeffer 2019). O'Keeffe (2020) noted that death care during the COVID-19 pandemic increased concerns about risks of infection from handling dead bodies, storing bodies, or from contact with family members and religious officials in the contexts of preparing the dead body, viewing the body, and engaging in other after-death funeral or memorial services.

Medical Examiners

Medical examiners (MEs) are often physicians who have chosen to specialize in after-death care. The staff in ME offices include investigators who go to the scene of death, examine the body, and construct a history for the deceased. The first author of this book used to take students for a tour of an ME's office. These tours were given by one of the investigators who was always open to student questions. When asked how he coped with working every day with dead people, he emphasized the positive aspects of his work, for example, finding the identity of the deceased and constructing an explanation and account of their death.

One investigator told the story of a woman they could not identify. The ME office kept her in their freezer long after they were legally obligated to do so. It bothered them that they could not give this person the identification that humanized the body as a unique individual with a life story and family. The investigator noted the importance of properly identifying the deceased. Besides providing an identity, he mentioned that the family of the deceased typically benefited from knowing how the person died and often welcomed the account of death that the investigator compiled.

When asked if any deaths were troubling, this investigator mentioned that he found having to process deceased children the most distressing. He had children of his own, so the deaths of children constituted a personal reminder for him of their vulnerability.

When asked how office staff coped with repeated exposure to death, he emphasized that they cultivated a respectful, reverential culture in which each body was treated with care and respect. While this may have been the intention and the ideal, realities can be compromised. In 2019, a news story appeared in the media of bodies being stored in a refrigerated truck and bodies in body bags being dragged on the floor of the truck rather than being moved and stored in a more respectful manner. This led to a provincial government investigation and recommendations to reassure the public of respectful and dignified after-death care (Rusnell 2019).

It is important to note that most deaths do not involve MEs. Deaths that are expected, explained, and under the care of a physician are not processed by the ME office. The ME must examine all deaths that are unexpected, unexplained, or that involve accident, trauma, homicide, or suicide. For unexplained deaths, the ME may conduct autopsies in an effort to determine the manner of death but does not conduct open-body autopsies on all deaths that come to the ME office. In some cases, causes of death may be determined by ultrasound scanning. This is of particular importance to some cultural groups, including Jewish and Islamic families, who prefer to have their loved one's body remain intact.

Funeral, Cemetery, and Crematory Workers

People who are involved in providing after-death care for the deceased and their families can also be expected to have some emotional reactions (Pfeffer 2019). Pfeffer reported for *CBC News* about Canadian funeral home workers and their mental health. They had established a peer-counselling group in Ottawa to help with their industry's mental health challenges. Pfeffer noted: "They [funeral home workers] say they're surrounded by trauma and it takes a toll." In addition to dealing with dead bodies, the funeral home workers also deal with the families of the dead. This creates a "vicarious trauma," as funeral home workers "deal with the trauma other people are experiencing."

The first author of this book asked a former student about her experience working during the summer in a cemetery. She titled her thoughts "Life and Death in the Cemetery":

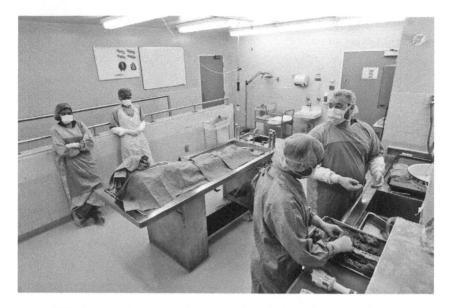

Image 7.5. A room where autopsies are performed. Note that the deceased is covered respectfully on the table.
Source: Kevin Van Passen/The Globe and Mail/The Canadian Press. All rights reserved.

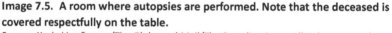

I've always loved cemeteries. To me they were and are peaceful, beautiful parks, with the added joy of being a gathering spot to remember and honour loved ones that I knew, and those who had gone long before. Somehow, being at the final resting place of a loved one, looking at their name engraved in stone, while sharing their stories makes these ancestors just a little more real to me.

Loving cemeteries and the out-of-doors made my choice to do grounds work for a local cemetery only natural. Mowing the grass among the endless rows of headstones gave me much time to wonder about those who lay there. What was their story, who did they leave behind, who went before them, how did they live, how did they die? Always the quick calculation in my head: did they die "too" young, die at my present age, or did they live a long life? Some graves were frequently visited, as evidenced by flowers, trinkets, and tokens left by visitors. Others seemed forgotten.

I loved it when family members of the deceased would stop me to tell me of their loved one instead of leaving me to wonder about them.

Headstones that were engraved with various images such as tractors, mountains, flowers, or cars, would give me a basis to imagine who may be resting there. In the infant and children's section of the cemetery I would wonder who these little angels would have been had they been given the chance to flourish on earth.

My work in the cemetery made me realize how much I hope that someone will always be there to visit my grave and to tell my story. Or at the very least that someone will always care enough to pull back the grass and dust off my headstone with a little kindness, and wonder to whom I had once mattered.

Working at the cemetery led to an interesting blend of the solemn and comical. While eating lunch a special delivery was made. The worker tossed the [mortuary] box casually in the middle of our table as our lead signed for the package. We all looked at the box, our lunches, and one another, and started laughing at the oddity that a cremated body was now at the centre of our table.

Participating in the cremation process became a part of my job duties. It was hard to wrap my mind around purposefully setting a body on fire, and furthermore, dropping the ash and chunks of bone afterwards into a blender. A blender! Seeing the process firsthand, it all seemed so absurd. More akin to a Wile E. Coyote vignette than reality.

I could never take on the task of crawling into the oven to sweep the corners out, as I could not get past the idea that someone could close the door behind me and start the fire. This task brought images of the Holocaust to my mind that I could not shake. The days we were processing bodies at the crematory left a different smell in the air that I tried not to think of too much, and wondered if visitors to the cemetery realized what it was.

What better place than a cemetery to reflect on life and death? One glorious summer day the sun filtered down through the trees shining upon a headstone illuminating a singing perky juvenile sparrow. Ah. Life. As I reflected on the beauty of the scene, a crow swooped down snatching the sparrow in its mouth, abruptly ending the tiny bird's song. And there it was. Death.

Jim was a seasoned year-round worker, not a summer employee like myself. He always spoke fondly of his time at the "bone-yard." He liked to tease about what odd goings-on might occur at night when no one was around. I enjoyed the fun of his tales. His attempts to make the cemetery seem "spooky" did not work on me. However, one day I was puzzled to see in the distance an uncovered freshly dug grave with no one in sight. We were never to leave a grave uncovered. I continued navigating my mower closer, squinting intently. I nearly had a heart attack when suddenly an arm popped up out of the hole and hooked over the edge, followed by another arm and then a head! Perhaps I had more concern over the existence of zombies than I thought! The "zombie" was really a worker who dropped an item into the grave and had gone in alone to retrieve it.

SUMMARY

This chapter focuses on first responders, health care workers, and death care workers. First responders such as police officers, firefighters, emergency medical technicians and paramedics; health care workers including doctors and nurses; and death care workers such as investigators in a medical examiner's office and funeral directors and their staff are all exposed to death, some on a regular basis and others on an occasional basis. Most find meaning and satisfaction in the work they do. Some, however, do not cope as well as others and find the exposure to dying and death stressful. Moreover, some deaths or dying processes are particularly difficult. These critical events or traumatic deaths, as they are called, can be disturbing and distressing. Reactions can include depression, anxiety, frustration, anger, despair, compassion fatigue, burnout, PTSD, alcohol and substance abuse, relationship problems, and suicidal thoughts and suicide. For many, these reactions are temporary. For some, however, these reactions can become chronic and can have serious impacts on their health and well-being.

In the past, first responder, health care, and death care occupations tended to share a culture that denied the legitimacy of emotional reactions. This is still true today, although to a lesser extent. Emotions were considered a sign of weakness. To show one's emotions was defined as unprofessional and considered "unmanly" in male-dominated professions; emotional expression was stigmatized. Professionals were and still are expected to keep their emotions under control. Today, however, emotional reactions to critical events such as traumatic death and to repeated exposure to dying and death are increasingly being acknowledged and normalized. It is recognized that care for the caregivers is not only needed but also must be provided.

Caring for the caregivers requires a culture that responds to the emotional needs of those who experience distress in dealing with the dying and the dead. A recurring and current notion is the importance of immediate, or as soon as possible, debriefing with colleagues following a traumatic death.

While formal support programs and professional counselling can also help, it appears that immediate informal support of colleagues tends to be the most effective first measure. It is important to be able to express one's feelings, perceptions, distress, frustration, anger, and so on to sympathetic and supportive colleagues who share workplace dilemmas, concerns, and risks. And it is important to find meaning and purpose in the work that is done to assist the dying, the dead, and their survivors.

QUESTIONS FOR REVIEW

1. Give some examples of traumatic deaths and critical incidents. Describe the range of possible reactions first responders and health care workers who experience a traumatic death or critical incident might have. What coping strategies do first responders and health care workers use?
2. Discuss difficulties that first responders and health care workers might have in coping with their personal exposure to a range of dying and death events, including post-traumatic stress disorder (PTSD) and other emotional and mental health issues. How can we best care for the caregivers?
3. Compare and contrast health care worker reactions to the death of a family member versus the death of a stranger in the ER, hospital ward, or long-term care facility.
4. First responders and health care workers care for the dying, while death care workers deal with those who are already dead. Examine the differences and similarities in the experiences of first responders, health care workers, and death care workers.
5. Discuss the roles played in the COVID-19 pandemic by first responders, health care workers, and death care workers. How were each of these groups affected by their work with COVID-19 victims, dead or alive? How did these people cope with uncertainty, fear, and other difficult circumstances?

KEY TERMS

burnout – Loss of motivation, interest, commitment, and empathy. (p. 273)
compassion fatigue – When health care workers lose compassion and empathy for clients over time as a result of ongoing stress at work. (p. 274)

critical incident – A traumatic event involving the occurrence or threat of death. (p. 258)

critical incident stress management (CISM) – A formal program that typically involves giving first responders a chance to talk over their experiences, feelings, and reactions with professional counsellors and co-workers following a traumatic death. (p. 250)

death care workers – People who process the dead body, including medical examiners, funeral directors, and those who work at cemeteries and crematoria. (p. 247)

first responders – Police officers, firefighters, paramedics and emergency medical technicians, and so on who are typically the first people called to the scene of an unexpected death. (p. 246)

health care workers – A wide range of health care personnel including physicians, nurses, aides, therapists, psychologists, and social workers. Does not include family members who act as unpaid caregivers. (p. 247)

medical examiner (ME) – A public official responsible for investigating sudden, suspicious, or unexplained deaths including accidents, suicides, and homicides. (p. 278)

moral distress – When health care workers feel conflicted or distressed about the ethics of providing care that may be futile, unnecessary, or harmful to a patient. (p. 273)

post-traumatic stress disorder (PTSD) – A pattern of symptoms and behaviours that are long-lasting and occur as a result of exposure to traumatic or repeated death(s). Associated with a variety of emotional and mental health issues such as anxiety, depression, relationship difficulties, and suicide. (p. 246)

primary trauma – Directly experiencing a death. For example, a police officer may deal with a death from a motor vehicle accident, murder, suicide, and so on. (p. 255)

secondary trauma – Exposure to the suffering of others who have experienced the death of a loved one. For example, a police officer may have to tell family and friends of the death of a loved one from a motor vehicle accident or murder and witness their anguish. (p. 256)

terminal sedation – Medication prescribed and administered during the active dying process to manage symptoms and make dying more comfortable. (p. 267)

Conclusion

Dying and death reflect the material and social conditions of society. Centuries ago, in the pre-contact era, living conditions for Indigenous peoples in Canada were such that life expectancy was perhaps 30 to 40 years, about the same as it was in Europe at that time. While death often came early for Indigenous peoples, some individuals survived to old age. Nevertheless, dying and death were common, visible, and expected occurrences. Indigenous social practices and cultural definitions reflected these realities and, in turn, shaped the experience of dying and death.

Contact with Europeans brought devastation to Indigenous peoples in Canada. Infectious diseases previously unknown in North America increased death rates and annihilated whole populations. The destruction of Indigenous economies and ways of life further contributed to high rates of death. In addition, European culture, first brought by missionaries and traders, had an impact on Indigenous social practices and cultural definitions and tended to transform the social and personal experience of dying and death. Christian religious views of life and death sharply contrasted with the values common among Indigenous groups. For Indigenous peoples, death was more likely to be a natural or unavoidable part of life, explained by their cosmology and given meaning by their spirituality. Death began to take on a new significance when viewed in the Christian context of heaven and hell.

While the infectious diseases brought to Canada by the Europeans were especially devastating for Indigenous peoples, they did not spare European explorers, traders, and settlers. The harsh climate, tough pioneer existence, low standards of living, and unsanitary practices contributed to many early deaths in the colonies. Infant mortality was high, as was maternal mortality, and life expectancy in general was low. Health care was relatively ineffective, and the few hospitals that existed were considered places of death. It was not until the late nineteenth century that the newly emerging public health movement began to have a positive impact on health and life expectancy by improving sanitation and the safety of food and water. Subsequent advances in health care in the twentieth century helped bring dramatic improvements in life expectancy. The causes of death shifted from infectious and acute illnesses to chronic diseases, and the timing of death shifted increasingly to later life. The care of the dying was transferred from family members to health care professionals, and dying and death were moved from the home and community to the hospital and nursing home. Death, which had been common and familiar, became unfamiliar and expected only in old age.

At the beginning of the twenty-first century, the most common causes of death are cancer and circulatory disease, although causes of death vary considerably depending on personal characteristics such as age, sex, and social class. Young adults are most likely to die of accidents, injuries, and suicide. In older age groups, cancer and circulatory disease dominate as causes of death. The timing of death has become noticeably discrepant for males and females, with females outliving males by several years on average. This sex differential in life expectancy emerged during the twentieth century, but in recent years it has begun to decrease. Disadvantaged individuals and groups such as Indigenous peoples continue to have life expectancies below the Canadian norm. Nevertheless, deaths occurring early in life have come to be unexpected and have been labelled premature.

Social institutions such as family, religion, the health care system, the legal system, and the funeral industry continue to influence views of dying and death, along with related practices. Families have become less likely to be involved as sole primary caregivers for the dying. Professional caregivers typically attend to the dying, often in institutional settings such as a nursing home for the oldest old, a hospice for those in need of palliative care, or a hospital for younger people. Furthermore, families have become much less involved with the processing of the dead body. Instead, processing of the dead body and management of the funeral or memorial rituals are now typically provided by the funeral industry, which has become "big business" consistent with a general trend toward the corporatization, bureaucratization, professionalization, and secularization of dying and death. Funeral rituals have moved from the home, community, and church to the profit-driven funeral industry.

Religion has played a significant part in giving meaning to dying and death and continues to do so for those who maintain a religious commitment. Furthermore, religion continues to play an active role in social debates about end-of-life issues such as assisted death. Nevertheless, the influence of religion for many has been replaced by secular trends.

The success of twentieth-century health care in curing diseases and forestalling death led to the dominance of a curative model in modern health care that emphasizes resisting death, viewing it as a failure of the health care system. Toward the end of the twentieth century, however, the hospice/palliative care movement gained momentum; it emphasizes quality of life for the dying by focusing on managing symptoms and facilitating a good death for the dying and their families rather than engaging in futile attempts to cure or prolong life. Further, advance directives that authorize the withholding or withdrawing of medical treatment have not only become legal but are now in common use. In 2015, the Supreme Court of Canada mandated changes to the Criminal Code of Canada, which in 2016 resulted in the legalization of Medical Assistance in Dying (MAID). Previously, the Criminal Code defined assisted death as illegal.

Despite the twentieth-century trends toward the hospitalization, bureaucratization, and professionalization of dying and death, there appears now to be a substantial move toward bringing dying and death back to the home and family, where family members once again may be the primary caregivers, functioning with the assistance of health care professionals in providing end-of-life care at home. And the advent of MAID in 2016 reveals an increasing emphasis on individuals gaining control over their end of life.

There is a diversity of views now as to what death is and what it means. For some, death is a transition to a better life. Others view it as the final end. For many, death is a mystery or, as Shakespeare put it in *Hamlet*, "the undiscovered country from whose bourn no traveller returns" (Act III, Scene I). People facing death tend to interpret it and give it meaning, but the specific meaning assigned to death varies from one individual to another, and from one social context to another. Those facing death often engage in a review of their life, examining their biography to give it meaning and to claim meaning in the face of death. Just as the specific meaning assigned to death tends to vary from one individual to another, so does the meaning of one's life.

Because each individual's biography is personal and unique, the construction of life's meaning and the construction of the meaning of dying and death are both personal and unique, even if shaped to a degree by the individual's culture and society.

The dying and the living tend to view the process of dying as more fearful and distressing than the prospect of death itself. Pain and suffering are not welcome. Furthermore, the dying do not welcome the various losses—of health, future, competence, independence, social roles, social status, and personal relationships—that they face in the course of dying. Although they may express concern for those who will survive them and for the relationships that will be disrupted by their death, they may welcome death itself as an end to a dying process marked by pain and prolonged losses.

There are many different kinds of deaths and many different ways of dying. Similarly, there are many different ways to grieve. While shock and numbness often attend the loss of a loved one, and while sadness is commonly experienced by the bereaved, individuals grieve in their own way and in their own time. While *intense* grieving does usually end, grieving may nevertheless last a lifetime.

Losing a loved one means losing, or more accurately changing, a relationship with that person, a relationship that is part of oneself. It follows that the loss of a significant other involves a transformation of the self. Loved ones are not forgotten; they are remembered from time to time with varying degrees of emotion, and as such the relationships between the living and the dead continue. In that sense, grieving does not end. Furthermore, the process of making sense of loss and of finding meaning in death and in life is often ongoing. Nevertheless, over time grieving is likely to become less "disruptive" to one's personal and social functioning.

While dying, death, bereavement, and grieving are intensely personal experiences, and while reactions vary from one individual to another, society and culture nevertheless provide definitions and guidelines for grieving. When personal grief violates these guidelines—for example, when a person continues to grieve intensely beyond the time allotted for grieving—then such grief becomes defined as complicated, prolonged, chronic, unresolved, deviant, abnormal, pathological, or a sign of individual failure and weakness. Definitions and normative guidelines such as these fail to legitimize individual differences in grieving and put pressure on people to hide their personal grief.

People may manage their emotions and behaviours in public to conform to social expectations, showing grief or hiding it when appropriate. Public displays of either grief or non-grief should not be mistaken for the private and the personal. Similarly, the homogeneity of public displays should not blind one to the heterogeneity of personal experiences. Dying and death, as well as bereavement and grieving are, in the end, both highly social and highly personal experiences.

Today the course of dying is shaped by decisions made by people who may or may not acknowledge they are dying, their family members, and any involved health care staff. Although the hospital continues to have a major role in dying and death, the primary location of dying and death has shifted from the hospital to continuing care facilities, the home, and other locations like hospices. Even in the hospital, the location of death is shifting from acute care wards to palliative care beds. Similarly, although health care workers may be primary caregivers for the dying in hospitals and nursing homes, the family is often heavily involved and participates in end-of-life care decisions and actual caregiving. It is reassuring to note that the dying and their family caregivers generally assess their experiences with end-of-life care in positive terms. Nevertheless, some express dissatisfaction and most, when pressed, can identify elements of care that they feel could have been better and that could have helped the deceased to experience a better death. Health care workers also wish to provide their dying patients with a good death and sometimes complain that family members make this difficult when they deny that their loved one is dying and demand futile care.

First responders such as police officers, firefighters, emergency medical technicians (EMTs), and paramedics; health care workers including doctors and nurses; and death care workers such as medical examiners and funeral directors often find meaning and satisfaction in the work they do in relation to dying and death. Some, however, do not cope as well as others and find the exposure to dying and death stressful. Reactions can include depression, anxiety, frustration, anger, despair, compassion fatigue, burnout, post-traumatic stress disorder (PTSD), alcohol and substance abuse, relationship problems, and suicidal thoughts, plans, and suicide. For many, these reactions are temporary. For some, however, these reactions are long-lasting. Today, emotional reactions to critical events such as traumatic death and to repeated exposure to dying and death are increasingly being acknowledged, and efforts are being made to care for the caregivers.

One of the recurring themes in this book is that dying and death have changed, continue to change, or need to change. For example, we have told the story of a former student's anger at "failing grief," as she put it, frustrated by unhelpful social rules that did not help her grieve the death of her mother. And the story of the father who lost two children to separate, bizarre accidents challenges the notion that grief is a series of linear and time-limited steps. Our understanding of grief is evolving and needs to continue to do so. We also included the story of a mother's long journey into dementia and her exclusion from Medical Assistance in Dying; her daughter argued that this exclusion has to change. An expectant mother told the story of her traumatic miscarriage and the social rule that disenfranchises the grief of mothers (and fathers and grandparents) when a miscarriage occurs, especially in the early months of a pregnancy. This has got to change, says the grieving mother. The increasing recognition and normalization of mental health in its many forms including depression, anxiety, anger, and PTSD is encouraging. The COVID-19 pandemic has laid bare the structural and institutional inadequacies of the long-term care sector where many frail elderly Canadians are housed. This has to change, is the echoing refrain. And the evening news at the time of writing highlights the unwarranted and continuing loss of Black lives and immigrant or visible minority lives in the context of institutionalized racism endemic in police forces and wider society, the missing and murdered Indigenous women and girls across the country, and the deaths of the mentally ill in violent encounters with police. These things, too, need to change.

Glossary

active dying   The process of dying leading to immediate and inevitable death.

advance directive   A legal document that allows competent individuals to indicate their preferences for care before care is actually needed and in anticipation of circumstances where the person might not be able to make or voice decisions. Also referred to as a living will, personal directive, health care directive, representation agreement, or power of attorney for personal care.

analgesic   A substance used to reduce pain.

asepsis   Keeping a clean, germ-free environment.

assisted death   Usually involves providing a lethal substance, at the patient's request (or at the request of the patient's designated decision maker), that the patient consumes or that is administered to the patient with the intent of causing death. Includes both assisted suicide and euthanasia.

assisted suicide   Helping someone to die by suicide.

bereaved   People who experience the death of a loved one.

bereavement   The bereaved go through a period of bereavement.

bureaucratization   The establishment of extensive formal rules to govern procedures and division of labour in a complex organization such as a hospital.

burnout   Loss of motivation, interest, commitment, and empathy.

cardiopulmonary resuscitation (CPR)   Efforts made to restart a heart that has ceased functioning and to restore breathing.

centenarian   A person who is 100 years of age or older.

chronic illness   Illnesses that are incurable and typically progressive.

compassion fatigue   When health care workers lose compassion and empathy for clients over time as a result of ongoing stress at work.

courtesy stigma   When a person is stigmatized because of a stigma attached to someone else with whom he or she is associated.

cremation   The process by which a very hot fire is used to reduce the body and its container to ash.

critical incident   A traumatic event involving the occurrence or threat of death.

critical incident stress management (CISM)   A formal program that typically involves giving first responders a chance to talk over their experiences, feelings, and reactions with professional counsellors and co-workers following a traumatic death.

cultural competence   Being aware of and responsive to cultural differences in ways that are sensitive, caring, and supportive.

dark tourism   The phenomenon of people travelling to places associated with death such as battlefields, cemeteries, memorials, and Second World War concentration camps. Also known as morbid tourism and death tourism.

death care workers   People who process the dead body, including medical examiners, funeral directors, and those who work at cemeteries and crematoria.

discourse   A widely shared set of beliefs, assumptions, values, and so on.

disenfranchised grief   Grief that is not recognized as socially legitimate. The bereaved person is not accorded the right to mourn openly.

do-not-resuscitate (DNR) order   A note on a patient's chart indicating that no attempt is to be made to restart the patient's heart if it stops.

edgework   Exploring the limits of safety, social convention, and so on. Usually associated with voluntary risk taking.

embalming   A process that replaces body fluids with liquid chemicals (such as formaldehyde) to preserve the body after death.

eulogy   A selective and idealized reconstruction of the life of the deceased. Presented at a funeral or memorial service.

euphemism   A word or phrase that is used when a more direct statement would make people uncomfortable.

euthanasia   Causing the death of another person. Sometimes referred to as "mercy killing" when done in the belief that the deceased was suffering and wanted to die.

first responders   Police officers, firefighters, paramedics and emergency medical technicians, and so on who are typically the first people called to the scene of an unexpected death.

folklore   The beliefs, customs, myths, legends, folk tales, stories, rumours, jokes, and sayings that are anonymously produced, collectively shared, and communicated in both oral and written forms (Clifton 1991).

frail elderly   Individuals in generally poor health due to advanced age. Usually aged 85 and older.

generativity   Making meaningful contributions to others and to society. Gerotranscendence is a related concept referring to generativity in old age.

good death   An optimal or ideal dying process and the end point of that process.

grief   Intense suffering caused by the death of a loved one.

health care workers   A wide range of health care personnel including physicians, nurses, aides, therapists, psychologists, and social workers. Does not include family members who act as unpaid caregivers.

healthy immigrant effect   Immigrants who come to Canada often have better health than native-born Canadians because people in ill health are less likely to immigrate.

hospice/palliative care   End-of-life care designed to relieve suffering and improve the quality of life for persons who are dying and their family members.

identifying moments   Experiences that make a person realize their current social status.

identity foreclosure   A change in social status (e.g., widowhood, retirement) resulting in the termination of one's former identity (e.g., as a wife, employee).

immunization   Injection of substances that create resistance to infectious pathogens.

mausoleum   A building containing tombs for dead bodies. A columbarium contains niches for the cremains (ashes) of cremated bodies.

medical examiner (ME)   A public official responsible for investigating sudden, suspicious, or unexplained deaths including accidents, suicides, and homicides.

medicalization   The process of defining and treating phenomena as medical pathology. Medicalized constructions contrast other possible constructions, such as criminalization, immorality, and normalization.

memorialization   Various ways of remembering the dead.

Métis   The descendants of European fur traders and their Indigenous wives.

moral distress   When health care workers feel conflicted or distressed about the ethics of providing care that may be futile, unnecessary, or harmful to a patient.

mourning   Public displays of grief conforming to social and cultural norms.

near-death experience (NDE)   Unusual experiences associated with almost dying that are remembered when the person recovers. May include perceptions of experiences that seem to occur out of one's body; hence the term "out-of-body" experience.

nonvoluntary euthanasia   When a person who cannot express his or her wishes is euthanized on the assumption or assertion that he or she would prefer to die.

orphan   A child whose parents are dead.

ossuary   A container or burial site for the bones of the dead.

pandemic   An infectious disease that is widely prevalent across multiple countries or that has spread worldwide, as contrasted with an epidemic, which is confined to one country or one region of a country.

perinatal death   The death of a baby before or soon after birth.

post-traumatic stress disorder (PTSD)   A pattern of symptoms and behaviours that are long-lasting and occur as a result of exposure to traumatic or repeated death(s). Associated with a variety of emotional and mental health issues such as anxiety, depression, relationship difficulties, and suicide.

potential years of life lost (PYLL)   An estimate of the additional years a person might have lived had premature death not intervened or if a particular cause of death was eliminated.

premature death   Death before the age of 75.

primary trauma   Directly experiencing a death. For example, a police officer may deal with a death from a motor vehicle accident, murder, suicide, and so on.

professionalization   Defining an occupation as professional involves extensive specialized training, licensure or certification, and adoption of the values and practices of the professional group.

psychogenic death   Giving up and dying in difficult or traumatic situations. Losing the will to live.

rites of intensification   Social rituals that intensify feelings and emotions and then provide a means by which individuals can express their sentiments.

secondary trauma   Exposure to the suffering of others who have experienced the death of a loved one. For example, a police officer may have to tell family and friends of the death of a loved one from a motor vehicle accident or murder and witness their anguish.

secularization   A decline in the importance of religion as a central social institution.

senescence   The wearing out of the body as a result of aging.

shaman   An Indigenous healer.

stigma   An attribute that disqualifies a person from full social acceptance (Goffman 1963). Stigmatization involves being socially excluded as a result of that stigma.

taboo   A widely and strongly held social rule that results in social sanctioning (punishment) when broken.

terminal sedation   Medication prescribed and administered during the active dying process to manage symptoms and make dying more comfortable.

traumatic death   A death that is out of the ordinary and may be particularly gruesome or disturbing. Includes unnatural and unexpected deaths such as some homicides, suicides, or motor vehicle accidents, for example.

urban legends   Stories that are not true but nevertheless circulate widely and are told as if they are true.

voluntary euthanasia   Euthanasia performed at the request of a person who asks for death and is competent to do so.

widow   A woman whose husband has died. She experiences widowhood.

widower   A man whose wife has died. He experiences widowerhood.

withdrawing treatment   Stopping treatment that has been initiated previously.

withholding treatment   Not initiating treatment that is available.

Appendix: Selected Visual Media Sources Dealing with Dying, Death, and End-of-Life Care

Websites

Canadian Hospice Palliative Care Association (https://www.chpca.ca/): This association is the national voice for hospice/palliative care within Canada. Advancing and advocating for quality hospice/palliative care in Canada, its work is oriented to public policy, public and professional education, and enhanced awareness of dying and death.

Canadian Institute for Health Information (www.cihi.ca): An extensive source of data on health care utilization.

Canadian Virtual Hospice (www.virtualhospice.ca): This site contains information and support on palliative care and grief.

Government of Canada COVID-19 daily epidemiology update: https://health -infobase.canada.ca/covid-19/epidemiological-summary-covid-19-cases.html.

Media Watch: A free, weekly emailed document of global hospice, palliative care, and end-of-life care information compiled and annotated by Barry R. Ashpole. Email: barryashpole@bell.net.

Statistics Canada (www.statcan.gc.ca): A rich source of data on life expectancy, death rates, causes of death, and much more.

Documentaries

Beyond Memory. 2007. A National Film Board of Canada documentary that features case studies of persons experiencing dementia and the challenges that their caregivers face.

The Boy Whose Skin Fell Off—Jonny Kennedy. 2004. A moving and memorable British documentary about the last days of Jonny Kennedy.

The Bridge. 2006. Documentary about people who die by suicide by jumping off the Golden Gate Bridge in San Francisco. A net is being installed to stop this long-standing pattern, due for completion in 2021.

The Caregivers Club. 2018. A CBC documentary about caregivers coping with a family member who has dementia.

Death: Trip of a Lifetime. 1993. A four-part series with episodes titled "The Chasm," "The Good Death," "Letting Go," and "Going for Glory." This documentary provides a cross-cultural tour of beliefs and customs about death. While this series was made years ago, it still works in the classroom today.

Dying at Grace. 2003. This film follows five terminally ill patients in the palliative care unit at the Salvation Army's Toronto Grace Health Centre.

Her Last Project. 2019. A CBC documentary about Dr. Shelly Sarwal's fatal disease and her decision to donate her organs following death using Medical Assistance in Dying (MAID).

How to Die in Oregon. 2011. This film is about assisted suicide in Oregon following its legalization there.

The Life and Death of Gloria Taylor. 2012. A documentary from CBC's *The Fifth Estate*. Gloria Taylor was the face of the movement to legalize assisted death in Canada, resulting in the 2015 Supreme Court ruling requiring that the Criminal Code be changed to allow for assisted death resulting in the implementation of Medical Assistance in Dying (MAID) in Canada in 2016.

Lost on Arrival: Me, the Mounties and PTSD. 2017. A CBC documentary that describes PTSD as experienced by veteran CBC journalist Curt Petrovich, as well as by the four Mounties involved in the death of Robert Djiekanski at the Vancouver International Airport in 2007.

Road to Mercy. 2016. A CBC documentary that explores the ethics of Medical Assistance in Dying (MAID).

The Suicide Tourist. 2007. An investigative piece from PBS's *Frontline* about travelling to Switzerland to obtain assisted suicide.

That's My Time. 2008. A CTV documentary about Irwin Barker's last year of life dying from cancer. Barker was a Canadian comedy writer and comedian.

The Undertaking. 2007. A PBS *Frontline* film about an undertaker/funeral director in a small town in Michigan.

Who Owns My Life? The Sue Rodriguez Story. 1993. A CBC film about Sue Rodriguez's dying from ALS and her campaign to legalize assisted suicide in Canada.

National Film Board of Canada

Aftermath: The Legacy of Suicide. 2001.
Bearing Witness: Luke Melchior (about a person with ALS). 2003.
Beyond Memory (about dementia). 2007.
Farewell Touch (about an undertaker). 2012.
Griefwalker (about palliative care). 2008.
Inhale Exhale (about birth and death). 2009.
My Healing Journey: Seven Years with Cancer. 1999.
Richard Cardinal: Cry from a Diary of a Métis Child. 1986.
Surviving Death: Stories about Grief. 1998.

Movies

Among the many movies that depict dying and death, some examples:

The Bucket List. 2007. A movie about two older men who carry out a plan to live life fully until death.
The Farewell. 2019. West meets East. The story of a Chinese-American granddaughter and her Chinese grandmother and extended family. Chinese culture requires that dying not be acknowledged openly, contrasting American values and practices.
God Said "Ha"! 1998. Starring *Saturday Night Live*'s Julia Sweeney and produced by Quentin Tarantino. Sweeney finds humour in the year when both she and her brother were diagnosed with rare forms of cancer and moved in with their parents.
Gravity. 2013. A movie about courage and bereavement.
Harold and Maude. 1971. A dark comedy.
Magnolia. 1999. Explores dying and grief from many perspectives.
Man Running. 2018. A Canadian film that features a medical doctor wrestling with the ethics of assisted death.
Me Before You. 2016. Despite finding love, a paralyzed man chooses to purchase assisted suicide.
Million Dollar Baby. 2004. Explores assisted dying.

My Girl. 1991. A coming-of-age movie about a young girl obsessed with death.

News of the World. 2020. A multilayered movie about loss and grief.

Passchendaele. 2008. A Canadian film about the involvement of Canadian troops in the First World War battles at Passchendaele.

Tuesdays with Morrie. 1999. Film starring Jack Lemmon about a man dying from ALS. Based on the bestselling book of the same title.

You Don't Know Jack: The Life and Deaths of Jack Kevorkian. 2010. An HBO film about American assisted suicide crusader Dr. Jack Kevorkian. Starring Al Pacino as Kevorkian along with Susan Sarandon and John Goodman.

Weekend at Bernie's. 1989. A dark comedy.

Wit. 2001. A television movie starring Emma Thompson and directed by Mike Nichols based on a play of the same title. Explores the experience of being treated for terminal cancer.

Television Series

After Life (2019–). Netflix. A dark comedy-drama following the life of a middle-aged widower.

The Big C (2010–13). Showtime. A series about a woman living with a diagnosis of terminal cancer.

Dead to Me (2019–). Netflix. A dark comedy about a recently widowed woman trying to come to terms with her loss.

Pushing Daisies (2007–9). ABC. A quirky "forensic fairy tale."

Six Feet Under (2001–5). HBO. A drama series that follows a family who runs a funeral home in Los Angeles.

YouTube

Brittany Maynard describes her decision to seek assisted death in the US. 2014. https://www.youtube.com/watch?v=1lHXH0Zb2QI

Dr. Donald Low, eight days before his death, advocates for assisted death in Canada. 2013. https://www.youtube.com/watch?v=q3jgSkxV1rw&t=10s

James Corden and Eric Idle sing "We Are Probably All Going to Die." 2018. https://www.youtube.com/watch?v=tAPceUSVLKM

Randy Pausch, "Last Lecture: Achieving Your Childhood Dreams." 2007. An outstanding, uplifting lecture about how to live given by a dying professor. https://www.youtube.com/watch?v=ji5_MqicxSo

References

Achille, M.A., and J.R.P. Ogloff. 2003–4. "Attitudes toward and Desire for Assisted Suicide among Persons with Amyotrophic Lateral Sclerosis." *Omega* 48 (1): 1–21. http://dx.doi.org/10.2190/G5TA-9KV0-MT3G-RWM0. Medline:15688543

Adelson, N. 2005. "The Embodiment of Inequity: Health Disparities in Aboriginal Canada." *Canadian Journal of Public Health* 96 (Supl 2): S45–S61. Medline:16078555

Agnew, G.H. 1974. *Canadian Hospitals, 1920–1970*. Toronto: University of Toronto Press.

Aiken, L.R. 2001. *Dying, Death, and Bereavement*, 4th ed. Mahwah, NJ: Lawrence Erlbaum.

Ajemian, I.C. 1990. "Palliative Care in Canada: 1990." *Journal of Palliative Care* 6 (4): 47–50. Medline:1704914

Ajemian, I.C. 1992. "Hospitals and Health Care Facilities." *Journal of Palliative Care* 8 (1): 33–7. Medline:1583566

Alam, R., M. Barrera, N. D'Agostino, D.B. Nicholas, and G. Schneiderman. 2012. "Bereavement Experiences of Mothers and Fathers over Time after the Death of a Child Due to Cancer." *Death Studies* 36 (1): 1–22. http://dx.doi.org/10.1080/07481187.2011.553312. Medline:24567992

Albom, M. 1997. *Tuesdays with Morrie*. New York: Doubleday.

Albuquerque, S., M. Pereira, and I. Narciso. 2016. "Couple's Relationship after the Death of a Child: A Systematic Review." *Journal of Child and Family Studies* 25 (1): 30–53. https://doi.org/10.1007/s10826-015-0219-2

Aljazeera. 2020. "Mother 'Reunites' with Dead Daughter in Virtual Reality." *Aljazeera*, February 14. https://www.aljazeera.com/news/2020/02/mother-reunites-dead-daughter-virtual-reality-200214112010283.html

Amyot, G.F. 1967. "Some Historical Highlights of Public Health in Canada." *Canadian Journal of Public Health* 58 (8): 337–41. Medline:4863397

Anderson, H. 1980. "The Death of a Parent: Its Impact on Middle-Aged Sons and Daughters." *Pastoral Psychology* 28 (3): 151–67. http://dx.doi.org/10.1007/BF01760282

Andriessen, K., K. Krysinska, D.A. Castelli Dransart, L. Dargis, and B.L. Mishara. 2019. "Grief after Euthanasia and Physician-Assisted Suicide: A Systematic Review." *Crisis: The Journal of Crisis Intervention and Suicide Prevention.* Advance online publication. https://doi.org/10.1027/0227-5910/a000630. Medline:31657640

Antonovsky, A. 1987. *Unraveling the Mystery of Health: How People Manage Stress and Stay Well.* San Francisco: Jossey-Bass.

Apelian, E., and O. Nesteruk. 2017. "Reflections of Young Adults on the Loss of a Parent in Adolescence." *International Journal of Child, Youth and Family Studies* 8 (3–4): 79–100. https://doi.org/10.18357/ijcyfs83/4201718002

Ariès, P. 1974. *Western Attitudes toward Death: From the Middle Ages to the Present.* Baltimore: Johns Hopkins University Press.

Ariès, P. 1981. *The Hour of Our Death.* New York: Knopf.

Arnup, K. 2013. "Death, Dying and Canadian Families." The Vanier Institute of the Family. http://www.vanierinstitute.ca/include/get.php?nodeid=3540

Asmundson, G.J.G., and J.A. Stapleton. 2008. "Associations between Dimensions of Anxiety Sensitivity and PTSD Symptom Clusters in Active-Duty Police Officers." *Cognitive Behaviour Therapy* 37 (2): 66–75. http://dx.doi.org/10.1080/16506070801969005. Medline:18470738

Audette, A. 1964. "Nursing Care in Cardiovascular Surgery." *Canadian Nurse* 60 (3): 259–70. Medline:14126087

Auger, J.A. 2003. *Passing Through: The End-of-Life Decisions of Lesbians and Gay Men.* Halifax: Fernwood Publishing.

Auger, J.A., and K. Krug. 2013. *Under the Rainbow: A Primer on Queer Issues in Canada.* Halifax: Fernwood Publishing.

Austin, W., G. Lemermeyer, L. Goldberg, V. Bergum, and M.S. Johnson. 2005. "Moral Distress in Healthcare Practice: The Situation of Nurses." *HEC Forum* 17 (1): 33–48. http://dx.doi.org/10.1007/s10730–005–4949–1. Medline:15957267

Aylsworth, L., and F. Trovato. 2015. "Demography of Native People." In *The Canadian Encyclopedia.* http://www.thecanadianencyclopedia.ca/en/article/aboriginal-people-demography/

Bablitz, C., A. Ahnadzadeh, and S.B. MacLeod. 2018. "Dying Alone: An Indigenous Man's Journey at the End of Life." *Canadian Family Physician* 64 (9): 667–8. https://www.ncbi.nlm.nih.gov/pmc/articles/PMC6135132/

Baptist, K.W. 2010. "Diaspora: Death without a Landscape." *Mortality* 15 (4): 294–307. http://dx.doi.org/10.1080/13576275.2010.513162

Barrera, M., K. O'Connor, N.M. D'Agostino, L. Spencer, D. Nicholas, V. Jovcevska, S. Tallet, and G. Schneiderman. 2009. "Early Parental Adjustment and Bereavement after Childhood Cancer Death." *Death Studies* 33 (6): 497–520. http://dx.doi.org/10.1080/07481180902961153. Medline:19565685

Bartel, B.T. 2020. "Families Grieving Together: Integrating the Loss of a Child through Ongoing Relational Connections." *Death Studies* 44 (8): 498–509. https://doi.org/10.1080/07481187.2019.1586794. Medline:30907697

Bartlett, S. (Director and Producer). 1994. *Who Owns My Life? The Sue Rodriguez Story*. From the television series *Witness* [Video]. Canadian Broadcasting Corporation.

Bayatrizi, Z. 2008. *Life Sentences: The Modern Ordering of Mortality*. Toronto: University of Toronto Press.

Becker, E. 1973. *The Denial of Death*. New York: Free Press.

Belicki, K., N. Gulko, K. Ruzycki, and J. Aristotle. 2003. "Sixteen Years of Dreams following Spousal Bereavement." *Omega* 47 (2): 93–106.

Betancourt, M.T., K.C. Roberts, T-L. Bennett, E.R. Driscoll, G. Jayaraman, and L. Pelletier. 2014. "Monitoring Chronic Diseases in Canada: The Chronic Disease Indicator Framework." *Chronic Diseases and Injuries in Canada* 34 (Supplement 1). http://www.phac-aspc.gc.ca/publicat/hpcdp-pspmc/34-1-supp/index-eng.php

Bettmann, O.L. 1956. *A Pictorial History of Medicine*. Springfield, IL: C.C. Thomas.

Betty, L.S. 2014. "Are They Hallucinations or Are They Real? The Spirituality of Deathbed and Near-Death Visions." In *Annual Editions: Dying, Death, and Bereavement*, 14th ed., edited by G.E. Dickinson and M.R. Leming, 87–93. New York: McGraw-Hill.

Beuthin, R., A. Bruce, M. Hopwood, W.D. Robertson, and K. Bertoni. 2020. "Rediscovering the Art of Medicine, Rewards, and Risks: Physicians' Experience of Providing Medical Assistance in Dying in Canada." *Sage Open Medicine* 8: 1–9. https://doi.org/10.1177/2050312120913452. Medline:32206313

Beuthin, R., A. Bruce, and M. Scaia. 2018. "Medical Assistance in Dying (MAiD): Canadian Nurses' Experiences." *Nursing Forum* 53: 511–20. https://doi.org/10.1111/nuf.12280. Medline:29972596

Blanchard-Boehm, R.D., and M.J. Cook. 2004. "Risk Communication and Public Education in Edmonton, Alberta, Canada on the 10th Anniversary of the 'Black Friday' Tornado." *International Research in Geographical and Environmental Education* 13 (1): 38–54. https://doi.org/10.1080/10382040408668791

Blanchard-Boehm, R.D., and M.J. Cook. 2015. "The 1987 Edmonton, Alberta Canada Tornado: Perception, Experience, and Response Then and Now." In *Evolving Approaches to Understanding Natural Hazards*, edited by G.A. Tobin and B.E. Montz, 360–72. Newcastle: Cambridge Scholars Publishing.

Bolton, J.M. W. Au, D. Chateau, R. Walld, W.D. Leslie, J. Enns, P.J. Martens, L.Y. Katz, S. Logsetty, J. Sareen. 2016. "Bereavement after Sibling Death: A Population-Based Longitudinal Case-Control Study." *World Psychiatry* 15 (1): 59–66. https://doi.org/10.1002/wps.20293. Medline:26833610

Bolton, J.M., W. Au, W.D. Leslie, P.J. Martens, M.W. Enns, L.L. Roos, L.Y. Katz, H.C. Wilcox, A. Erlangsen, D. Chateau, et al. 2013. "Parents Bereaved by Offspring Suicide: A Population-Based Longitudinal Case-Control Study." *JAMA*

Psychiatry 70 (2): 158–67. http://dx.doi.org/10.1001/jamapsychiatry.2013.275. Medline:23229880

Bolton, J.M., W. Au, R. Walld, D. Chateau, P.J. Martens, W.D. Leslie, M.W. Enns, and J. Sareen. 2014. "Parental Bereavement after the Death of an Offspring in a Motor Vehicle Collision: A Population-Based Study." *American Journal of Epidemiology* 179 (2): 177–85. http://dx.doi.org/10.1093/aje/kwt247. Medline:24186971

Bonoti, F., A. Leondari, and A. Mastora. 2013. "Exploring Children's Understanding of Death: Through Drawings and the Death Concept Questionnaire." *Death Studies* 37 (1): 47–60. http://dx.doi.org/10.1080/07481187.2011.623216. Medline:24600720

Bowman, K.W., and P.A. Singer. 2001. "Chinese Seniors' Perspectives on End -of-Life Decisions." *Social Science & Medicine* 53 (4): 455–64. http://dx.doi .org/10.1016/S0277–9536(00)00348–8. Medline:11459396

Bradley, Leonard O. 1958. "The Changed Role of Hospitals." *Canadian Nurse* 54 (6): 550–8. Medline:13570650

Bradley, Louise. 2015. "A Silent Killer: Giving a Voice to the Quiet Mental Health Crisis among First-Responders." *Psynopsis* 37 (2): 10.

Branswell, H. 2013. "Ten Years Later, SARS Still Haunts Survivors and Health-Care Workers." *The Globe and Mail*, March 6. http://www.theglobeandmail.com/life /health-and-fitness/health/ten-years-later-sars-still-haunts-survivors-and -health-care-workers/article9363178/

Braun, M.J. 1992. "Meaning Reconstruction in the Experience of Parental Bereavement." Unpublished master's thesis, University of Manitoba, Winnipeg.

Brazil, K., D. Bainbridge, J. Ploeg, P. Krueger, A. Taniguchi, and D. Marshall. 2012. "Family Caregiver Views on Patient-Centred Care at the End of Life." *Scandinavian Journal of Caring Sciences* 26 (3): 513–18. http://dx.doi.org /10.1111/j.1471–6712.2011.00956.x. Medline:22117607

Brazil, K., P. Krueger, M. Bedard, L. Kelley, C. McAiney, C. Justice, and A. Taniguchi. 2006. "Quality of Care for Residents Dying in Ontario Long-Term Care Facilities: Findings from a Survey of Directors of Care." *Journal of Palliative Care* 22 (1): 18–25. Medline:16689411

Brondolo, E., P. Eftekharzadeh, C. Clifton, J.E. Schwartz, and D. Delahanty. 2018. "Work-Related Trauma, Alienation, and Posttraumatic and Depressive Symptoms in Medical Examiner Employees." *Psychological Trauma: Theory, Research, Practice, and Policy* 10 (6): 689–97. https://doi.org/10.1037/tra0000323. Medline:28981313

Brooks, L. 2019. "Health Care Provider Experiences of and Perspectives on Medical Assistance in Dying: A Scoping Review of Qualitative Studies." *Canadian Journal on Aging* 38 (3): 384–96. https://doi.org/10.1017/S0714980818000600. Medline:30626453

Brown, J.S.H. 1980. *Strangers in Blood: Fur Trade Company Families in Indian Country*. Vancouver: University of British Columbia Press.

Bryce, G. 1902. *The Remarkable History of the Hudson's Bay Company*, 2nd ed. London: Sampson Low Marston.

Buckle, J.L. 2013. "University Students' Perspectives on a Psychology of Death and Dying Course: Exploring Motivation to Enroll, Goals, and Impact." *Death Studies* 37 (9): 866–82. http://dx.doi.org/10.1080/07481187.2012.699911. Medline:24517595

Buckley, S. 1988. "The Search for the Decline in Maternal Mortality: The Place of Hospital Records." In *Essays in the History of Canadian Medicine*, edited by W. Mitchinson and J.D. McGinnis, 148–63. Toronto: McClelland and Stewart.

Burch, E.S. 1988. *The Eskimos*. Norman: University of Oklahoma Press.

Burton, H., F. Rabito, L. Danielson, and T.K. Takaro. 2016. "Health Effects of Flooding in Canada: A 2015 Review and Description of Gaps in Research." *Canadian Water Resources Journal* 41 (1–2): 238–49. https://doi.org/10.1080/07011784.2015.1128854

Bushnik, T. 2016. "The Health of Girls and Women in Canada." Statistics Canada Report Number 89-503-X. https://www150.statcan.gc.ca/n1/pub/89-503-x/2015001/article/14324-eng.htm

Cable-Williams, B.E., and D.M. Wilson. 2014. "Awareness of Impending Death for Residents of Long-Term Care Facilities." *International Journal of Older People Nursing* 9 (2): 169–79. http://dx.doi.org/10.1111/opn.12045. Medline:24433366

Cable-Williams, B.E., and D.M. Wilson. 2017. "Dying and Death within the Culture of Long-Term Care Facilities in Canada." *International Journal of Older People* 12 (1): 1–11. https://doi.org/10.1111/opn.12125. Medline:27431427

Cable-Williams, B.E., D.M. Wilson, and N. Keating. 2014. "Advance Directives in the Context of Uncertain Prognosis for Residents of Nursing Homes." *Open Journal of Nursing* 4 (4): 321–9. http://dx.doi.org/10.4236/ojn.2014.44037

Campbell, M.L. 2013. "Should We Be Asking about Preferred Place for Dying Care?" *Journal of Palliative Medicine* 16 (5): 462. http://dx.doi.org/10.1089/jpm.2013.9511. Medline:23822209

Campion, B. 1994. "Is There a Place for Good Death?" *Catholic Health Association of Canada Review* 22 (1): 4–5. Medline:10146007

Canadian Cancer Society. 2020a. "Cancer Statistics." https://www.cancer.ca/en/cancer-information/cancer-101/cancer-statistics-at-a-glance/?region=on

Canadian Cancer Society. 2020b. "6 Statistics That Reveal the Impact of Cancer in Canada for 2020." https://www.cancer.ca/en/about-us/our-stories/6-statistics-about-cancer-in-canada-for-2020/?region=bc

Canadian Frailty Network. n.d. "What Is Frailty?" Accessed June 9, 2021. https://www.cfn-nce.ca/frailty-matters/what-is-frailty/

Canadian Hospice Palliative Care Association. n.d. "What Is Hospice Palliative Care?" Accessed June 9, 2021. https://www.chpca.ca/about-hpc/

Canadian Hospice Palliative Care Association. 2013. "A Model to Guide Hospice Palliative Care: Based on National Principles and Norms of Practice: Revised and Condensed Edition." https://www.chpca.ca/wp-content/uploads/2019/12/norms-of-practice-eng-web.pdf

Canadian Institute for Health Information. n.d. "Health Spending – Nursing Homes." Accessed July 14, 2020. https://secure.cihi.ca/free_products/infosheet_Residential_LTC_Financial_EN.pdf

Canadian Institute for Health Information. 2014. "National Health Expenditure Trends, 1975–2014." http://www.cihi.ca/web/resource/en/nhex_2014 _report_en.pdf

Canadian Institute for Health Information. 2016. *Canada's International Health System Performance Over 50 Years: Examining Potential Years of Life Lost*. Ottawa: CIHI. https://www.cihi.ca/en/health-system-performance /performance-reporting/international/pyll

Canadian Institute for Health Information. 2018. "Access to Palliative Care in Canada." https://www.cihi.ca/sites/default/files/document/access-palliative -care-2018-en-web.pdf

Canadian Institute for Health Information. 2018–19. "Profile of Residents in Residential and Hospital-Based Continuing Care, 2018–2019." https://www.cihi .ca/en/profile-of-residents-in-residential-and-hospital-based-continuing-care -2018-2019

Canadian Institute for Health Information. 2019. "Organ Replacement in Canada: CORR Annual Statistics, 2019." https://www.cihi.ca/en/organ-replacement -in-canada-corr-annual-statistics-2019

Canadian Institute for Health Information. 2020a. "Nursing in Canada, 2019." https://www.cihi.ca/en/nursing-in-canada-2019

Canadian Institute for Health Information. 2020b. "Hospital Stays in Canada." https://www.cihi.ca/en/hospital-stays-in-canada

Canadian Institute for Health Information. 2020c. "Inpatient Hospitalization, Surgery and Newborn Statistics, 2018–2019." https://www.cihi.ca/en/quick-stats

Canadian Medical Association. 1995. "Joint Statement on Resuscitative Interventions (update 1995): CMA Policy Summary." *Canadian Medical Association Journal* 153 (11): 1652A–52F. http://www.ncbi.nlm.nih.gov/pmc /articles/PMC1488016/

Canadian Nurses Association. 2020. "Nursing Statistics." Accessed July 13, 2020. https://www.cna-aiic.ca/en/nursing-practice/the-practice-of-nursing/health -human-resources/nursing-statistics

Canadian Nurses Association (CNA), Canadian Medical Association (CMA), and Canadian Hospital Association (CHA). 1984. "Joint Statement on Terminal Illness." *Canadian Medical Association Journal* 130 (10): 1357–8. http://www .ncbi.nlm.nih.gov/pmc/articles/PMC1488016/

Canadian Press. 2015. "Group Draws Attention to Paramedic Suicides, Says Professional Help Needed." *Huffington Post*, January 28. http://www .huffingtonpost.ca/2015/01/28/group-draws-attention-to-_n_6567956.html

Carleton, R.N., T.O. Afifi, T. Taillieu, S. Turner, R. Krakauer, G.S. Anderson, R.S. MacPhee, R. Ricciardelli, H.A. Cramm, D. Groll, et al. 2019. "Exposures to Potentially Traumatic Events among Public Safety Personnel in Canada." *Canadian Journal of Behavioural Science* 51 (1): 37–52. https://doi.org/10.1037 /cbs0000115

Carleton, R.N., T.O. Afifi, S. Turner, T. Taillieu, S. Duranceau, D.M. LeBouthillier, J. Sareen, R. Ricciardelli, R.S. MacPhee, D. Groll, et al. 2018a. "Mental Disorder

Symptoms among Public Safety Personnel in Canada." *The Canadian Journal of Psychiatry* 63 (1): 54–64. https://doi.org/10.1177/0706743717723825

Carleton, R.N., T.O. Afifi, S. Turner, T. Taillieu, S. Duranceau, D.M. LeBouthillier, J. Sareen, R. Ricciardelli, R.S. MacPhee, D. Groll, et al. 2018b. "Suicidal Ideation, Plans, and Attempts among Public Safety Personnel in Canada." *Canadian Psychology* 59 (3): 220–31. https://doi.org/10.1037/cap0000136

Caron, C.D., J. Griffith, and M. Arcand. 2005. "Decision Making at the End of Life in Dementia: How Family Caregivers Perceive Their Interactions with Health Care Providers in Long-Term-Care Settings." *Journal of Applied Gerontology* 24 (3): 231–47. http://dx.doi.org/10.1177/0733464805275766

Carstairs, S. 2000. *Quality End-of-Life Care: The Right of Every Canadian. Final Report of the Subcommittee to Update "Of Life and Death" of the Standing Senate Committee on Social Affairs, Science and Technology.* Ottawa: Parliament of Canada.

Carter, W.H. 1973. *Medical Practices and Burial Customs of North American Indians.* London, ON: Namind.

Castleden, H., V.A. Crooks, N. Hanlon, and N. Schuurman. 2010. "Providers' Perceptions of Aboriginal Palliative Care in British Columbia's Rural Interior." *Health and Social Care in the Community* 18 (5): 483–91. http://dx.doi.org /10.1111/j.1365–2524.2010.00922.x. Medline:20500225

Caxaj, C.S., K. Schill, and R. Janke. 2017. "Priorities and Challenges for a Palliative Approach to Care for Rural Indigenous Populations: A Scoping Review." *Health and Social Care in the Community* 26: e329–e36. https://doi.org/10.1111 /hsc.12469. Medline:28703394

CBC. 2012. *The Fifth Estate.* Season 38, "Assisted Suicide: The Life and Death of Gloria Taylor," October 12. https://www.cbc.ca/fifth/episodes/2012-2013 /the-life-and-death-of-gloria-taylor

Chai, H., D.N. Guerriere, B. Zagorski, and P.C. Coyte. 2014. "The Magnitude, Share and Determinants of Unpaid Care Costs for Home-Based Palliative Care Service Provision in Toronto, Canada." *Health & Social Care in the Community* 22 (1): 30–9. http://dx.doi.org/10.1111/hsc.12058. Medline:23758771

Chakraborty, C., A. Dean, and A. Failler. 2017. "The Art of Public Mourning: An Introduction." In *Remembering Air India: The Art of Public Mourning*, edited by A.R. Dean, C. Chakraborty, and A. Failler, xiii–xxxii. Edmonton: University of Alberta Press.

Chappell, N. 1992. *Social Support and Aging.* Toronto: Butterworths.

Chasteen, A.L., and S.F. Madey. 2003. "Belief in a Just World and the Perceived Injustice of Dying Young or Old." *Omega* 47 (4): 313–26.

Chochinov, H.M., T. Hack, T. Hassard, L.J. Kristjanson, S. McClement, and M. Harlos. 2002. "Dignity in the Terminally Ill: A Cross-Sectional, Cohort Study." *Lancet* 360 (9350): 2026–30. http://dx.doi.org/10.1016/S0140–6736(02)12022–8. Medline:12504398

Choudhry, N.K., J. Ma, I. Rasooly, and P.A. Singer. 1994. "Long-Term Care Facility Policies on Life-Sustaining Treatments and Advance Directives in Canada."

Journal of the American Geriatrics Society 42 (11): 1150–3. http://dx.doi.org
/10.1111/j.1532–5415.1994.tb06980.x. Medline:7963200

Chow, H.P.H. 2017. "A Time to Be Born and a Time to Die: Exploring the
Determinants of Death Anxiety among University Students in a Western
Canadian City." *Death Studies* 41 (6): 345–52. https://doi.org/10.1080/07481187
.2017.1279240. Medline:28060575

Clamageran, A. 1964. "Submission on Aging." *Canadian Nurse* 60 (8): 741–4.
Medline:14178668

Clark, G.T. 1993. "Personal Meanings of Grief and Bereavement." Doctoral
dissertation, University of Alberta, Edmonton.

Clarke, J.N. 2004. "A Comparison of Breast, Testicular and Prostate Cancer in Mass
Print Media (1996–2001)." *Social Science & Medicine* 59 (3): 541–51. http://
dx.doi.org/10.1016/j.socscimed.2003.11.018. Medline:15144763

Clarke, J.N. 2006. "Death under Control: The Portrayal of Death in Mass Print
English Language Magazines in Canada." *Omega* 52 (2): 153–67.

Clarke, L.H., A. Korotchenko, and A. Bundon. 2012. "'The Calendar Is Just about
Up': Older Adults with Multiple Chronic Conditions Reflect on Death and
Dying." *Ageing and Society* 32 (8): 1399–417. http://dx.doi.org/10.1017
/S0144686X11001061. Medline:24976657

Claxton-Oldfield, S., J. Tomes, M. Brennan, C. Fawcett, and J. Claxton-Oldfield.
2005. "Palliative Care Volunteerism among College Students in Canada."
American Journal of Hospice and Palliative Medicine 22 (2): 111–18. http://
dx.doi.org/10.1177/104990910502200206. Medline:15853088

Clifton, J.A. 1991. "Folklore." In *The Encyclopedic Dictionary of Sociology*, 4th ed.,
edited by R. Lachmann, 115. Guilford, CT: Dushkin.

Cohen, J., D.M. Wilson, A. Thurston, R. MacLeod, and L. Deliens. 2012. "Access
to Palliative Care Services in Hospital: A Matter of Being in the Right Hospital.
Hospital Charts Study in a Canadian City." *Palliative Medicine* 26 (1): 89–94.
http://dx.doi.org/10.1177/0269216311408992. Medline:21680750

Colarusso, C.A. 1999. "The Development of Time Sense in Middle Adulthood."
Psychoanalytic Quarterly 68 (1): 52–83. http://dx.doi.org/10.1002/j.2167
–4086.1999.tb00636.x. Medline:10029973

Coleman, V. 1985. *The Story of Medicine*. London: Robert Hale.

Commission on the Future of Health Care in Canada. 2002. *Building on Values:
The Future of Health Care in Canada—Final Report*. Cat. CP32-85/2002E-IN.
Government of Canada. http://publications.gc.ca/collections/Collection/CP32
-85-2002E.pdf

Conn, S.M., and L.D. Butterfield. 2013. "Coping with Secondary Traumatic Stress
by General Duty Police Officers: Practical Implications." *Canadian Journal of
Counselling and Psychotherapy* 47 (2): 272–98.

Corlett, W.T. 1935. *The Medicine-Man of the American Indians and His Cultural
Background*. Springfield, IL: Charles C. Thomas.

Corr, C.A., and D.M. Corr. 2013. *Death and Dying, Life and Living*, 7th ed.
Independence, KY: Cengage Learning.

Corr, C.A., D.M. Corr, and K.J. Doka. 2019. *Death and Dying, Life and Living*, 8th ed. Independence, KY: Cengage Learning.

Counts, D.R., and D.A. Counts. 1991. "Conclusions: Coping with the Final Tragedy." In *Coping with the Final Tragedy: Cultural Variation in Dying and Grieving*, edited by D.R. Counts and D.A. Counts, 277–91. Amityville, NY: Baywood.

Cox, G.R., J. Robinson, M. Williamson, A. Lockley, Y.T.D. Cheung, and J. Pirkis. 2012. "Suicide Clusters in Young People: Evidence for the Effectiveness of Postvention Strategies." *Crisis* 33 (4): 208–14. https://doi.org/10.1027/0227 -5910/a000144. Medline:22713976

Creighton, G., J.L. Oliffe, S. Butterwick, and E. Saewyc. 2013. "After the Death of a Friend: Young Men's Grief and Masculine Identities." *Social Science & Medicine* 84: 35–43. http://dx.doi.org/10.1016/j.socscimed.2013.02.022. Medline:23517702

Creighton, G., J.L. Oliffe, J. Matthews, and E. Saewyc. 2016. "'Dulling the Edges': Young Men's Use of Alcohol to Deal with Grief following the Death of a Male Friend." *Health Education and Behaviour* 43 (1): 54–60. https://doi.org /10.1177/1090198115596164. Medline:26202615

Cremation Association of North America. 2015. "Industry Statistical Information." http://www.cremationhfassociation.org/?page=IndustryStatistics

Curran, W.J., and S.M. Hyg. 1984. "Quality of Life and Treatment Decisions: The Canadian Law Reform Report." *New England Journal of Medicine* 310 (5): 297–8. http://dx.doi.org/10.1056/NEJM198402023100506. Medline:6690953

Cystic Fibrosis Canada. 2018. "Growing Older with CF." *Cystic Fibrosis Canada Blog*, July 3. https://www.cysticfibrosis.ca/blog/growing-older-with-cf/

Dallaire, R. 2003. *Shake Hands with the Devil: The Failure of Humanity in Rwanda*. Toronto: Random House.

Daschuk, J.W., P. Hackett, and S. MacNeil. 2006. "Treaties and Tuberculosis: First Nations People in Late 19th-Century Western Canada, a Political and Economic Transformation." *Canadian Bulletin of Medical History* 23 (2): 307–30. https:// doi.org/10.3138/cbmh.23.2.307. Medline:17214120

Davidson, D. 2018. "Sibling Loss: Disenfranchised Grief and Forgotten Mourners." *Bereavement Care* 37 (3): 124–30. https://doi.org/10.1080/02682621.2018.1535882

Davidson, D., and G. Letherby. 2014. "Griefwork Online: Perinatal Loss, Lifecourse Disruption and Online Support." *Human Fertility* 17 (3): 214–17. http://dx.doi .org/10.3109/14647273.2014.945498. Medline:25122092

Davis, C.G., C. Harasymchuk, and M.J.A. Wohl. 2012. "Finding Meaning in a Traumatic Loss: A Families Approach." *Journal of Traumatic Stress* 25 (2): 142–9. http://dx.doi.org/10.1002/jts.21675. Medline:22522727

Death with Dignity. 2020. "Oregon Death with Dignity Act: Annual Reports." https://www.deathwithdignity.org/oregon-death-with-dignity-act-annual-reports/

de Beauvoir, S. 1973. *Old Age*. Translated by Patrick O'Brien. London: Deutsch.

Decker, J.F. 1991. "Depopulation of the Northern Plains Natives." *Social Science & Medicine* 33 (4): 381–93. http://dx.doi.org/10.1016/0277–9536(91)90319–8. Medline:1948151

Decker, J.F. 1997. "The York Factory Medical Journals, 1846–52." *Canadian Bulletin of Medical History* 14 (1): 107–31. Medline:11619769

Department of Justice Canada. 2020. "Government of Canada Proposes Changes to Medical Assistance in Dying Legislation." News Release, February 24. https://www.canada.ca/en/department-justice/news/2020/02/government-of-canada-proposes-changes-to-medical-assistance-in-dying-legislation.html

Department of Justice Canada. 2021a. "New Medical Assistance in Dying Legislation Becomes Law." News Release, March 17. https://www.canada.ca/en/department-justice/news/2021/03/new-medical-assistance-in-dying-legislation-becomes-law.html

Department of Justice Canada. 2021b. "Canada's New Medical Assistance in Dying (MAID) Law." Accessed 9 June 2021. https://www.justice.gc.ca/eng/cj-jp/ad-am/bk-di.html

Dermody, E. 2017. "Dark Tourism." In *Handbook of the Sociology of Death, Grief, and Bereavement: A Guide to Theory and Practice*, edited by N. Thompson and G.R. Cox, 194–209. New York: Routledge.

DeSpelder, L.A., and A.L. Strickland. 2011. *The Last Dance: Encountering Death and Dying*, 9th ed. New York: McGraw-Hill.

Dickason, O.P. 1984. *The Myth of the Savage and the Beginnings of French Colonialism in the Americas*. Edmonton: University of Alberta Press.

Didion, J. 2007. *The Year of Magical Thinking*. New York: Vintage International.

Dierickx, S., L. Deliens, J. Cohen, and K. Chambaere. 2016. "Euthanasia in Belgium: Trends in Reported Cases between 2003 and 2013." *Canadian Medical Association Journal* 188 (16): E407–E14. https://doi.org/10.1503/cmaj.160202. Medline:27620630

Doka, K.J. 1995. "Disenfranchised Grief." In *The Path Ahead: Readings in Death and Dying*, edited by L.A. DeSpelder and A.L. Strickland, 271–5. Mountain View, CA: Mayfield.

Dolgoy, R. (Director), and D. Phillips (Producer). 1991. *Living with Dying* [Video]. National Film Board of Canada.

Dong, T., Z. Zhu, M. Guo, P. Du, and B. Wu. 2019. "Association between Dying Experience and Place of Death: Urban–Rural Differences among Older Chinese Adults." *Journal of Palliative Medicine* 22 (11): 1386–93. https://doi.org/10.1089/jpm.2018.0583. Medline:31120357

Donnelly, S.M., N. Michael, and C. Donnelly. 2006. "Experience of the Moment of Death at Home." *Mortality* 11 (4): 352–67. http://dx.doi.org/10.1080/13576270600945410

Durkheim, E. [1915] 1965. *The Elementary Forms of Religious Life*. New York: Free Press.

Easson, A., A. Agarwal, S. Duda, and K. Bennett. 2014. "Portrayal of Youth Suicide in Canadian News." *Journal of the Canadian Academy of Child and Adolescent Psychiatry* 23 (3): 167–73. Medline:25320610

Emke, I. 2002. "Why the Sad Face? Secularization and the Changing Function of Funerals in Newfoundland." *Mortality* 7 (3): 269–84. http://dx.doi.org/10.1080/1357627021000025432

Ennis, J., and U. Majid. 2019. "'Death from a Broken Heart': A Systematic Review of the Relationship between Spousal Bereavement and Physical and Physiological Health Outcomes." *Death Studies*. Advance online publication. https://doi.org/10.1080/07481187.2019.1661884. Medline:31535594

Ens, C., and J.B. Bond, Jr. 2005. "Death Anxiety and Personal Growth in Adolescents Experiencing the Death of a Grandparent." *Death Studies* 29 (2): 171–8. http://dx.doi.org/10.1080/07481180590906192. Medline:15822244

Ens, C., and J.B. Bond, Jr. 2007. "Death Anxiety in Adolescents: The Contributions of Bereavement and Religiosity." *Omega* 55 (3): 169–84. http://dx.doi.org /10.2190/OM.55.3.a. Medline:18214066

Erichsen-Brown, C. 1979. *Use of Plants for the Past 500 Years*. Aurora, ON: Breezy Creeks Press.

Erikson, E.H. 1959. *Identity and the Life Cycle*. New York: W.W. Norton.

Erikson, E.H., J.M. Erikson, and H.Q. Kivnick. 1986. *Vital Involvement in Old Age*. New York: W.W. Norton.

Erikson, K.T. 1976. *Everything in Its Path: Destruction of Community in the Buffalo Creek Flood*. New York: Simon and Schuster.

Estabrooks, C.A., S. Straus, C.M. Flood, J. Keefe, P. Armstrong, G. Donner, V. Boscart, F. Ducharme, J. Silvius, and M. Wolfson. 2020. *Restoring Trust: COVID-19 and the Future of Long-Term Care*. Ottawa: Royal Society of Canada.

European Institute of Bioethics. 2020. Report 2016: Euthanasia in Netherlands. https://www.ieb-eib.org/en/report/end-of-life/unclassified/report-2016-euthanasia -in-netherlands-488.html

Evans, R.G., M.L. Barer, C. Hertzman, G.M. Anderson, I.R. Pulcins, and J. Lomas. 1989. "The Long Good-Bye: The Great Transformation of the British Columbia Hospital System." *Health Services Research* 24 (4): 435–59. Medline:2807932

Ewart, W.B. 1983. "Causes of Mortality in a Subarctic Settlement (York Factory, Man.), 1714–1946." *Canadian Medical Association Journal* 129 (6): 571–4. Medline:6349770

Failler, A. 2009. "Remembering the Air India Disaster: Memorial and Counter-Memorial." *The Review of Education, Pedagogy, and Cultural Studies* 31 (2–3): 150–76. https://doi.org/10/1080/10714410902827168

Fair, M. 1994. "The Development of National Vital Statistics in Canada: Part 1—From 1605 to 1945." *Health Reports* 6 (3): 355–75. Medline:7756573

Falconer, J., F. Couture, K.K. Demir, M. Lang, Z. Shefman, and M. Woo. 2019. "Perceptions and Intentions toward Medical Assistance in Dying among Canadian Medical Students." *BMC Medical Ethics* 20 (22): 1–7. https://doi .org/10.1186/s12910-019-0356-z. Medline:30940195

Farand, L., F. Chagnon, J. Renaud, and M. Rivard. 2004. "Completed Suicides among Quebec Adolescents Involved with Juvenile Justice and Child Welfare Services." *Suicide & Life-Threatening Behavior* 34 (1): 24–35. http://dx.doi .org/10.1521/suli.34.1.24.27774. Medline:15106885

Flynn, D. 1993. *The Truth about Funerals: How to Beat the High Cost of Dying (An Insider's Perspective)*. Burlington, ON: Funeral Consultants International.

Forsey, C. 2012. *Men on the Edge: Taking Risks and Doing Gender among BASE Jumpers*. Black Point, NS: Fernwood Publishing.

Fraess-Phillips, A., S. Wagner, and R.L. Harris. 2017. "Firefighters and Traumatic Stress: A Review." *International Journal of Emergency Services* 6 (1): 67–80. https://doi.org/10.1108/IJES-10-2016-0020

Frank, A.W. 1991. *At the Will of the Body: Reflections on Illness*. Boston: Houghton Mifflin.

Frank, A.W. 2013. *The Wounded Storyteller: Body, Illness, and Ethics*, 2nd ed. Chicago: University of Chicago Press.

Frank, R. 2011. *Newslore: Contemporary Folklore on the Internet*. Jackson, MS: University Press of Mississippi.

Fries, J.F. 1980. "Aging, Natural Death, and the Compression of Morbidity." *New England Journal of Medicine* 303 (3): 130–5. http://dx.doi.org/10.1056/NEJM198007173030304. Medline:7383070

Fruch, V., L. Monture, H. Prince, and M.L. Kelley. 2016. "Coming Home to Die: Six Nations of the Grand River Territory Develops Community-Based Palliative Care." *International Journal of Indigenous Health* 11 (1): 50–74. https://doi.org/10.18357/ijih111201615303

Fry, P.S. 1997. "Grandparents' Reactions to the Death of a Grandchild: An Exploratory Factor Analytic Study." *Omega* 35: 119–40.

Fulton, A.E., and J. Drolet. 2018. "Responding to Disaster-Related Loss and Grief: Recovering from the 2013 Flood in Southern Alberta, Canada." *Journal of Loss and Trauma* 23 (2): 140–58. https://doi.org/10.1080/15325024.2018.1423873

Funk, L.M., K.I. Stajduhar, S. Robin Cohen, D.K. Heyland, and A. Williams. 2012. "Legitimising and Rationalising in Talk about Satisfaction with Formal Healthcare among Bereaved Family Members." *Sociology of Health & Illness* 34 (7): 1010–24. http://dx.doi.org/10.1111/j.1467–9566.2011.01457.x. Medline:22384989

Funk, L.M., S. Waskiewich, and K.I. Stajduhar. 2013–14. "Meaning-Making and Managing Difficult Feelings: Providing Front-Line End-of-Life Care." *Omega* 68 (1): 23–43. http://dx.doi.org/10.2190/OM.68.1.b. Medline:24547663

Gallagher, R., and M. Krawczyk. 2013. "Family Members' Perceptions of End-of-Life Care across Diverse Locations of Care." *BMC Palliative Care* 12 (1): 25. http://dx.doi.org/10.1186/1472–684X-12–25. Medline:23870101

Garner, R., P. Tanuseputro, D.G. Manuel, and C. Sanmartin. 2018. "Transitions to Long-Term and Residential Care among Older Canadians." Statistics Canada: Health Reports. https://www150.statcan.gc.ca/n1/pub/82-003-x/2018005/article/54966-eng.htm

Gee, E.M., and M.M. Kimball. 1987. *Women and Aging*. Toronto: Butterworths.

Gélinas, C., L. Fillion, M.A. Robitaille, and M. Truchon. 2012. "Stressors Experienced by Nurses Providing End-of-Life Palliative Care in the Intensive Care Unit." *Canadian Journal of Nursing Research* 44 (1): 18–39. Medline:22679843

Généreux, M., D. Maltais, G. Petit, and M. Roy. 2019. "Monitoring Adverse Psychosocial Outcomes One and Two Years after the Lac-Mégantic Train Derailment Tragedy (Eastern Townships, Quebec, Canada)." *Prehospital and Disaster Medicine* 34 (3): 251–9. https://doi.org/10.1017/S1049023X19004321

Gibson, M., and E. Gorman. 2010. "Contextualizing End-of-Life Care for Ageing Veterans: Family Members' Thoughts." *International Journal of Palliative Nursing* 16 (7): 339–43. http://dx.doi.org/10.12968/ijpn.2010.16.7.49062

Gilbert, K.R. 2017. "Death, Grief, and Virtual Connections." In *Handbook of the Sociology of Death, Grief, and Bereavement: A Guide to Theory and Practice*, edited by N. Thompson and G.R Cox, 291–305. New York: Routledge.

Gilmour, H. 2018. "Unmet Home Care Needs in Canada." Statistics Canada: Health Report. https://www150.statcan.gc.ca/n1/pub/82-003-x/2018011/article/00002-eng.htm

Gilson, M. (Director), and T. Daly (Producer). 1980. *The Last Days of Living* [Video]. National Film Board of Canada.

Gina, K.G.G., E. Fukushima, R.B. Abu-Laban, and D.D. Sweet. 2012. "Prevalence of Advance Directives among Elderly Patients Attending an Urban Canadian Emergency Department." *Canadian Journal of Emergency Medical Care* 14 (2): 90–6. Medline:22554440

Glaser, B.G., and A.L. Strauss. 1965. *Awareness of Dying*. Chicago: Aldine.

Glaser, B.G., and A.L. Strauss. 1968. *Time for Dying*. Chicago: Aldine.

Goffman, E. 1963. *Stigma*. Englewood Cliffs: Prentice-Hall.

Gollom, M. 2014. "Why Emergency Services Need a 'Culture Change' to Deal with PTSD." *CBC News*, September 29. http://www.cbc.ca/news/canada/why-emergency-services-need-a-culture-change-to-deal-with-ptsd-1.2781733

Goodridge, D., J.B. Bond, Jr., C. Cameron, and E. McKean. 2005. "End-of-Life Care in a Nursing Home: A Study of Family, Nurse and Healthcare Aide Perspectives." *International Journal of Palliative Nursing* 11 (5): 226–32. http://dx.doi.org/10.12968/ijpn.2005.11.5.226. Medline:15944496

Gorman, E. 2019. "Children and Death in the Canadian Context." In *Contextualizing Childhoods: Growing Up in Europe and North America*, edited by S. Frankel and S. McNamee, 197–218. Cham, Switzerland: Palgrave Macmilllan. eBook. https://doi.org/10.1007/978-3-319-94926-0

Goto, C. 2006. "Prevalence of Post-Traumatic Stress Disorder in the Royal Canadian Mounted Police." Master's thesis, University of British Columbia.

Government of Canada. 2017. "Compassionate Care Leave." https://www.canada.ca/en/employment-social-development/services/labour-standards/reports/compassionate-care.html

Government of Canada. 2018. "Framework for Palliative Care in Canada." https://www.canada.ca/en/health-canada/services/health-care-system/reports-publications/palliative-care/framework-palliative-care-canada.html

Government of Canada. 2019. "Palliative Care." https://www.canada.ca/en/health-canada/services/palliative-care.html

Government of Canada. 2020a. "Medical Assistance in Dying." https://www.canada
.ca/en/health-canada/services/medical-assistance-dying.html

Government of Canada. 2020b. "EI Caregiving Benefits and Leave: What Caregiving
Benefits Offer." https://www.canada.ca/en/services/benefits/ei/caregiving.html

Government of Canada. 2020c. "Coronavirus Disease 2019 (COVID-19): Epidemiology
Update." Accessed June 29, 2020. https://health-infobase.canada.ca/covid-19
/epidemiological-summary-covid-19-cases.html?stat=num&measure=deaths#a2

Government of Canada. 2020d. "Canada's Response to Ukraine International
Airlines Flight PS752 Tragedy." https://www.international.gc.ca/world-monde
/issues_development-enjeux_developpement/response_conflict-reponse_conflits
/crisis-crises/flight-vol-ps752.aspx?lang=eng

Government of Canada. 2021. "Medical Assistance in Dying." Accessed March 20,
2021. https://www.canada.ca/en/health-canada/services/medical-assistance
-dying.html

Granek, L. 2010. "Grief as Pathology: The Evolution of Grief Theory in Psychology
from Freud to the Present." *History of Psychology* 13 (1): 46–73. http://dx.doi
.org/10.1037/a0016991. Medline:20499613

Granek, L. 2017. "Is Grief a Disease? The Medicalization of Grief by the Psy-
Disciplines in the Twenty-First Century." In *Handbook of the Sociology of
Death, Grief, and Bereavement: A Guide to Theory and Practice*, edited by
N. Thompson and G.R Cox, 264–77. New York: Routledge.

Granek, L., M. Barrera, K. Scheinemann, and U. Bartels. 2016. "Pediatric
Oncologists' Coping Strategies for Dealing with Patient Death." *Journal of
Psychosocial Oncology* 34 (1–2): 39–59. https://doi.org/10.1080/07347332.2015
.1127306. Medline:26865337

Granek, L., M.K. Krzyzanowska, R. Tozer, and P. Mazzotta. 2012. "Difficult Patient
Loss and Physician Culture for Oncologists Grieving Patient Loss." *Journal of
Palliative Medicine* 15 (11): 1254–60. http://dx.doi.org/10.1089/jpm.2012.0245.
Medline:23016965

Granek, L., M.K. Krzyzanowska, R. Tozer, and P. Mazzotta. 2013. "Oncologists'
Strategies and Barriers to Effective Communication about the End of Life."
Journal of Oncology Practice / American Society of Clinical Oncology 9 (4):
e129–35. http://dx.doi.org/10.1200/JOP.2012.000800. Medline:23942929

Grant, J.H.B. 1946. "Immunization in Children." *Canadian Medical Association
Journal* 55 (5): 493–7. Medline:20323952

Grant Kalischuk, R., and V.E. Hayes. 2003. "Grieving, Mourning, and Healing
following Youth Suicide: A Focus on Health and Well Being in Families." *Omega*
48 (1): 45–67.

The Grey Nuns of Montreal. 2014. "History of the Grey Nuns of Montreal." http://
www.sgm.qc.ca/data/soeursgrises/files/file/history_of_the_grey_nun_of
_montreal.pdf

Gunn, J.F., III, and D. Lester. 2012. "Media Guidelines in the Internet Age." *Crisis*
33 (4): 187–9. https://doi.org/10.1027/0227-5910/a000171. Medline:22820640

Haas, J. 1977. "Learning Real Feelings: A Study of High Steel Ironworkers' Reactions to Fear and Danger." *Sociology of Work and Occupations* 4 (2): 147–70. http://dx.doi.org/10.1177/073088847700400202

Hadad, M. 2009. *The Ultimate Challenge: Coping with Death, Dying, and Bereavement.* Toronto: Nelson Education.

Hafferty, F.W. 1988. "Cadaver Stories and the Emotional Socialization of Medical Students." *Journal of Health and Social Behavior* 29 (4): 344–56. http://dx.doi.org/10.2307/2136868. Medline:3253325

Hall, E. 1947. "Health Problems of an Aging Population." *Canadian Nurse* 43 (8): 591–4. Medline:20256311

Hall, G.S. 1922. *Senescence: The Last Half of Life.* New York: Appleton and Company. http://dx.doi.org/10.1037/10896-000

Hall, P., C. Schroder, and L. Weaver. 2002. "The Last 48 Hours of Life in Long-Term Care: A Focused Chart Audit." *Journal of the American Geriatrics Society* 50 (3): 501–6. http://dx.doi.org/10.1046/j.1532-5415.2002.50117.x. Medline:11943047

Hall, P., L. Weaver, F. Fothergill-Bourbonnais, S. Amos, N. Whiting, P. Barnes, and F. Legault. 2006. "Interprofessional Education in Palliative Care: A Pilot Project Using Popular Literature." *Journal of Interprofessional Care* 20 (1): 51–9. http://dx.doi.org/10.1080/13561820600555952. Medline:16581639

Hall, S., A. Legault, and J. Côté. 2010. "Dying Means Suffocating: Perceptions of People Living with Severe COPD Facing the End of Life." *International Journal of Palliative Nursing* 16 (9): 451–7. http://dx.doi.org/10.12968/ijpn.2010.16.9.78640. Medline:20871500

Halpern, J., M. Gurevich, B. Schwartz, and P. Brazeau. 2009a. "Interventions for Critical Incident Stress in Emergency Medical Services: A Qualitative Study." *Stress and Health* 25 (2): 139–49. http://dx.doi.org/10.1002/smi.1230

Halpern, J., M. Gurevich, B. Schwartz, and P. Brazeau. 2009b. "What Makes an Incident Critical for Ambulance Workers? Emotional Outcomes and Implications for Intervention." *Work and Stress* 23 (2): 173–89. http://dx.doi.org/10.1080/02678370903057317

Halpern, J., R.G. Maunder, B. Schwartz, and M. Gurevich. 2012. "The Critical Incident Inventory: Characteristics of Incidents Which Affect Emergency Medical Technicians and Paramedics." *BMC Emergency Medicine* 12 (10). https://doi.org/10.1186/1471-227X-12-10

Halpin, M., M. Phillips, and J.L. Oliffe. 2009. "Prostate Cancer Stories in the Canadian Print Media: Representations of Illness, Disease and Masculinities." *Sociology of Health & Illness* 31 (2): 155–69. http://dx.doi.org/10.1111/j.1467-9566.2008.01122.x. Medline:18983423

Hammond, M.L. 2020. *Epidemics and the Modern World.* Toronto: University of Toronto Press.

Hampton, M., A. Baydala, C. Bourassa, K. McKay-McNabb, C. Placsko, K. Goodwill, B. McKenna, P. McNabb, and R. Boekelder. 2010. "Completing the Circle: Elders Speak about End-of-Life Care with Aboriginal Families in Canada." *Journal of Palliative Care* 26 (1): 6–14. Medline:20402179

Harding le Riche, W. 1979. "Seventy Years of Public Health in Canada." *Canadian Journal of Public Health* 70 (3): 155–63. Medline:387201

Harris, D. 2009–10. "Oppression of the Bereaved: A Critical Analysis of Grief in Western Society." *Omega* 60 (3): 241–53. http://dx.doi.org/10.2190/OM.60.3.c. Medline:20361724

Hartling, R.N. 1993. *Nahanni: River of Gold, River of Dreams*. Hyde Park, ON: The Canadian Recreational Canoeing Association.

Hauser, D.J. 1974. "Seat Belts: Is Freedom of Choice Worth 800 Deaths a Year?" *Canadian Medical Association Journal* 110 (12): 1418–22. Medline:4834532

Haw, C., K. Hawton, C. Niedzwiedz, and S. Platt. 2013. "Suicide Clusters: A Review of Risk Factors and Mechanisms." *Suicide and Life-Threatening Behavior* 43 (1): 97–108. https://doi.org/10.1111/j.1943-278X.2012.00130.x. Medline:23356785

Hayter, J. 1968. "Organ Transplants—A New Type of Nursing?" *Canadian Nurse* 64 (11): 49–53. Medline:4176918

Heagerty, J.J. 1928. *Four Centuries of Medical History in Canada*. Toronto: Macmillan.

Heagerty, J.J. 1940. *The Romance of Medicine in Canada*. Toronto: Ryerson Press.

Health Canada. 2003. *Learning from SARS: Renewal of Public Health in Canada— Report of the National Advisory Committee on SARS and Public Health*. Cat. H21-220/2003E. Ottawa: Her Majesty the Queen in Right of Canada. https://www.canada.ca/en/public-health/services/reports-publications/learning-sars-renewal-public-health-canada.html

Health Canada. 2019. *Fourth Interim Report on Medical Assistance in Dying in Canada*. Cat. H14-230/4-2019E-PDF. Ottawa: Her Majesty the Queen in Right of Canada. https://www.canada.ca/en/health-canada/services/publications/health-system-services/medical-assistance-dying-interim-report-april-2019.html

Health Canada. 2020. *First Annual Report on Medical Assistance in Dying in Canada, 2019*. Cat. H22-1/6E-PDF. Ottawa: Her Majesty the Queen in Right of Canada. https://www.canada.ca/en/health-canada/services/medical-assistance-dying-annual-report-2019.html

Heart and Stroke Foundation of Canada. n.d. "Heart Failure." Accessed June 9, 2021. https://www.heartandstroke.ca/heart/conditions/heart-failure

Hebert, M.P. 1998. "Perinatal Bereavement in Its Cultural Context." *Death Studies* 22 (1): 61–78. http://dx.doi.org/10.1080/074811898201731. Medline:10179835

Hegg-Deloye, S., P. Brassard, N. Jauvin, J. Prairie, D. Larouche, P. Poirier, A. Tremblay, and P. Corbeil. 2014. "Current State of Knowledge of Post-Traumatic Stress, Sleeping Problems, Obesity and Cardiovascular Disease in Paramedics." *Emergency Medicine Journal* 31 (3): 242–7. http://dx.doi.org/10.1136/emermed-2012–201672. Medline:23314206

Henry, M., B. Trickey, L.N. Huang, and S.R. Cohen. 2012. "How Is Cancer Recently Portrayed in Canadian Newspapers Compared to 20 Years Ago?" *Supportive Care in Cancer* 20 (1): 49–55. http://dx.doi.org/10.1007/s00520-010-1049-9. Medline:21132331

Heyland, D.K., C. Frank, J. Tranmer, N. Paul, D. Pichora, X. Jiang, and A.G. Day. 2009. "Satisfaction with End-of-Life Care: A Longitudinal Study of Patients and Their Family Caregivers in the Last Months of Life." *Journal of Palliative Care* 25 (4): 245–56. Medline:20131581

Hindmarch, S., M. Orsini, and M. Gagnon. 2018. "Conclusion." In *Seeing Red: HIV/AIDS and Public Policy in Canada*, edited by S. Hindmarch, M. Orsini, and M. Gagnon, 334–47. Toronto: University of Toronto Press.

Ho, H.C., A. Knudby, B.B. Walker, and S.B. Henderson. 2017. "Delineation of Spatial Vulnerability in the Temperature-Mortality Relationship on Extremely Hot Days in Greater Vancouver, Canada." *Environmental Health Perspectives* 125 (1): 66–75. https://doi.org/10.1289/EHP224. Medline:27346526

Holmes, S., E. Wiebe, J. Shaw, A. Nuhn, A. Just, and M. Kelly. 2018. "Exploring the Experience of Supporting a Loved One through a Medically Assisted Death in Canada." *Canadian Family Physician* 64 (9): e387–e93. https://www.ncbi.nlm.nih.gov/pmc/articles/PMC6135137/

Holtslander, L.F., J.M.G. Bally, and M.L. Steeves. 2011. "Walking a Fine Line: An Exploration of the Experience of Finding Balance for Older Persons Bereaved after Caregiving for a Spouse with Advanced Cancer." *European Journal of Oncology Nursing* 15 (3): 254–9. http://dx.doi.org/10.1016/j.ejon.2010.12.004. Medline:21247803

Holtslander, L.F., and W.D. Duggleby. 2009. "The Hope Experience of Older Bereaved Women Who Cared for a Spouse with Terminal Cancer." *Qualitative Health Research* 19 (3): 388–400. http://dx.doi.org/10.1177/1049732308329682. Medline:19224881

Holtslander, L., and W. Duggleby. 2010. "The Psychosocial Context of Bereavement for Older Women Who Were Caregivers for a Spouse with Advanced Cancer." *Journal of Women & Aging* 22 (2): 109–24. http://dx.doi.org/10.1080/08952841003716147. Medline:20408032

Howarth, G. 2007. *Death and Dying: A Sociological Introduction*. Cambridge: Polity Press.

Howlett, J., L. Morrin, M. Fortin, G. Heckman, P.H. Strachan, N. Suskin, J. Shamian, R. Lewanczuk, and H.M. Aurthur. 2010. "End-of-Life Planning in Heart Failure: It Should Be the End of the Beginning." *Canadian Journal of Cardiology* 26 (3): 135–41. http://dx.doi.org/10.1016/S0828-282X(10)70351-2. Medline:20352133

Hsu, C., M. O'Connor, and S. Lee. 2009. "Understandings of Death and Dying for People of Chinese Origin." *Death Studies* 33 (2): 153–74. https://doi.org/10.1080/07481180802440431. Medline:19143109

Hu, W., Y. Yasui, J. White, and M. Winget. 2014. "Aggressiveness of End-of-Life Care for Patients with Colorectal Cancer in Alberta, Canada: 2006–2009." *Journal of Pain and Symptom Management* 47 (2): 231–44. http://dx.doi.org/10.1016/j.jpainsymman.2013.03.021. Medline:23870414

Hughes, R. 1999. "In Death's Throat: After a Car Crash, Our Art Critic Learns the Challenge—and Meaning—of Survival." *Time* 154 (15): 78–9. Medline:10620935

Humphry, D. 1991. *Final Exit: The Practicalities of Self-Deliverance and Assisted Suicide for the Dying.* Eugene, OR: Hemlock Society.

IbisWorld. 2020. "Funeral Homes in Canada – Market Research Report." https://www.ibisworld.com/canada/market-research-reports/funeral-homes-industry/

Industry Canada. 2015. "Canadian Industry Statistics." Government of Canada. https://www.ic.gc.ca/app/scr/sbms/sbb/cis/definition.html?code=81221&lang=eng

Jack, D. 1981. *Rogues, Rebels, and Geniuses: The Story of Canadian Medicine.* Toronto: Doubleday.

Jalland, P. 2006. *Changing Ways of Death in Twentieth-Century Australia.* Sydney, AU: University of New South Wales Press.

Jeannette, J.M., and A. Scoboria. 2008. "Firefighter Preferences Regarding Post-Incident Intervention." *Work and Stress* 22 (4): 314–26. http://dx.doi.org/10.1080/02678370802564231

John, A., K. Hawton, K. Lloyd, A. Luce, S. Platt, J. Scourfield, A.L. Marchant, P.A. Jones, and M.S. Dennis. 2014. "PRINTQUAL—A Measure for Assessing the Quality of Newspaper Reporting of Suicide." *Crisis* 35 (6): 431–5. https://doi.org/10.1027/0227-5910/a000276. Medline:25231856

Joseph, S.E. 1994. "Coast Salish Perceptions of Death and Dying: An Ethnographic Study." Unpublished master's thesis, University of Victoria, British Columbia.

Kastenbaum, R.J. 2007. *Death, Society, and Human Experience*, 9th ed. Boston: Allyn and Bacon.

Kastenbaum, R.J. 2009. *Death, Society, and Human Experience*, 10th ed. Boston: Allyn and Bacon.

Kastenbaum, R.J. 2012. *Death, Society, and Human Experience*, 11th ed. Boston: Allyn and Bacon.

Kaufert, J.M., and J.D. O'Neil. 1991. "Cultural Mediation of Dying and Grieving among Native Canadian Patients in Urban Hospitals." In *Coping with the Final Tragedy: Cultural Variation in Dying and Grieving*, edited by D.R. Counts and D.A. Counts, 231–51. Amityville, NY: Baywood.

Kellehear, A. 2007. *A Social History of Dying.* Cambridge: Cambridge University Press. http://dx.doi.org/10.1017/CBO9780511481352

Kelley, M.L., H. Prince, S. Nadin, K. Brazil, M. Crow, G. Hanson, L. Maki, L. Monture, C.J. Mushquash, V. O'Brien, et al. 2018. "Developing Palliative Care Programs in Indigenous Communities Using Participatory Action Research: A Canadian Application of the Public Health Approach to Palliative Care." *Annals of Palliative Medicine* 7 (Supplement 2): S52–S72. https://doi.org/10.21037/apm.2018.03.06. Medline:29764173

Kelly, E., and J. Nisker. 2010. "Medical Students' First Clinical Experiences of Death." *Medical Education* 44 (4): 421–8. http://dx.doi.org/10.1111/j.1365-2923.2009.03603.x. Medline:20236239

Kelm, M., and L. Townsend, eds. 2006. *In the Days of Our Grandmothers: A Reader in Aboriginal Women's History in Canada.* Toronto: University of Toronto Press.

Kendall, D., J.L. Murray, and R. Linden. 2000. *Sociology in Our Times*, 2nd Canadian ed. Scarborough, ON: Nelson.

Kent, G. 1996. "Robson: A Climber's Baptism." *Explore*, 15th Anniversary Issue, June/July, 80–3.

Knaak, S., D. Luong, R. McLean, A. Szeto, and K.S. Dobson. 2019. "Implementation, Uptake, and Culture Change: Results of a Key Informant Study of a Workplace Mental Health Training Program in Police Organizations in Canada." *The Canadian Journal of Psychiatry* 64 (Supplement 1): 30S–38S. https://doi.org/10.1177/0706743719842565. Medline:31056932

Kouwenhoven, W.B., J.R. Jude, and G.G. Knickerbocker. 1960. "Closed-Chest Cardiac Massage." *Journal of the American Medical Association* 173 (10): 1064–7. http://dx.doi.org/10.1001/jama.1960.03020280004002. Medline:14411374

Kübler-Ross, E. 1969. *On Death and Dying*. New York: Macmillan.

Kuhl, D. 2006. *Facing Death, Embracing Life: Understanding What Dying People Want*. Toronto: Doubleday.

Kyriakopoulos, P., M. Fedyk, and M. Shamy. 2017. "Translating Futility." *Canadian Medical Association Journal* 189 (23): E805–E806. https://doi.org/10.1503/cmaj.161354. Medline:28606979

Lalonde, M. 1978. *A New Perspective on the Health of Canadians: A Working Document*. Ottawa: Minister of Supply and Services.

Lang, A., A.R. Fleiszer, F. Duhamel, W. Sword, K.R. Gilbert, and S. Corsini-Munt. 2011. "Perinatal Loss and Parental Grief: The Challenge of Ambiguity and Disenfranchised Grief." *Omega* 63 (2): 183–96. http://dx.doi.org/10.2190/OM.63.2.e. Medline:21842665

Langham, P. "Medical Intervention and Effectiveness of the Health Care Delivery System: A Canadian Perspective." *Holistic Nursing Practice* 5 (3): 77–84. http://dx.doi.org/10.1097/00004650-199104000-00013. Medline:2045442

Langham, P., and D. Flagel. 1991. "Medical Intervention and the Effectiveness of the Health Care Delivery System: A Canadian Perspective." *Holistic Nursing Practice* 5 (3): 77–84. http://dx.doi.org/10.1097/00004650-199104000-00013. Medline:2045442

Laugrand, F. 2019. "The Beauty of the Afterlife among the Inuit of Nunavut." In *Death Across Cultures: Death and Dying in Non-Western Cultures*, edited by H. Selin and R.M. Rakoff, 351–67. Cham, Switzerland: Springer Nature.

Laurence, M. 1964. *The Stone Angel*. Toronto: McClelland and Stewart.

Lawson, E. 2014. "Disenfranchised Grief and Social Inequality: Bereaved African Canadians and Oppositional Narratives about the Violent Deaths of Friends and Family Members." *Ethnic and Racial Studies* 37 (11): 2092–109. http://dx.doi.org/10.1080/01419870.2013.800569.

Leach, J. 2011. "Survival Psychology: The Won't to Live." *The Psychologist* 24: 26–9. https://thepsychologist.bps.org.uk/volume-24/edition-1/survival-psychology-wont-live

Lehto, R.H., and K.F. Stein. 2009. "Death Anxiety: An Analysis of an Evolving Concept." *Research and Theory for Nursing Practice: An International Journal* 23 (1): 23–41. http://dx.doi.org/10.1891/1541–6577.23.1.23. Medline:19418886

Leming, M.R., and G.E. Dickinson. 2007. *Understanding Dying, Death, and Bereavement*, 6th ed. Belmont, CA: Thomson Wadsworth.

Leming, M.R., and G.E. Dickinson. 2016. *Understanding Dying, Death, and Bereavement*, 8th ed. Stamford, CT: Cengage Learning.

Lessard, R. 1991. *Health Care in Canada during the Seventeenth and Eighteenth Centuries*. Ottawa: Canadian Museum of Civilization.

Leung, D., M.J. Esplen, E. Peter, D. Howell, G. Rodin, and M. Fitch. 2012. "How Haematological Cancer Nurses Experience the Threat of Patients' Mortality." *Journal of Advanced Nursing* 68 (10): 2175–84. http://dx.doi.org/10.1111 /j.1365–2648.2011.05902.x. Medline:22150339

Lévy, J.J., A. Dupras, and J. Samson. 1985. "La religion, la mort et la sexualité au Québec." *Cahiers de Recherches en Sciences de la Religion* 6: 25–34.

Li, M., S. Watt, M. Escaf, M. Gardam, A. Heesters, G. O'Leary, and G. Rodin. 2017. "Medical Assistance in Dying—Implementing a Hospital-Based Program in Canada." *The New England Journal of Medicine* 376: 2082–8. https://doi.org /10.1056/NEJMms1700606. Medline:28538128

Lindsay, C. 1999. "Seniors: A Diverse Group Aging Well." *Canadian Social Trends* 52 (Summer): 24–6.

Linkletter, M., K. Gordon, and J. Dooley. 2010. "The Choking Game and YouTube: A Dangerous Combination." *Clinical Pediatrics* 49 (3): 274–9. http://dx.doi .org/10.1177/0009922809339203. Medline:19596864

Lowe, M.E., and S.E. McClement. 2010–11. "Spousal Bereavement: The Lived Experience of Young Canadian Widows." *Omega* 62 (2): 127–48. http://dx.doi .org/10.2190/OM.62.2.c. Medline:21375118

Lu, C., and E. Ng. 2019. "Healthy Immigrant Effect by Immigrant Category in Canada." Statistics Canada: Heath Reports. https://www150.statcan.gc.ca/n1 /pub/82-003-x/2019004/article/00001-eng.htm

Lucas, R.A. 1968. "Social Implications of the Immediacy of Death." *Canadian Review of Sociology and Anthropology* 5 (1): 1–16. http://dx.doi.org/10.1111 /j.1755–618X.1968.tb01165.x

Lyng, S. 1990. "Edgework: A Social Psychological Analysis of Voluntary Risk Taking." *American Journal of Sociology* 95 (4): 851–86. http://dx.doi.org /10.1086/229379

Lyng, S., ed. 2005a. *Edgework: The Sociology of Risk-Taking*. New York: Routledge.

Lyng, S. 2005b. "Edgework and the Risk-Taking Experience." In *Edgework: The Sociology of Risk-Taking*, edited by S. Lyng, 3–14. New York: Routledge.

MacDougall, H. 1994. "Sexually Transmitted Diseases in Canada, 1800–1992." *Genitourinary Medicine* 70 (1): 56–63. Medline:8300103

MacKillop, H.I. 1978. "Effects of Seatbelt Legislation and Reduction of Highway Speed Limits in Ontario." *Canadian Medical Association Journal* 119 (10): 1154–8. Medline:743655

MacNeil, M.S. 2008. "An Epidemiologic Study of Aboriginal Adolescent Risk in Canada: The Meaning of Suicide." *Journal of Child and Adolescent Psychiatric Nursing* 21 (1): 3–12. https://doi.org/10.1111/j.1744-6171.2008.00117.x. Medline:18269407

Macy, M.A. 2013. "Through the Eyes of a Child: Reflections on My Mother's Death from Cancer." *Journal of Pain & Palliative Care Pharmacotherapy* 27 (2): 176–8. http://dx.doi.org/10.3109/15360288.2013.782938. Medline: 23621174

Maddalena, V., W.T. Bernard, S. Davis-Murdoch, and D. Smith. 2013. "Awareness of Palliative Care and End-of-Life Options among African Canadians in Nova Scotia." *Journal of Transcultural Nursing* 24 (2): 144–52. http://dx.doi.org /10.1177/1043659612472190. Medline:23341407

Major, R.J., W.J. Whelton, J. Schimel, and D. Sharpe. 2016. "Older Adults and the Fear of Death: The Protective Function of Generativity." *Canadian Journal on Aging* 35 (2): 261–72. https://doi.org/10.1017/S0714980816000143. Medline:27118066

Malcom, N.L. 2010–11. "Images of Heaven and the Spiritual Afterlife: Qualitative Analysis of Children's Storybooks about Death, Dying, Grief, and Bereavement." *Omega* 62 (1): 51–76. http://dx.doi.org/10.2190/OM.62.1.c. Medline:21138070

Malette v. Schulman. 1992. 72 OR (2d) 417 (Ont CA).

Marchand, A., R. Boyer, C. Nadeau, and M. Martin. 2013. "Predictors of Posttraumatic Stress Disorder in Police Officers: Prospective Study. Report R-786." Montreal: The Institute de recherche Robert-Sauvé en santé et en sécurité du travail (IRSST). http://www.irsst.qc.ca/media/documents /PubIRSST/R-786.pdf

Marchenski, S. 2004. "Parental Grief and Trauma: An Exposure Comparison Study of Injury versus Non-Injury Child Deaths." Unpublished master's thesis, University of Manitoba, Winnipeg.

Marion, N., and J. Scanlon. 2011. "Mass Death and Mass Illness in an Isolated Canadian Town: Coping with Pandemic Influenza in Kenora, Ontario, in 1918–1921." *Mortality* 16 (4): 325–42. http://dx.doi.org/10.1080/13576275.201 1.613268

Marsh, J.H. 1985. "Disease." In *The Canadian Encyclopedia*, ed. J.H. Marsh, 833–4. Edmonton: Hurtig.

Marshall, V.W. 1986. "A Sociological Perspective on Aging and Dying." In *Later Life: The Social Psychology of Aging*, edited by V.W. Marshall, 125–46. Beverly Hills: Sage.

Marshall, V.W. 2013. "Death and Dying." In *The Canadian Encyclopedia*. http:// www.thecanadianencyclopedia.ca/en/article/death-and-dying/

Martin, K. 1998. *When a Baby Dies of SIDS: The Parents' Grief and Search for Reason*. Edmonton: Qual Institute Press (International Institute for Qualitative Methodology).

Martin, K., and S. Elder. 1993. "Pathways through Grief: A Model of the Process." In *Personal Care in an Impersonal World: A Multidimensional Look at Bereavement*, edited by J.D. Morgan, 73–86. Amityville, NY: Baywood.

Martin, M., A. Marchand, R. Boyer, and N. Martin. 2009. "Predictors of the Development of Posttraumatic Stress Disorder among Police Officers." *Journal of Trauma & Dissociation* 10 (4): 451–68. http://dx.doi.org/10.1080 /15299730903143626. Medline:19821179

Martin Matthews, A. 1987. "Widowhood as an Expectable Life Event." In *Aging in Canada: Social Perspectives*, 2nd ed., edited by V.W. Marshall, 343–66. Markham, ON: Fitzhenry and Whiteside.

Martin Matthews, A. 1991. *Widowhood in Later Life*. Toronto: Butterworths.

Martin Matthews, A. 2011. "Revisiting Widowhood in Later Life: Changes in Patterns and Profiles, Advances in Research and Understanding." *Canadian Journal on Aging* 30 (3): 339–54. http://dx.doi.org/10.1017 /S0714980811000201. Medline:21787444

Matthews, L.R., M.G. Quinlan, and P. Bohle. 2019. "Posttraumatic Stress Disorder, Depression, and Prolonged Grief Disorder in Families Bereaved by a Traumatic Workplace Death: The Need for Satisfactory Information and Support." *Frontiers in Psychiatry* 10 (609). https://doi.org/10.3389/fpsyt.2019.00609. Medline: 31543835

McClement, S., M. Lobchuk, H.M. Chochinov, and R. Dean. 2010. "'Broken Covenant': Healthcare Aides' 'Experience of the Ethical' in Caring for Dying Seniors in a Personal Care Home." *Journal of Clinical Ethics* 21 (3): 201–11. Medline:21089989

McEwen, R.N., and K. Scheaffer. 2013. "Virtual Mourning and Memory Construction on Facebook: Here Are the Terms of Use." *Bulletin of Science, Technology & Society* 33 (3–4): 64–75. http://dx.doi.org/10.1177 /0270467613516753

McGinnis, J.D. 1985. "Public Health." In *The Canadian Encyclopedia*, ed. J.H. Marsh, 1507–8. Edmonton: Hurtig.

McGregor, M.J., J. Slater, J. Sloan, K.M. McGrail, A. Martin-Matthews, S. Berg, A. Plecash, L. Sloss, J. Trimble, and J.M. Murphy. 2017. "How's Your Health at Home: Frail Homebound Patients Reported Health Experience and Outcomes." *Canadian Journal on Aging* 36 (3): 273–85. https://doi.org/10.1017 /S0714980817000186. Medline:28558857

McPhail, A., S. Moore, J. O'Connor, and C. Woodward. 1981. "One Hospital's Experience with a 'Do Not Resuscitate' Policy." *Canadian Medical Association Journal* 125 (8): 830–6. Medline:7306894

McPherson, B.D. 2004. *Aging as a Social Process: Canadian Perspectives*, 4th ed. Toronto: Oxford University Press.

McPherson, C.J., K.G. Wilson, and M.A. Murray. 2007. "Feeling Like a Burden: Exploring the Perspectives of Patients at the End of Life." *Social Science & Medicine* 64 (2): 417–27. http://dx.doi.org/10.1016/j.socscimed.2006.09.013. Medline:17069943

McPherson, K. 1996. *Bedside Matters: The Transformation of Canadian Nursing, 1900–1990*. Toronto: Oxford University Press.

McWhinney, I.R., and M.A. Stewart. 1994. "Home Care of Dying Patients: Family Physicians' Experience with a Palliative Care Support Team." *Canadian Family Physician* 40: 240–6. Medline:7510562

McWhirter, J.E., L. Hoffman-Goetz, and J.N. Clarke. 2012. "Can You See What They Are Saying? Breast Cancer Images and Text in Canadian Women's and

Fashion Magazines." *Journal of Cancer Education* 27 (2): 383–91. https://doi
.org/10.1007/s13187-011-0305-0. Medline: 22228485

Mealer, M., E.L. Burnham, C.J. Goode, B. Rothbaum, and M. Moss. 2009. "The
Prevalence and Impact of Post Traumatic Stress Disorder and Burnout Syndrome
in Nurses." *Depression and Anxiety* 26 (12): 1118–26. http://dx.doi.org/10.1002
/da.20631. Medline:19918928

Miele, R., and J. Clarke. 2014. "'We Remain Very Much the Second Sex': The
Constructions of Prostate Cancer in Popular News Magazines, 2000–2010."
American Journal of Men's Health 8 (1): 15–25. https://doi.org/10.1177
/1557988313487922. Medline:23660236

Millar, W.J. 1995. "Life Expectancy of Canadians." *Health Reports* 7 (3): 23–6.
Medline:8652800

Millar, W.J., and G.B. Hill. 1995. "The Elimination of Disease: A Mixed Blessing."
Health Reports 7 (3): 7–13. Medline:8652803

Miller, L.G. 1960. "Geriatric Nursing in the Home." *Canadian Nurse* 56 (7):
606–69.

Mirabelli, A. 2018. *What's in a Name? Defining Family in a Diverse Society.*
Ottawa: Vanier Institute of the Family. https://vanierinstitute.ca/whats-in
-a-name-defining-family-in-a-diverse-society/

Mirowsky, J., and C.E. Ross. 1989. *The Social Causes of Psychological Distress.*
New York: Aldine de Gruyter.

Mishara, B.L., and N. Martin. 2012. "Effects of a Comprehensive Police Suicide
Prevention Program." *Crisis* 33 (3): 162–8. https://doi.org/10.1027/0227-5910
/a000125. Medline:22450038

Mitchell, I., J.R. Guichon, and S. Wong. 2015. "Caring for Children, Focusing on
Children." *Paediatrics & Child Health* 20 (6): 293–5. https://doi.org/10.1093
/pch/20.6.293. Medline:26435666

Mitchell, L.M., P.H. Stephenson, S. Cadell, and M.E. Macdonald. 2012. "Death and
Grief Online: Virtual Memorialization and Changing Concepts of Childhood
Death and Parental Bereavement on the Internet." *Health Sociology Review*
21 (4): 413–31. http://dx.doi.org/10.5172/hesr.2012.21.4.413

Mitchell, W.O. 1947. *Who Has Seen the Wind.* Agincourt, ON: Macmillan.

Molzahn, A.E., A. Bruce, and L. Sheilds. 2008. "Learning from Stories of People
with Chronic Kidney Disease." *Nephrology Nursing Journal* 35 (1):
13–20.

Molzahn, A.E., L. Sheilds, A. Bruce, K. Schick-Makaroff, M. Antonio, and
A.M. Clark. 2020. "Life and Priorities before Death: A Narrative Inquiry of
Uncertainty and End of Life in People with Health Failure and Their Family
Members." *European Journal of Cardiovascular Nursing* 19 (4): 1–9. https://doi
.org/10.1177/1474515120918355. Medline:32340476

Molzahn, A.E., L. Sheilds, A. Bruce, K. Schick-Makaroff, M. Antonio, and L.
White. 2019. "Living with Dying: A Narrative Inquiry of People with Chronic
Kidney Disease and Their Family Members." *Journal of Advanced Nursing* 75
(1): 129–37. https://doi.org/10.1111/jan.13830. Medline:30132956

Molzahn, A., L. Sheilds, A. Bruce, K.I. Stajduhar, K.S. Makaroff, R. Beuthin, and S. Shermak. 2012. "Perceptions Regarding Death and Dying of Individuals with Chronic Kidney Disease." *Nephrology Nursing Journal* 39 (3): 197–204. Medline:22866359

Molzahn, A.E., R. Starzomski, M. McDonald, and C. O'Loughlin. 2004. "Aboriginal Beliefs about Organ Donation: Some Coast Salish Viewpoints." *Canadian Journal of Nursing Research* 36 (4): 110–28. Medline:15739940

Molzahn, A.E., R. Starzomski, M. McDonald, and C. O'Loughlin. 2005. "Chinese Canadian Beliefs toward Organ Donation." *Qualitative Health Research* 15 (1): 82–98. http://dx.doi.org/10.1177/1049732304270653. Medline:15574717

Monette, M. 2012. "Senior Suicide: An Overlooked Problem." *Canadian Medical Association Journal* 184 (17): E885–6. http://dx.doi.org/10.1503/cmaj.109–4287. Medline:23091186

Montreal Gazette. 2019. "Cadotte Relieved by Manslaughter Verdict." February 24. https://montrealgazette.com/news/michel-cadotte-found-guilty-of-manslaughter-in-death-of-ailing-wife

Morris, S., K. Fletcher, and R. Goldstein. 2019. "The Grief of Parents after the Death of a Young Child." *Journal of Clinical Psychology in Medical Settings* 26 (3): 321–38. https://doi.org/10.1007/s10880-018-9590-7. Medline:30488260

Morton, D. 1997. *A Short History of Canada*, 3rd ed. Toronto: McClelland and Stewart.

Morton, D. 2006. *A Short History of Canada*, 6th ed. Toronto: McClelland and Stewart.

Moss, M.S., N. Resch, and S.Z. Moss. 1997. "The Role of Gender in Middle-Age Children's Responses to Parent Death." *Omega* 35 (1): 43–65.

Murray, M.E. 1981. "Palliative Care." *Canadian Nurse* 77 (5): 16–17. Medline:6163520

Muskat, B., D. Brownstone, and A. Greenblatt. 2017. "The Experiences of Pediatric Social Workers Providing End-of-Life Care." *Social Work in Health Care* 56 (6): 505–23. https://doi.org/10.1080/00981389.2017.1302034. Medline:28398174

Nayfeh, A., I. Marcoux, and J. Jutai. 2019. "Advance Care Planning for Mechanical Ventilation: A Qualitative Study on Health-Care Providers' Approaches to Cross-Cultural Care." *Omega* 80 (2): 305–30. https://doi.org/10.1177/0030222817732467. Medline:28946842

Nicholas, D.B., L. Beaune, M. Barrera, J. Blumberg, and M. Belletrutti. 2016. "Examining the Experiences of Fathers of Children with a Life-Limiting Illness." *Journal of Social Work in End-of-Life and Palliative Care* 12 (1–2): 126–44. https://doi.org/10.1080/15524256.2016.1156601. Medline:27143577

Nichols, D. 2005. "*Dying at Grace*: A Documentary Video." *Gerontologist* 45 (1): 141–3. http://dx.doi.org/10.1093/geront/45.1.141-a

Nielsen, L.S., J.E. Angus, D. Gastaldo, D. Howell, and A. Husain. 2013. "Maintaining Distance from a Necessary Intrusion: A Postcolonial Perspective on Dying at Home for Chinese Immigrants in Toronto, Canada." *European Journal of Oncology Nursing* 17 (5): 649–56. http://dx.doi.org/10.1016/j.ejon.2013.06.006. Medline:23891386

Niezen, R. 2009. "Suicide as a Way of Belonging: Causes and Consequences of Cluster Suicides in Aboriginal Communities." https://doi.org/10.2139/ssrn.3075644

Nissim, R., L. Gagliese, and G. Rodin. 2009. "The Desire for Hastened Death in Individuals with Advanced Cancer: A Longitudinal Qualitative Study." *Social Science & Medicine* 69 (2): 165–71. http://dx.doi.org/10.1016 /j.socscimed.2009.04.021. Medline:19482401

Nissim, R., D. Rennie, S. Fleming, S. Hales, L. Gagliese, and G. Rodin. 2012. "Goals Set in the Land of the Living/Dying: A Longitudinal Study of Patients Living with Advanced Cancer." *Death Studies* 36 (4): 360–90. http://dx.doi.org /10.1080/07481187.2011.553324. Medline:24567991

Norris, J. 1994. "Widowhood in Later Life." In *Late-Life Marital Disruptions: Writings in Gerontology*, Vol. 14. Ottawa: National Advisory Council on Aging.

Northcott, H.C., and M.D. Harvey. 2012. "Public Perceptions of Key Performance Indicators of Healthcare in Alberta, Canada." *International Journal for Quality in Health Care* 24 (3): 214–23. http://dx.doi.org/10.1093/intqhc/mzs012. Medline:22461204

Nota, P.M.D., G.S. Anderson, R. Ricciardelli, R.N. Carleton, and D. Groll. 2020. "Mental Disorders, Suicidal Ideation, Plans and Attempts among Canadian Police." *Occupational Medicine* 70: 183–90. https://doi.org/10.1093/occmed /kqaa026. Medline:32154872

Nouvet, E., P.H. Strachan, J. Kryworuchko, J. Downar, and J.J. You. 2016. "Waiting for the Body to Fail: Limits to End-of-Life Communication in Canadian Hospitals." *Mortality* 21(4), 340–56. https://doi.org/10.1080/13576275.2016.1140133

Novak, M., H.C. Northcott, and K. Kobayashi. 2021. *Aging and Society: Canadian Perspectives*, 9th ed. Toronto: Top Hat.

Nowatzki, N.R., and R. Grant Kalischuk. 2009. "Post-Death Encounters: Grieving, Mourning, and Healing." *Omega* 59 (2): 91–111. http://dx.doi.org/10.2190/OM .59.2.a. Medline:19697714

O'Connor, K., and M. Barrera. 2014. "Changes in Parental Self-Identity following the Death of a Child to Cancer." *Death Studies* 38 (6): 404–11. http://dx.doi.org /10.1080/07481187.2013.801376. Medline:24666147

Ogden, R. 1994. "The Right to Die: A Policy Proposal for Euthanasia and Aid in Dying." *Canadian Public Policy* 20 (1): 1–25. http://dx.doi.org/10.2307/3551832. Medline:11652969

O'Keeffe, J. 2020. "Death Care during the COVID-19 Pandemic: Understanding the Public Health Risks." *Environmental Health Review* 3 (2): 40–7. https://doi .org/10.5864/d2020-009

Oneschuk, D., N. MacDonald, S. Bagshaw, N. Mayo, H. Jung, and J. Hanson. 2002. "A Pilot Survey of Medical Students' Perspectives on Their Educational Exposure to Palliative Care in Two Canadian Universities." *Journal of Palliative Medicine* 5 (3): 353–61. http://dx.doi.org/10.1089/109662102320135243. Medline:12133241

Organisation for Economic Co-operation and Development (OECD). 2014. "Obesity Update." http://www.oecd.org/els/health-systems/Obesity-Update-2014.pdf

Organisation for Economic Co-operation and Development (OECD). 2019. *Health at a Glance 2019: OECD Indicators*. Paris: OECD Publishing. https://doi.org/10.1787/4dd50c09-en

Orsini, M., S. Hindmarch, and M. Gagnon. 2018. "Introduction." In *Seeing Red: HIV/AIDS and Public Policy in Canada*, edited by S. Hindmarch, M. Orsini, and M. Gagnon, 3–23. Toronto: University of Toronto Press.

Palda, V.A., K.W. Bowman, R.F. McLean, and M.G. Chapman. 2005. "'Futile' Care: Do We Provide It? Why? A Semistructured, Canada-Wide Survey of Intensive Care Unit Doctors and Nurses." *Journal of Critical Care* 20 (3): 207–13. http://dx.doi.org/10.1016/j.jcrc.2005.05.006. Medline:16253788

Pannuti, F., and S. Tanneberger. 1992. "The Bologna Eubiosia Project: Hospital-at-Home Care for Advanced Cancer Patients." *Journal of Palliative Care* 8 (2): 11–17. Medline:1378893

Patterson, R.M. [1954] 1989. *Dangerous River*. Toronto: Stoddart.

Penz, K., and L. Tipper. 2019. "Who Cares for the Caregiver? Professional Quality of Life in Palliative Care." In *Hospice Palliative Home Care and Bereavement Support: Nursing Interventions and Supportive Care*, edited by L. Holtslander, S. Peacock, and J. Bally, 1–16. Cham, Switzerland: Springer Nature.

Petrovich, C., and H. Slinger (Director). 2017. *Lost on Arrival: Me, the Mounties & PTSD* [Video]. CBC Documentary Film.

Pfeffer, A. 2019. "Funeral Workers Launch Peer Support Group to Help Their Mental Health." *CBC News*, February 6. https://www.cbc.ca/news/canada/ottawa/funeral-mental-health-support-peers-1.5007428

Phillips, J.R. 1992. "Choosing and Participating in the Living-Dying Process: A Research Emergent." *Nursing Science Quarterly* 5 (1): 4–5. http://dx.doi.org/10.1177/089431849200500103. Medline:1538854

Pirkis, J., R.W. Blood, A. Beautrais, P. Burgess, and J. Skehan. 2006. "Media Guidelines on the Reporting of Suicide." *Crisis* 27 (2): 82–7. https://doi.org/10.1027/0227-5910.27.2.82. Medline:16913330

Posner, J. 1976. "Death as a Courtesy Stigma." *Essence* 1: 39–49.

Powell, K.A., and A. Matthys. 2013. "Effects of Suicide on Siblings: Uncertainty and the Grief Process." *Journal of Family Communication* 13 (4): 321–9. http://dx.doi.org/10.1080/15267431.2013.823431

Preston, R.J., and S.C. Preston. 1991. "Death and Grieving among Northern Forest Hunters: An East Cree Example." In *Coping with the Final Tragedy: Cultural Variation in Dying and Grieving*, edited by D.R. Counts and D.A. Counts, 135–55. Amityville, NY: Baywood.

Préville, M., R. Hébert, R. Boyer, G. Bravo, and M. Seguin. 2005. "Physical Health and Mental Disorder in Elderly Suicide: A Case-Control Study." *Aging & Mental Health* 9 (6): 576–84. http://dx.doi.org/10.1080/13607860500192973. Medline:16214706

Pritchard, M., E.A. Burghen, J.S. Gattuso, N.K. West, P. Gajjar, D.K. Srivastava, S.L. Spunt, J.N. Baker, J.R. Kane, W.L. Furman, et al. 2010. "Factors That Distinguish Symptoms of Most Concern to Parents from Other Symptoms of

Dying Children." *Journal of Pain and Symptom Management* 39 (4): 627–36. http://dx.doi.org/10.1016/j.jpainsymman.2009.08.012. Medline:20413052

Public Health Agency of Canada. 2019. "Prevalence of Chronic Diseases among Canadian Adults." https://www.canada.ca/en/public-health/services/chronic-diseases/prevalence-canadian-adults-infographic-2019.html

Quill, T., and G.K. Kimsma. 2006. "How Much Suffering Is Enough?" *Medical Ethics* 13 (2): 10–11. Medline:17111512

Radin, P. 2006. "'To Me, It's My Life': Medical Communication, Trust, and Activism in Cyberspace." *Social Science & Medicine* 62 (3): 591–601. http://dx.doi.org/10.1016/j.socscimed.2005.06.022. Medline:16039031

Rallison, L.B., and S. Raffin-Bouchal. 2012. "Living in the In-Between: Families Caring for a Child with a Progressive Neurodegenerative Illness." *Qualitative Health Research* 23 (2): 194–206. http://dx.doi.org/10.1177/1049732312467232. Medline:23175537

Ramos, H., and K. Gosine. 2002. "'The Rocket': Newspaper Coverage of the Death of a Québec Cultural Icon, a Canadian Hockey Player." *Journal of Canadian Studies* 36 (4): 9–31.

Rando, T.A., K.J. Doka, S. Fleming, M.H. Franco, E.A. Lobb, C.M. Parkes, and R. Steele. 2012. "A Call to the Field: Complicated Grief in the DSM-5." *Omega* 65 (4): 251–5. http://dx.doi.org/10.2190/OM.65.4.a. Medline:23115891

Rasooly, I., J.V. Lavery, S. Urowitz, S. Choudhry, N. Seeman, E.M. Meslin, F.H. Lowy, and P.A. Singer. 1994. "Hospital Policies on Life-Sustaining Treatments and Advance Directives in Canada." *Canadian Medical Association Journal* 150 (8): 1265–70. Medline:8162549

Rawlings, D., C. Lister, L. Miller-Lewis, J. Tieman, and K. Swetenham. 2020. "The Voices of Death Doulas about Their Role in End-of-Life Care." *Health and Social Care in the Community* 28: 12–21. https://doi.org/10.1111/hsc.12833. Medline:31448464

Rawlings, D., J. Tieman, L. Miller-Lewis, and K. Swetenham. 2019. "What Role to Death Doulas Play in End-of-Life Care? A Systematic Review." *Health and Social Care in the Community* 27: e82–e94. https://doi.org/10.1111/hsc.12660. Medline:30255588

Rawlings, D., J.J. Tieman, C. Sanderson, D. Parker, and L. Miller-Lewis. 2017. "Never Say Die: Death Euphemisms, Misunderstandings and Their Implications for Practice." *International Journal of Palliative Nursing* 23 (7): 112–18. https://doi.org/10.12968/ijpn.2017.23.7.324. Medline:28756754

Regehr, C., M.G. Carey, S. Wagner, L.E. Alden, N. Buys, W. Corneil, T. Fyfe, L. Matthews, C. Randall, M. White, et al. 2019. "A Systematic Review of Mental Health Symptoms in Police Officers following Extreme Traumatic Exposures." *Police Practice and Research* 22 (1): 225–39. https://doi.org/10.1080/15614263.2019.1689129

Regehr, C., G. Goldberg, G.D. Glancy, and T. Knott. 2002. "Posttraumatic Symptoms and Disability in Paramedics." *Canadian Journal of Psychiatry* 47 (10): 953–8. Medline:12553131

Reutter, L.I., and H.C. Northcott. 1993. "Making Risk Meaningful: Developing Caring Relationships with AIDS Patients." *Journal of Advanced Nursing* 18 (9): 1377–85. http://dx.doi.org/10.1046/j.1365–2648.1993.18091377.x. Medline:8258595

Reutter, L.I., and H.C. Northcott. 1994. "Achieving a Sense of Control in a Context of Uncertainty: Nurses and AIDS." *Qualitative Health Research* 4 (1): 51–71. http://dx.doi.org/10.1177/104973239400400104

Reutter, L.I., and H.C. Northcott. 1995. "Managing Occupational HIV Exposures: A Canadian Study." *International Journal of Nursing Studies* 32 (5): 493–505. http://dx.doi.org/10.1016/0020–7489(95)00010-U. Medline:8550309

Ribkoff, F. 2012. "Bharati Mukherjee's 'The Management of Grief' and the Politics of Mourning in the Aftermath of the Air India Bombing." In *Literature for Our Times: Postcolonial Studies in the Twenty-First Century*, edited by B. Ashcroft, R. Mendis, J. McGonegal, and A Mukherjee, 507–22. New York: Rodopi.

Robinson, C.A., J.L. Bottorff, E. McFee, L.J. Bissell, and G. Fyles. 2017. "Caring at Home until Death: Enabled Determination." *Supportive Care in Cancer* 25 (4): 1229–36. https://doi.org/10.1007/s00520-016-3515-5. Medline:27924357

Rodabough, T., and K. Cole. 2003. "Near-Death Experiences as Secular Eschatology." In *Handbook of Death and Dying, Volume One: The Presence of Death*, edited by C.D. Bryant, 137–47. Thousand Oaks, CA: Sage. http://dx.doi.org/10.4135/9781412914291.n15

Roland, C. 1985. "History of Medicine." In *The Canadian Encyclopedia*, ed. J.H. Marsh, 1112–14. Edmonton: Hurtig.

Rosenberg, M.W., and E.G. Moore. 1997. "The Health of Canada's Elderly Population: Current Status and Future Implications." *Canadian Medical Association Journal* 157 (8): 1025–32. Medline:9347773

Rusnell, C. 2019. "Storage of Bodies in Rented Trailer Leads to Probe of Medical Examiner's Space Shortage." *CBC News*, September 10. https://www.cbc.ca/news/canada/edmonton/bodies-stored-rented-trailer-medical-examiner-1.5278243

Rutty, C., and S.C. Sullivan. 2010. *This Is Public Health: A Canadian History*. Ottawa: Canadian Public Health Association. https://www.cpha.ca/sites/default/files/assets/history/book/history-book-print_all_e.pdf

Sadler, E., B. Hales, B. Henry, W. Xiong, J. Myers, L. Wynnychuk, R. Taggar, D. Heyland, and R. Fowler. 2014. "Factors Affecting Family Satisfaction with Inpatient End-of-Life Care." *PLoS One* 9 (11): e110860. http://dx.doi.org/10.1371/journal.pone.0110860. Medline:25401710

Sankaran, K., E. Hedin, and H. Hodgson-Viden. 2016. "Neonatal End of Life Care in a Tertiary Care Centre in Canada: A Brief Report." *The Chinese Journal of Contemporary Pediatrics* 18 (5): 379–85. https://doi.org/10.7499/j.issn.1008-8830.2106.05.001

Sax Institute. 2017. "Tools to Aide Clinical Identification of End of Life." https://www.saxinstitute.org.au/wp-content/uploads/Tools-to-aid-clinical-identification-of-end-of-life.pdf

Scalena, A. 2006. "Defining Quackery: An Examination of the Manitoba Medical Profession and the Early Development of Professional Unity." *Journal of the Canadian Chiropractic Association* 50 (3): 209–18. Medline:17549158

Schick-Makaroff, K.L., L. Sheilds, and A. Molzahn. 2013. "Stories of Chronic Kidney Disease: Listening for the Unsayable." *Journal of Advanced Nursing* 69 (12): 2644–53. https://doi.org/10.1111/jan.12149. Medline:23594086

Schormans, A.F. 2004. "Experiences following the Deaths of Disabled Foster Children: 'We Don't Feel Like "Foster" Parents.'" *Omega* 49 (4): 347–69.

Schriever, S.H. 1990. "Comparison of Beliefs and Practices of Ethnic Viet and Lao Hmong Concerning Illness, Healing, Death and Mourning: Implications for Hospice Care with Refugees in Canada." *Journal of Palliative Care* 6 (1): 42–9. Medline:2332823

Schultz, L.E. 2007. "The Influence of Maternal Loss on Young Women's Experience of Identity Development in Emerging Adulthood." *Death Studies* 31 (1): 17–43. http://dx.doi.org/10.1080/07481180600925401. Medline:17131560

Senate of Canada. 1995. *Of Life and Death: Report of the Special Senate Committee on Euthanasia and Assisted Suicide.* Ottawa: Minister of Supply and Services Canada.

Service Corporation International (SCI). n.d. "Who We Are." Accessed June 9, 2021. https://investors.sci-corp.com/

Sheilds, L., A. Molzahn, A. Bruce, K. Schick-Makaroff, K. Stajduhar, R. Beuthin, and S. Shermak. 2015. "Contrasting Stories of Life-Threatening Illness: A Narrative Inquiry." *International Journal of Nursing Studies* 52 (1): 207–15. https://doi.org/10/1016/j.ijnurstu.2014.10.0080020-7489. Medline:25457877

Shor, E., D.J. Roelfs, M. Curreli, L. Clemow, M.M. Burg, and J.E. Schwartz. 2012. "Widowhood and Mortality: A Meta-Analysis and Meta-Regression." *Demography* 49 (2): 575–606. http://dx.doi.org/10.1007/s13524–012–0096-x. Medline:22427278

Silverman, P.R., S. Nickman, and J.W. Worden. 1995. "Detachment Revisited: The Child's Reconstruction of a Dead Parent." In *The Path Ahead: Readings in Death and Dying*, edited by L.A. DeSpelder and A.L. Strickland, 260–70. Mountain View, CA: Mayfield.

Simons, K., and E. Park-Lee. 2009. "Social Work Students' Comfort with End-of-Life Care." *Journal of Social Work in End-of-Life & Palliative Care* 5 (1–2): 34–48. http://dx.doi.org/10.1080/15524250903173884

Sirois, F. 2012. "Psychiatric Aspects of Chronic Palliative Care: Waiting for Death." *Palliative & Supportive Care* 10 (3): 205–11. http://dx.doi.org/10.1017/S1478951511000885. Medline:22935080

Smith, D. 2007. *Big Death: Funeral Planning in the Age of Corporate Deathcare.* Halifax: Fernwood Publishing.

Sneiderman, B. 1993. "The Case of Nancy B: A Criminal Law and Social Policy Perspective." *Health Law Journal* 1: 25–38. Medline:10569857

Sookram, S., H. Borkent, G. Powell, W.D. Hogarth, and L. Shepherd. 2001. "Tornado at Pine Lake, Alberta—July 14, 2000: Assessment of the Emergency

Medicine Response to a Disaster." *Canadian Journal of Emergency Medicine* 3 (1): 34–7. https://doi.org/10.1017/S1481803500005133. Medline:17612439

Stajduhar, K.I., D.E. Allan, S.R. Cohen, and D.K. Heyland. 2008. "Preferences for Location of Death of Seriously Ill Hospitalized Patients: Perspectives from Canadian Patients and Their Family Caregivers." *Palliative Medicine* 22 (1): 85–8. http://dx.doi.org/10.1177/0269216307084612. Medline:18216081

Stajduhar, K.I., L. Funk, S.R. Cohen, A. Williams, D. Bidgood, D. Allan, L. Norgrove, and D. Heyland. 2011. "Bereaved Family Members' Assessments of the Quality of End-of-Life Care: What Is Important?" *Journal of Palliative Care* 27 (4): 261–9. Medline:22372280

Stajduhar, K.I., L. Funk, and L. Outcalt. 2013. "Family Caregiver Learning—How Family Caregivers Learn to Provide Care at the End of Life: A Qualitative Secondary Analysis of Four Datasets." *Palliative Medicine* 27 (7): 657–64. http://dx.doi.org/10.1177/0269216313487765. Medline:23695826

Staniloiu, A., and A. Feinstein. 2017. "Post-Traumatic Stress Disorder (PTSD) in Canada." In *The Canadian Encyclopedia*. https://www.thecanadianencyclopedia.ca/en/article/post-traumatic-stress-disorder-ptsd-in-canada

Stanley, I.H., M.A. Hom, and T.E. Joiner. 2016. "A Systematic Review of Suicidal Thoughts and Behaviours among Police Officers, Firefighters, EMTs, and Paramedics." *Clinical Psychology Review* 44: 25–44. https://doi.org/10.1016/j.cpr.2015.12.002. Medline:26719976

Statistics Canada. 2014a. "2011 National Household Survey: Data Tables." http://www12.statcan.gc.ca/nhs-enm/2011/dp-pd/dt-td/Rp-eng.cfm?LANG=E&APATH=3&DETAIL=0&DIM=0&FL=A&FREE=0&GC=0&GID=0&GK=0&GRP=0&PID=105399&PRID=0&PTYPE=105277&S=0&SHOWALL=0&SUB=0&Temporal=2013&THEME=95&VID=0&VNAMEE=&VNAMEF=

Statistics Canada. 2014b. "Deaths in Hospital and Elsewhere, Canada, Provinces and Territories." Table 102-0509. http://www5.statcan.gc.ca/cansim/a26?lang=eng&id=1020509

Statistics Canada. 2017a. "Immigration and Ethnocultural Diversity." https://www150.statcan.gc.ca/n1/daily-quotidien/171025/dq171025b-eng.htm?indid=14428-1&indgeo=0

Statistics Canada. 2017b. "Canada Day ... by the Numbers." https://www.statcan.gc.ca/eng/dai/smr08/2017/smr08_219_2017

Statistics Canada. 2019. "Deaths and Age-Specific Mortality Rates, by Selected Grouped Causes." Table 13-10-0392-01. https://doi.org/10.25318/1310039201-eng

Statistics Canada. 2020a. "History of Vital Statistics." https://www.statcan.gc.ca/eng/about/relevant/vscc/history

Statistics Canada. 2020b. "Deaths and Mortality Rates, by Age Group." https://www150.statcan.gc.ca/t1/tbl1/en/tv.action?pid=1310071001

Statistics Canada. 2020c. "Leading Causes of Death, Total Population, by Age Group." https://www150.statcan.gc.ca/t1/tbl1/en/tv.action?pid=1310039401

Statistics Canada. 2020d. "Deaths Subject to Autopsy." https://www150.statcan.gc.ca/t1/tbl1/en/tv.action?pid=1310071601

Statistics Canada. 2020e. "Leading Causes of Death, Infants." https://www150
.statcan.gc.ca/t1/tbl1/en/tv.action?pid=1310039501

Statistics Canada. 2020f. "Employment Insurance Beneficiaries by Type of Income
Benefits, Monthly, Unadjusted for Seasonality." https://www150.statcan.gc.ca/t1
/tbl1/en/tv.action?pid=1410000901

Statistics Canada. 2020g. "Population Estimates on July 1st, by Age and Sex."
https://www150.statcan.gc.ca/t1/tbl1/en/tv.action?pid=1710000501

Statistics Canada. 2020h. "Life Expectancy and Other Elements of the Life Table,
Canada, All Provinces except Prince Edward Island." Table 13-10-0114-01.
https://doi.org/10.25318/1310011401-eng

Statistics Canada. 2020i. "Deaths, by Month." https://www150.statcan.gc.ca/t1/tbl1
/en/tv.action?pid=1310070801

Statistics Canada. 2020j. "Support Received by Caregivers in Canada." https://
www150.statcan.gc.ca/n1/pub/75-006-x/2020001/article/00001-eng.htm

Statistics Canada. 2020k. "Estimates of Population as of July 1st, by Marital Status
or Legal Marital Status, Age and Sex." Table 17-10-0060-01. https://doi.org
/10.25318/1710006001-eng

Stein, D.J., K.A. McLaughlin, K.C. Koenen, L. Atwoli, M.J. Friedman, E.D. Hill, A.
Maercker, M. Petukhova, V. Shahly, M. van Ommeren, et al. 2014. "DSM-5 and
ICD-11 Definitions of Posttraumatic Stress Disorder: Investigating 'Narrow' and
'Broad' Approaches." *Depression and Anxiety* 31 (6): 494–505. http://dx.doi
.org/10.1002/da.22279. Medline:24894802

Stelnicki, A.M., L. Jamshidi, A. Angehrn, and R.N. Carleton. 2020. "Suicidal
Behaviors among Nurses in Canada." *Canadian Journal of Nursing Research* 52
(3): 226–36. https://doi.org/10.1177/0844562120934237

Stephenson, P.H. 1992. "'He Died Too Quick!' The Process of Dying in a Hutterian
Colony." In *Grief in Cross-Cultural Perspective: A Casebook*, edited by L.A.
Platt and V.R. Persico, Jr., 293–303. New York: Garland Publishing.

Stone, E. 1962. *Medicine among the American Indians*. New York: Hafner.

Stroebe, M., M.M. Gergen, K.G. Gergen, and W. Stroebe. 1995. "Broken Hearts or
Broken Bonds: Love and Death in Historical Perspective." In *The Path Ahead:
Readings in Death and Dying*, edited by L.A. DeSpelder and A.L. Strickland,
231–41. Mountain View, CA: Mayfield.

Subedi, R., T.L. Greenberg, and S. Roshanafshar. 2019. "Does Geography Matter in
Mortality? An Analysis of Potentially Avoidable Mortality by Remoteness Index
in Canada." Statistics Canada: Health Reports. https://www150.statcan.gc.ca/n1
/pub/82-003-x/2019005/article/00001-eng.htm

Sudnow, D. 1967. *Passing On: The Social Organization of Dying*. Englewood Cliffs,
NJ: Prentice-Hall.

Supreme Court of Canada. 2013. *Cuthbertson v. Rasouli*, SCC 53, 34362. October
18. https://scc-csc.lexum.com/scc-csc/scc-csc/en/item/13290/index.do

Supreme Court of Canada. 2015. *Carter v. Canada*, SCC5, 35591. February 6.
https://scc-csc.lexum.com/scc-csc/scc-csc/en/item/14637/index.do

Symbaluk, D.G., and T.M. Bereska. 2019. *Sociology in Action: A Canadian
Perspective*, 3rd ed. Toronto: Nelson.

Tan, A., and D. Manca. 2013. "Finding Common Ground to Achieve a 'Good Death': Family Physicians Working with Substitute Decision-Makers of Dying Patients. A Qualitative Grounded Theory Study." *BMC Family Practice* 14 (1): 14. http://dx.doi.org/10.1186/1471–2296–14–14. Medline:23339822

Tatterton, M.J., and C. Walshe. 2019. "Understanding the Bereavement Experience of Grandparents following the Death of a Grandchild from a Life-Limiting Condition: A Meta-Ethnography." *Journal of Advanced Nursing* 75: 1406–17. https://doi.org/10.1111/jan.13927. Medline:30536458

Thomas, D. 1971. *The Poems*. Edited with an introduction and notes by D. Jones. London: Dent.

Thompson, G.N., V.H. Menec, H.M. Chochinov, and S.E. McClement. 2008. "Family Satisfaction with Care of a Dying Loved One in Nursing Homes: What Makes the Difference?" *Journal of Gerontological Nursing* 34 (12): 37–44. http://dx.doi.org/10.3928/00989134–20081201–10. Medline: 19113002

Thompson, N. 2017a. "Culturally Competent Practice." In *Handbook of the Sociology of Death, Grief, and Bereavement: A Guide to Theory and Practice*, edited by N. Thompson and G.R. Cox, 237–50. New York: Routledge.

Thompson, N. 2017b. "The Role of Religion and Spirituality in Grieving." In *Handbook of the Sociology of Death, Grief, and Bereavement: A Guide to Theory and Practice*, edited by N. Thompson and G.R. Cox, 337–50. New York: Routledge.

Thompson, N., and K.J. Doka. 2017. "Disenfranchised Grief." In *Handbook of the Sociology of Death, Grief, and Bereavement: A Guide to Theory and Practice*, edited by N. Thompson and G.R. Cox, 177–90. New York: Routledge.

Thurston, A.J., D.M. Wilson, and J.A. Hewitt. 2012. "Current End-of-Life Care Needs and Care Practices in Acute Care Hospitals." *Nursing Research and Practice*. Medline:22315678

Tjepkema, M., T. Bushnik, and E. Bougie. 2019. "Life Expectancy of First Nations, Métis and Inuit Household Populations in Canada." Statistics Canada: Health Reports. https://www150.statcan.gc.ca/n1/pub/82-003-x/2019012/article/00001-eng.htm

Topf, L., C.A. Robinson, and J.L. Bottorff. 2013. "When a Desired Home Death Does Not Occur: The Consequences of Broken Promises." *Journal of Palliative Medicine* 16 (8): 875–80. http://dx.doi.org/10.1089/jpm.2012.0541. Medline:23808644

Tornstam, L. 2005. *Gerotranscendence: A Developmental Theory of Positive Aging*. New York: Springer.

Tousignant, M., B.L. Mishara, A. Caillaud, V. Fortin, and D. St-Laurent. 2005. "The Impact of Media Coverage of the Suicide of a Well-Known Quebec Reporter: The Case of Gaëtan Girouard." *Social Science and Medicine* 60 (9): 1919–26. https://doi.org/10.1016/j.socscimed.2004.08.054. Medline:15743643

Trovato, F. 2015. *Canada's Population in a Global Context: An Introduction to Social Demography*, 2nd ed. Toronto: Oxford University Press.

Tucker, S., and A. Keefe. 2019. "2019 Report on Work Fatality and Injury Rates in Canada, April 25, 2019." https://www.uregina.ca/business/faculty-staff/faculty /file_download/2019-Report-on-Workplace-Fatalities-and-Injuries.pdf

Turner, K., R. Chye, G. Aggarwal, J. Philip, A. Skeels, and J.N. Lickiss. 1996. "Dignity in Dying: A Preliminary Study of Patients in the Last Three Days of Life." *Journal of Palliative Care* 12 (2): 7–13. Medline:8708856

United Nations. 2020. *World Mortality 2019*. New York: United Nations. https:// www.un.org/en/development/desa/population/publications/pdf/mortality /WMR2019/World_Mortality_2019.pdf

Vachon, M., L. Fillion, and M. Achille. 2012. "Death Confrontation, Spiritual-Existential Experience and Caring Attitudes in Palliative Care Nurses: An Interpretative Phenomenological Analysis." *Qualitative Research in Psychology* 9 (2): 151–72. http://dx.doi.org/10.1080/14780881003663424

van den Hoonaard, D.K. 1997. "Identity Foreclosure: Women's Experiences of Widowhood as Expressed in Autobiographical Accounts." *Ageing and Society* 17 (5): 533–51. http://dx.doi.org/10.1017/S0144686X97006582

van den Hoonaard, D.K. 1999. "No Regrets: Widows' Stories about the Last Days of Their Husbands' Lives." *Journal of Aging Studies* 13 (1): 59–72. http://dx.doi .org/10.1016/S0890-4065(99)80006-1

van den Hoonaard, D.K. 2001. *The Widowed Self: The Older Women's Journey through Widowhood*. Waterloo, ON: Wilfrid Laurier University Press.

van den Hoonaard, D.K. 2010. *By Himself: The Older Man's Experience of Widowhood*. Toronto: University of Toronto Press.

van den Hoonaard, D.K., K.M. Bennett, and E. Evans. 2014. "'I Was There When She Passed': Older Widowers' Narratives of the Death Their Wife." *Ageing and Society* 34 (6): 974–91. http://dx.doi.org/10.1017/S0144686X12001353

Veatch, R.M. 1989. *Death, Dying, and the Biological Revolution: Our Last Quest for Responsibility*, rev. ed. New Haven, CT: Yale University Press.

Venema, K. 2018. "'And Then Nothing': Alzheimer's Archives and the Good (Enough) Death." *Death Studies* 42 (5): 298–305. https://doi.org/10.1080 /07481187.2017.1396408. Medline:29267143

Venema, K. 2019. "My Mother Couldn't Choose Her Story's End. This Needs to Change." *The Globe and Mail*, May 9. https://www.theglobeandmail.com /opinion/article-my-mother-couldnt-choose-her-storys-end-this-needs-to -change/

Veterans Affairs Canada. 2015. "Learn about PTSD." http://www.veterans.gc.ca /eng/services/health/mental-health/publications/learn-ptsd

Viszmeg, J. (Director, Writer, and Editor), and J. Krepakevich (Producer). 1998. *My Healing Journey: Seven Years with Cancer* [Video]. National Film Board of Canada.

Wagner, S.L., and R. Pasca. 2020. "Recruit Firefighters: A Longitudinal Investigation of Mental Health and Work." *International Journal of Emergency Services* 9 (2): 143–52. https://doi.org/10/1108/IJES-01-2018-0005. Medline:32419181

Wagner, S.L., N. White, T. Fyfe, L.R. Matthews, C. Randall, C. Regehr, M. White, L.E. Alden, N. Buys, and M.G. Carey. 2020. "Systematic Review of Posttraumatic Stress Disorder in Police Officers Following Routine Work-Related Critical Incident Exposure." *American Journal of Industrial Medicine* 63: 600–15. https://doi.org/10.1002/ajim.23120

Wagner, S.L., N. White, C. Randall, C. Regehr, M. White, L.E. Alden, N. Buys, M.G. Carey, W. Corneil, and T. Fyfe. 2020. "Mental Disorders in Firefighters following Large-Scale Disaster." *Disaster Medicine and Public Health Preparedness*. Advance online publication. https://doi.org/10.1017/dmp.2020.61

Wagner, S.L., N. White, C. Regehr, M. White, L.E. Alden, N. Buys, M.G. Carey, W. Corneil, and T. Fyfe. 2020. "Ambulance Personnel Systematic Review of Mental Health Symptoms." *Traumatology*. Advance online publication. https://doi.org/10.1037/trm0000251

Waskowic, T.D., and B.M. Chartier. 2003. "Attachment and the Experience of Grief following the Loss of a Spouse." *Omega* 47 (1): 77–91.

Watford, M.L. 2008. "Bereavement of Spousal Suicide: A Reflective Self-Exploration." *Qualitative Inquiry* 14 (3): 335–59. http://dx.doi.org/10.1177/1077800407309325

Watson, J., A. Simmonds, M. La Fontaine, and M.E. Fockler. 2019. "Pregnancy and Infant Loss: A Survey of Families' Experiences in Ontario Canada." *BMC Pregnancy and Childbirth* 19 (1): 129. https://doi.org/10.1186/s12884-019-2270-2. Medline:30991981

Waugh, E. 2013. "Funeral Practices." In *The Canadian Encyclopedia*. http://www.thecanadianencyclopedia.ca/en/article/funeral-practices/

Webb, M. 1997. *The Good Death: The New American Search to Reshape the End of Life*. New York: Bantam Books.

Widger, K., and C. Picot. 2008. "Parents' Perceptions of the Quality of Pediatric and Perinatal End-of-Life Care." *Pediatric Nursing* 34 (1): 53–8. Medline:18361087

Wiersma, E., J. Marcella, J. McAnulty, and M.L. Kelley. 2019. "'That Just Breaks My Heart': Moral Concerns of Direct Care Workers Providing Palliative Care in LTC Homes." *Canadian Journal on Aging* 38 (3): 268–80. https://doi.org/10.1017/S0714980800000624. Medline:30632479

Wilinsky, C.F. 1943. "Hospitals Have Place in Public Health Programme." *Canadian Hospital* 36 (January): 12.

Williamson, J.B., L. Evans, and A. Munley. 1980. *Aging and Society*. New York: Holt, Rinehart and Winston.

Willison, K.D. 2006. "Integrating Self-Care and Chronic Disease Management through a Community Based Research Approach." Ontario Health Promotion E-Bulletin. http://www.ohpe.ca/:/index.php?option=com_contentandtask=viewandid=7747andItemid=77

Wilson, D.M. 1996. "Highlighting the Role of Policy in Nursing Practice through a Comparison of 'DNR' Policy Influences and 'No CPR' Decision Influences." *Nursing Outlook* 44 (6): 272–9. http://dx.doi.org/10.1016/S0029-6554(96)80083-2. Medline:8981497

Wilson, D.M. 1997. "A Report of an Investigation of End-of-Life Care Practices
in Health Care Facilities and the Influences on Those Practices." *Journal of
Palliative Care* 13 (4): 34–40. Medline:9447810

Wilson, D.M. 2002. "The Duration and Degree of End-of-Life Dependency of Home
Care Clients and Hospital Inpatients." *Applied Nursing Research* 15 (2): 81–6.
http://dx.doi.org/10.1053/apnr.2002.29526. Medline:11994824

Wilson, D.M., F. Anafi, S. Roh, and B. Errasti-Ibarrondo. 2020. "A Scoping
Research Literature Review to Identify Contemporary Evidence on the Incidence,
Causes, and Impacts of End-of-Life Intra-Family Conflict." https://doi.org/10
.1080/10410236.2020.1775448

Wilson, D.M., M.C. Anderson, R.L. Fainsinger, H.C. Northcott, S.L. Smith, and
M.J. Stingl. 1998. *Social and Health Care Trends Influencing Palliative Care
and the Location of Death in Twentieth-Century Canada. NHRDP Final Report.*
Edmonton: University of Alberta.

Wilson, D.M., S. Birch, R. MacLeod, N. Dhanji, J. Osei-Waree, and J. Cohen. 2013.
"The Public's Viewpoint on the Right to Hastened Death in Alberta, Canada:
Findings from a Population Survey Study." *Health & Social Care in the Community*
21 (2): 200–8. http://dx.doi,org/10.1111/hsc.12007. Medline:23216961

Wilson, D.M., R. Brow, R. Playfair, and B. Errasti-Ibarrondo. 2018. "What Is the
'Right' Number of Hospital Beds for Palliative Population Health Needs?"
Societies 8 (4): 108. https://doi.org/10.3390/soc8040108

Wilson, D.M., J. Cohen, L. Deliens, J.A. Hewitt, and D. Houttekier. 2013. "The
Preferred Place of Last Days: Results of a Representative Population-Based
Public Survey." *Journal of Palliative Medicine* 16 (5): 502–8. https://doi
.org/10.1089/jpm.2012.0262. Medline:23421538

Wilson, D.M., J. Cohen, R. MacLeod, and D. Houttekier. 2018. "Bereavement Grief:
A Population-Based Foundational Evidence Study." *Death Studies* 42 (7):
463–9. https://doi.org/10.1080/07481187.2017.1382609. Medline:28985143

Wilson, D.M., L. Fillion, R. Thomas, C. Justice, P.P. Bhardwaj, and A.M. Veillette.
2009. "The 'Good' Rural Death: A Report of an Ethnographic Study in Alberta,
Canada." *Journal of Palliative Care* 25 (1): 21–9. Medline:19445339

Wilson, D.M., B.L. Goodwin, and J.A. Hewitt. 2011. "An Examination of Palliative
or End-of-Life Care Education in Introductory Nursing Programs across
Canada." *Nursing Research and Practice.* http://dx.doi.org/10.1155/2011/907172

Wilson, D.M., and J.A. Hewitt. 2018. "A Scoping Research Literature Review
to Assess the State of Existing Evidence on the 'Bad' Death." *Palliative &
Supportive Care* 16 (1): 90–106. https://doi.org/10.1017/S1478951517000530.
Medline:28655363

Wilson, D.M., J.A. Hewitt, R.E. Thomas, and B. Woytowich. 2014. "Why Did
an Out-of-Hospital Shift of Death and Dying Occur in Canada after 1994?"
International Journal of Palliative Care 2014: 1–11. http://dx.doi.org
/10.1155/2014/157536

Wilson, D.M., D. Houttekier, S.A. Kunju, S. Birch, J. Cohen, R. MacLeod, and J.A.
Hewitt. 2013. "A Population-Based Study on Advance Directive Completion

and Completion Intention among Citizens of the Western Canadian Province of Alberta." *Journal of Palliative Care* 29 (1): 5–12. Medline:23614165

Wilson, D.M., J. Kinch, C. Justice, R. Thomas, D. Shepherd, and K. Froggatt. 2005. "A Review of the Literature on Hospice or Palliative Day Care." *European Journal of Palliative Care* 12 (5): 198–202.

Wilson, D.M., H.C. Northcott, C.D. Truman, S.L. Smith, M.C. Anderson, R.L. Fainsinger, and M.J. Stingl. 2001. "Location of Death in Canada: A Comparison of 20th-Century Hospital and Nonhospital Locations of Death and Corresponding Population Trends." *Evaluation & the Health Professions* 24 (4): 385–403. http://dx.doi.org/10.1177/01632780122034975. Medline:11817198

Wilson, D.M., and R. Playfair. 2016. "Bereavement Programs and Services in the Province of Alberta: A Mapping Report." *Canadian Journal on Aging* 35 (2): 273–8. https://doi.org/10.1017/S0714980816000271. Medline:27098597

Wilson, D.M., Y. Shen, and S. Birch. 2017. "New Evidence on End-of-Life Hospital Utilization for Enhanced Health Policy and Services Planning." *Journal of Palliative Medicine* 20 (7): 752–8. https://doi.org/10.1089/jpm.2016.0490. Medline:28282256

Wilson, D.M., Y. Shen, and S. Birch. 2019. "Who Are High Users of Hospitals in Canada? Findings from a Population-Based Study." *Canadian Journal of Nursing Research* 51 (4): 245–54. https://doi.org/10.1177/0844562119833584. Medline:30845831

Wilson, D.M., S.L. Smith, M.C. Anderson, H.C. Northcott, R.L. Fainsinger, M.J. Stingl, and C.D. Truman. 2002. "Twentieth-Century Social and Health-Care Influences on Location of Death in Canada." *Canadian Journal of Nursing Research* 34 (3): 141–61. Medline:12425015

Wilson, D.M., C.D. Truman, J. Huang, S. Sheps, S. Birch, R. Thomas, and T. Noseworthy. 2007. "Home Care Evolution in Alberta: How Have Palliative Clients Fared?" *Healthcare Policy* 2 (4): 58–69. Medline:19305733

Wilson, D.M., C.D. Truman, J. Huang, S. Sheps, R. Thomas, and T. Noseworthy. 2005. "The Possibilities and the Realities of Home Care." *Canadian Journal of Public Health* 96 (5): 385–9. Medline:16238160

Wilson, D.M., C.D. Truman, R. Thomas, R. Fainsinger, K. Kovacs-Burns, K. Froggatt, and C. Justice. 2009. "The Rapidly Changing Location of Death in Canada, 1994–2004." *Social Science & Medicine* 68 (10): 1752–8. http://dx.doi.org/10.1016/j.socscimed.2009.03.006. Medline:19342137

Wilson, D.M., and B. Woytowich. 2014. "What Proportion of Terminally Ill and Dying People Require Specialist Palliative Care Services?" *International Journal of Palliative Care* 2014: 1–7. http://dx.doi.org/10.1155/2014/529681

Wilson, K. 1983. *The Fur Trade in Canada*. Toronto: Grolier.

Wilson, K., K. Kortes-Miller, and A. Stinchcombe. 2018. "Staying Out of the Closet: LGBT Older Adults' Hopes and Fears in Considering End-of-Life." *Canadian Journal on Aging* 37 (1): 22–31. https://doi.org/10.1017/S0714980817000514. Medline:29335034

Winick, S.D. 2018. "Rumors of Our Deaths: Fake News, Folk News, and Far Away Moses." *The Journal of American Folklore* 131 (522): 388–97. https://doi .org/10.5406/jamerfolk.131.522.0388

Winterfeldt, E. 1991. "Historical Perspective, Part 1: Dietary Management of Diabetes Mellitus, 1675–1950." *Topics in Clinical Nutrition* 7 (1): 1–8.

Wood, C. 1994. "The Legacy of Sue Rodriguez." *Maclean's*, February 28, 21–5.

Woodgate, R.L. 2006. "Living in a World without Closure: Reality for Parents Who Have Experienced the Death of a Child." *Journal of Palliative Care* 22 (2): 75–82. Medline:17265659

World Bank. 2020. "Death Rate, Crude (per 1,000 People)." https://data.worldbank .org/indicator/SP.DYN.CDRT.IN

World Health Organization. 2020. "Chronic Diseases and Health Promotion." https:// www.who.int/chp/about/integrated_cd/en/

You, J.J., J. Downar, R.A. Fowler, F. Lamontagne, I.W.Y. Ma, D. Jayaraman, J. Kryworuchko, P.H. Strachan, R. Ilan, A.P. Nijjar, et al. 2015. "Barriers to Goals of Care Discussions with Seriously Ill Hospitalized Patients and Their Families." *JAMA Internal Medicine* 175 (4): 549–56. http://dx.doi.org/10.1001 /jamainternmed.2014.7732

Young, T.K. 2015. "Health of Aboriginal People." In *The Canadian Encyclopedia.* http://www.thecanadianencyclopedia.ca/en/article/aboriginal-people-health/

Zabjek, A. 2015. "A Final Farewell to an Edmonton Fire Captain." *Edmonton Journal*, July 10. http://edmontonjournal.com/news/local-news/a-final -farewell-to-an-edmonton-fire-captain

Zilm, G., and E. Warbinek. 1995. "Early Tuberculosis Nursing in British Columbia." *Canadian Journal of Nursing Research* 27 (3): 65–81. Medline:8556669

Zimmermann, C. 2004. "Denial of Impending Death: A Discourse Analysis of the Palliative Care Literature." *Social Science & Medicine* 59 (8): 1769–80. http:// dx.doi.org/10.1016/j.socscimed.2004.02.012. Medline:15279932

Zimmermann, C. 2012. "Acceptance of Dying: A Discourse Analysis of Palliative Care Literature." *Social Science & Medicine* 75 (1): 217–24. http://dx.doi .org/10.1016/j.socscimed.2012.02.047. Medline:22513246

Index

Tables, figures, and images indicated by page numbers in *italics*.